SMART HEALTHCARE MONITORING USING IOT WITH 5G

Internet of Everything (IoE): Security and Privacy Paradigm

Series Editors: Vijender Kumar Solanki, Raghvendra Kumar, and Le Hoang Son

Securing IoT and Big Data
Next Generation Intelligence
Edited by Vijayalakshmi Saravanan, Anpalagan Alagan, T. Poongodi, and Firoz Khan

Distributed Artificial Intelligence
A Modern Approach
Edited by Satya Prakash Yadav, Dharmendra Prasad Mahato, and Nguyen Thi Dieu Linh

Security and Trust Issues in Internet of Things
Blockchain to the Rescue
Edited by Sudhir Kumar Sharma, Bharat Bhushan, and Bhuvan Unhelkar

Internet of Medical Things
Paradigm of Wearable Devices
Edited by Manuel N. Cardona, Vijender Kumar Solanki, and Cecilia García Cena

Integration of WSNs into Internet of Things
A Security Perspective
Edited by Sudhir Kumar Sharma, Bharat Bhushan, Raghvendra Kumar, Aditya Khamparia, and Narayan C. Debnath

IoT Applications, Security Threats, and Countermeasures
Edited by Padmalaya Nayak, Niranjan Ray, and P. Ravichandran

Multimodal Biometric Systems
Security and Applications
Edited by Rashmi Gupta and Manju Khari

Smart Healthcare Monitoring Using IoT with 5G
Challenges, Directions, and Future Predictions
Edited by Meenu Gupta, Gopal Chaudhary, Victor Hugo C. de Albuquerque

For more information about this series, please visit: https://www.routledge.com/Internet-of-Everything-IoE/book-series/CRCIOESPP

SMART HEALTHCARE MONITORING USING IOT WITH 5G

Challenges, Directions, and Future Predictions

Edited by
Meenu Gupta, Gopal Chaudhary,
Victor Hugo C. de Albuquerque

CRC Press
Taylor & Francis Group
Boca Raton London New York

CRC Press is an imprint of the
Taylor & Francis Group, an **informa** business

First edition published 2022
by CRC Press
2385 NW Executive Center Drive, Suite 320, Boca Raton FL 33431

and by CRC Press
4 Park Square, Milton Park, Abingdon, Oxon, OX14 4RN

ISBN: 978-0-367-77529-2 (hbk)
ISBN: 978-0-367-77530-8 (pbk)
ISBN: 978-1-003-17182-9 (ebk)

DOI: 10.1201/9781003171829

Typeset in Times
by MPS Limited, Dehradun

Contents

Preface

Before Internet of Things (IoT), patients' interactions with doctors were limited to visits, and tele and text communications. There were no ways doctors or hospitals could monitor patients' health continuously and make recommendations accordingly. IoT-enabled devices have made remote monitoring in the healthcare sector possible, unleashing the potential to keep patients safe and healthy, and empowering physicians to deliver superlative care. It has also increased patient engagement and satisfaction as interactions with doctors have become easier and more efficient. Furthermore, remote monitoring of patient's health helps in reducing the length of hospital stay and prevents re-admissions. IoT also has a major impact on reducing healthcare costs significantly and improving treatment outcomes. IoT is undoubtedly transforming the healthcare industry by redefining the space of devices and people interaction in delivering healthcare solutions. IoT has applications in healthcare that benefit patients, families, physicians, hospitals, and insurance companies.

In parallel, 5G will enhance many existing use cases while creating new ones unfulfilled by current technologies, such as remotely performed patient examinations and even operations. What is also certain is that critical healthcare services require reliable connections. 5G networks will provide near-instantaneous data transfer speeds, which will make a massive impact on all connected devices in healthcare. Huge data files of medical imagery could be transported quickly and reliably, leading to improved quality of care.

The objective of this book is to provide a wide variety of topics as they pertain to knowledge management, decision science, inclusion of IoT, and 5G techniques with upgraded technologies. This publication will impact the field of business, organizations, management and information technology, healthcare industries, and hospitals because there is scant extant literature on IoT and 5G in smart healthcare as it pertains to business world.

Editor biographies

Meenu Gupta completed her PhD in computer science and engineering with an emphasis on traffic accident severity problem from the Ansal University, Gurugram, India (2020), an MTech in computer science and engineering from the M.D.U. University, Rohtak, India (2010), and she graduated in information technology at the K.U.K. University, Kurukshetra, India (2006). She is currently associate professor in Chandigarh University. She has 13 years of teaching experience. Her areas of research are machine learning, intelligent systems, data mining, with specific interest in artificial intelligence, image processing and analysis, smart cities, data analysis, and human/brain-machine interaction. She also completed two edited books of CRC press on healthcare and cancer diseases. She also has four authored books on engineering streams. She worked as a reviewer of many journals like *Big Data*, *CMC*, *Scientific Report*, *TSP*. She is a life member of ISTE and IAENG. She has authored or coauthored over 50 papers in refereed international journals (*SCI*/*SCIE*/*WoS*/Scopus/etc.), conferences, and more than 20 book chapters. She also chaired IEEE international Conference and convened many workshops/FDP.

Gopal Chaudhary is currently working as an assistant professor in Bharati Vidyapeeth's College of Engineering, Guru Gobind Singh Indraprastha University, Delhi, India. He holds a PhD in biometrics at the division of Instrumentation and Control Engineering, Netaji Subhas Institute of Technology, University of Delhi, India. He received a BE degree in electronics and communication engineering in 2009 and the MTech degree in microwave and optical communication from Delhi Technological University (formerly known as Delhi College of Engineering), New Delhi, India, in 2012. He has 30 publications in refereed national/international journals and conferences (e.g. Elsevier, Springer, Inderscience) in the area of biometrics and its applications. His current research interests include soft computing, intelligent systems, information fusion, and pattern recognition. He has organized many conferences and contributed to special issues.

Victor Hugo C. de Albuquerque has a PhD in mechanical engineering with an emphasis on materials from the Federal University of Paraíba (UFPB, 2010), an MSc in teleinformatics engineering from the Federal University of Ceará (UFC, 2007), and he graduated in mechatronics technology at the Federal Center of Technological Education of Ceará (CEFETCE, 2006). He is currently full professor of the graduate program in applied informatics, and coordinator of the Laboratory of Industrial Informatics, Electronics and Health at the University of Fortaleza (UNIFOR) and data science director at the Superintendency for Research and Public Safety Strategy of Ceará State (SUPESP/CE), Brazil. He has experience in computer systems, mainly in the research fields of applied computing, intelligent systems, visualization and interaction, with specific interest in pattern recognition, artificial intelligence, image processing, and analysis, as well as automation with respect to biological signal/image processing, image segmentation, biomedical circuits, and human/brain-machine interaction, including augmented and virtual reality simulation modeling for animals and humans. Additionally, he has done research on the microstructural characterization through the combination of non-destructive techniques with signal/image processing and analysis and pattern recognition. Prof. Victor is the leader of the Industrial Informatics, Electronics and Health Research Group. He is editor-in-chief of the *Journal of Artificial Intelligence and Systems* and associate editor of the *IEEE Access, Applied Soft Computing, Frontiers in Communications and Networks, Computational Intelligence and Neuroscience, Journal of Nanomedicine and Nanotechnology Research, Computational Physiology and Medicine*, and *Journal of Mechatronics Engineering*, and he has been a lead guest editor of several highly reputed journals, and TPC member of many international conferences.

1 The Internet of Things in Healthcare Management: Potential Applications and Challenges

P. Bajdor and M. Starostka-Patyk

CONTENTS

1.1   INTRODUCTION

The Internet of Things (IoT) concept has revolutionized the digital world. This idea was introduced and has been followed in many different areas. It has completely changed the way of many processes. The IoT's applicability, scope, and diversity are endless and can permeate all aspects of everyday life [1]. One such application area is healthcare informatics of multidisciplinary characteristics, which uses information engineering in healthcare management. Traditionally, health information is derived from various sources, including a system that uses informatics solutions. However, the emergence of IoT meant that this information is often spread across various IoT devices. The use of the IoT concept is slowly becoming the norm in this area.

Increasing spending on healthcare, demographic changes, especially the aging of societies, the threat of infectious diseases, and the increasingly multifaceted disease make innovation in healthcare provision a necessity. e-Health technologies are a promising innovative tool to tackle these problems [2]. Thanks to these technologies, it becomes possible to manage and monitor the health condition essential for the elderly constantly, and to monitor physical activity and patients' safety at home and in healthcare institutions.

The IoT will be conducive to better management of healthcare facilities and the improvement of communication between them. In 2005, the World Health Organization (WHO) recognized the potential of e-health in improving health

DOI: 10.1201/9781003171829-1

systems management and their safety and the quality and effectiveness [3]. The WHO perceives the e-health as the use of information with the IT technologies for proper management of health [4]. A similar definition states that e-health covers all types of activities affecting the health sector. In detail this definition states that e-health includes tools that are or can be used by health authorities (administrations) and professionals (medical staff), as well as personalized (individual) healthcare services for patients and citizens [5]. e-Health refers to applying information and communication technologies to services, products, and management processes related to health. It also includes organizational changes in healthcare systems and their modern management. All this is done to improve citizens' health and increase the efficiency and quality of healthcare services.

The concept of e-health is therefore understood as, among other things, interactions between patients and suppliers of medical services, data transmission between healthcare providers, peer-to-peer communication, including communication with patients or healthcare professionals [6]. The term also includes the interactions and connectivity of health information; electronic health records—EHR; telemedicine services (providing health services at a distance using information and communication technologies, so-called online medical consultations); and personal, portable devices that, thanks to the possibility of communication with each other, regardless of the human being, can support prevention, diagnosis, treatment of disease, health monitoring, and even manage the patient's lifestyle [5].

The purpose of applying ICT in health management is to expand geographic access to healthcare services, improve data management, accelerate diagnosis and treatment, facilitate patient-to-doctor contact outside the office, and minimize fraud and abuse [7].

IoT in healthcare applications has a lot of different requirements, mostly regarding the real-time recording of medical data, security and privacy of this data, and others, depending on the specific medical nature. Therefore, a good understanding of IoT's basic applications in healthcare, opportunities, and threats is essential.

1.2   INTERNET OF THINGS IN THE HEALTHCARE MANAGEMENT

The healthcare IoT technology [8] ensures access to data associated with healthcare and analysis regarding the functioning of informatics and smart medical devices and networks of these [9]. It works based on the architectural structure base, because IoT depends on many interconnected devices, as mentioned in some literature [10], and the general architecture of IoT in healthcare is shown in Figure 1.1. These devices send data via the network, mainly the Internet, to the cloud, which health workers can access [11].

IoT in healthcare management presents a whole range of essential benefits to health and people's well-being, offering improved quality of life and reducing healthcare costs. The most substantial bare elements in this technology's construction are wireless sensors used for remote monitoring of patients' health status, together with communication systems and applications that send the necessary information about patients to their caregivers' medical.

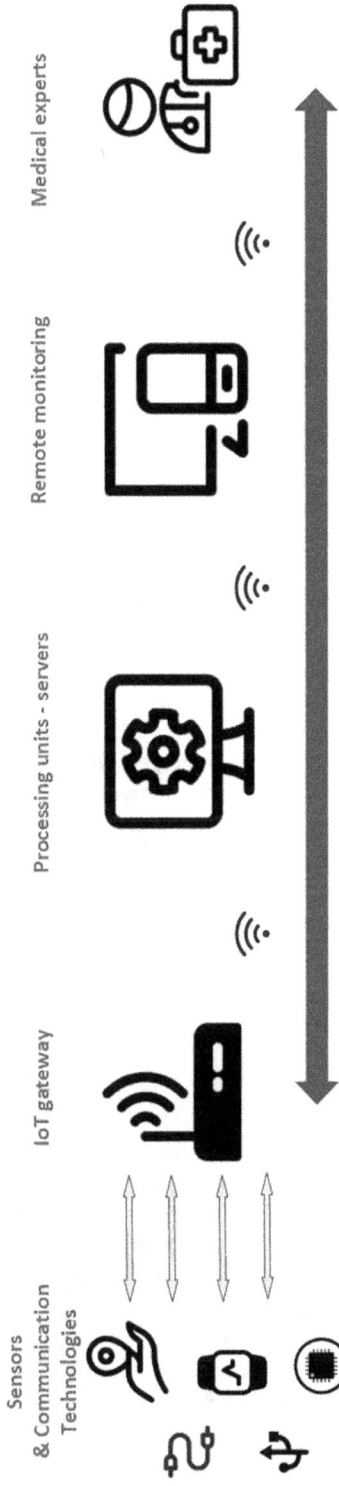

FIGURE 1.1 General architecture of IoT in healthcare.

The concept of IoT in healthcare management focuses on the concept of personal area networks (PAN), that is, a small network centered around a sensor connected to a machine or a human. PAN means a computer network connected to the devices that are used by the people [12]. A PAN network ensures data exchange between various computers, smartphones, tablets, etc. These networks are used to connect IT tools with a server gateway.

The basic assumptions of the PAN for IoT in healthcare management are as follows [13]:

- IT tools and people are equipped with sensors
- IT tools report their status with the Internet connection
- The established network is created when the need occurs and that is why it might be limited to some functions
- While some IT tools might not have limitless power banks, their functions are possible to be cut off
- The bordering power may cause the low bandwidth
- It must be well secured as health data is fragile

The range of applications present in healthcare IoT covers data collection using remote monitoring systems, which might be analyzed after the activity (e.g., sleep activity) and during their occurrence (e.g., heartbeat reports).

IT tools such as Fitbit, Garmin, or Xiaomi Misfit, used for health reporting, analyze the persons' health performance [14]. Because of some functionality limitations, most data of IT tools is exchanged with the use of LAN and/or WAN [15], which places high demands on the network. Also, IoT in healthcare management that evolves in real time in combination with a simultaneous development contributes to the different challenges [16]. They refer to some issues like security and privacy of data, efficient data maintaining and transferring, and large amounts of data management [17]. Such challenges and development of IT technologies connected to advanced sensors, mobile applications, artificial intelligence, big data, 3D printing, and mobility led to an increase in modern ways to support the medical business with the creation of new features of smart healthcare solutions [18].

Requirements for the use of IoT in smart healthcare management are divided into two: functional and non-functional [19]. The functional specification refers to the details of smart healthcare architecture. A temperature reporting system is an example. Hence, functional requirements are specific to each component used in this healthcare system based on their application. Non-functional requirements seem not to be specific. Non-functional details relate to features of healthcare quality. In a broader perspective, non-functional healthcare specifications are broken down into functional and ethical details [20].

There are many divisions of smart healthcare management systems, but here it is worth to mention how these specifications are broken down with regard to the software and hardware. The overarching criteria for an effective, intelligent healthcare management system are [21]:

- Energy
- Possibilities of use in housing
- Solidity of the system
- Service assurance
- Better perception by users
- Better productivity
- Possibilities for a broader exchange of information
- Ease of use
- The wide use of healthcare management tools that provide continuous support
- System scalability for developing solutions
- Wide inter-functioning

Modern smart healthcare management systems are developed to provide fast medical help and care. Some higher sophisticated applications, with regard to these details [22], must possess environmental intelligence to improve service quality.

It is possible to point out two critical aspects of IoT in healthcare management: services, such as devices to be worn on the body, and applications such as ECG or blood pressure monitoring [23]. Some examples of effective services and applications in IoT in healthcare management are mentioned in the literature [24], and Figure 1.2 shows the primary services and applications examples in an IoT in healthcare.

When analyzing the figure, you can notice that the services are used to create IoT in healthcare applications, while the applications are used directly by patients. In addition to their usefulness in supervising and managing the everyday health and well-being, the IoT devices in healthcare were designed to use with chronic diseases and their prevention, life and intervention remote assistants, improved management of drugs and healthcare, and prevention of disease in remote sites [25].

Now, there are various wearable devices available for people, such as activity monitors, automatic external defibrillators, blood pressure monitors, glucometers, fall sensors, fitness and heart rate monitors, multi-parameter monitors, programmable syringe pumps, pulse oximeters, smart pill dispensers, smartwatches, and the

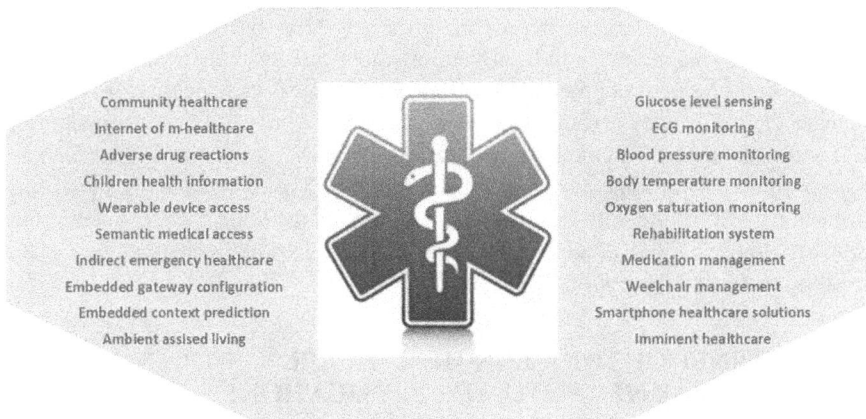

Community healthcare
Internet of m-healthcare
Adverse drug reactions
Children health information
Wearable device access
Semantic medical access
Indirect emergency healthcare
Embedded gateway configuration
Embedded context prediction
Ambient assised living

Glucose level sensing
ECG monitoring
Blood pressure monitoring
Body temperature monitoring
Oxygen saturation monitoring
Rehabilitation system
Medication management
Weelchair management
Smartphone healthcare solutions
Imminent healthcare

FIGURE 1.2 Primary services and applications examples in an IoT in healthcare.

handy injectors [1,3,26]. The IoMT application domain can include chronic disease (CD), health condition management (HCM), home medical care (HMH), hospital monitoring (HM), human activity recognition (HAR), medical nursing (MN), patient physiology (PPC), patient wear IoMT devices, pediatric and senior care (PEC), remote patient monitoring (RPM), concurrent reporting and monitoring (CRM), and patient drug tracking (TPM) [27].

In addition to these fields of application, remote telemedicine monitoring consulting (TMRC) stands for a modern way of medical services based on the historical data and current reports exchanged between parties through Internet communication to improve patients' healthcare [28]. The definition of telemedicine is strongly tied up with the telehealth (remote healthcare) [29]. In medical practice many of the applications use telemedicine. Based on the studies [14] that analyze the market of IT tools in medicine it is predicted that it will grow from $14.9 billion in 2017 to $52.2 billion in 2022. Currently, there are more than 500,000 different types of medical devices, including wearable external medical devices, implanted medical devices, and stationary medical devices.

Thanks to the use of telemedicine, patients' lives can be better. Telemonitoring services can improve the quality of life of chronically ill patients and reduce the need for hospitalization. Teleconsultation and teleradiology can reduce queues, optimize resource utilization, and increase efficiency [30]. It is estimated that the possibility of providing remote care for patients staying in their own homes, using telecommunications networks, will increase the survival rate by 15%, and decrease the length of hospitalization by 26%. On the contrary, the cost of nursing care can be reduced by around 10%. The introduction of e-prescriptions may reduce medical errors by 15%, resulting in inadequate dosing of the drug. Despite the aging of the EU countries' population, e-health services can keep treatment costs similar [31].

Technology IoT in healthcare management has now become an integral part of the same products, and—turning them into computers—provide four areas of benefits [32]. The benefits of using intelligent products in IoT in healthcare management are presented in Table 1.1.

According to the European Commission, by using the advantages of new technologies, e-health can solve healthcare problems. The use of information and communication technologies in health and medical care systems, which will allow the provision of electronic medical services, can improve their quality. It will also increase their efficiency and management, increase and improve citizens' quality of life, and open medical markets to innovation [33]. The quality of life for people with disabilities or chronic diseases will be promoted. The digital agenda's goal was to ensure by 2015 the safe access to health data to facilitate the treatment from anywhere in the EU [34]. Failure to achieve this goal does not mean that there is no need to create such an option in the future.

1.3 INTERNET OF THINGS IN HEALTHCARE MANAGEMENT—POTENTIAL APPLICATIONS

The foremost step toward an intelligent healthcare system is to use the potential of existing technologies to deliver the best services to users and make their lives better.

TABLE 1.1
Benefits of using intelligent products in IoT in healthcare management

Area	Benefits
MONITORING—the product can inform about its condition or external conditions.	• Knowledge about the condition of the product • Information about the external environment • Product performance data
CONTROL—the product can be monitored through commands sent to it, or the user can learn by himself or herself using algorithms built into it.	• Product function check • User learning
OPTIMIZATION—an intelligent product based on algorithms collecting data in real time and comparing it with historical data, increase its efficiency, and conduct diagnostics.	• Increasing product performance • Prognostics, diagnostics, repair, and service
AUTONOMY—the product can recognize needs by itself, connect with other objects, and even repair itself.	• Self-performance enhancement • Self-connection with other devices or systems • Auto-diagnosis and auto-repair

IoT is a technology supporting healthcare management, which can help in professional medicine in almost every area where a clinical decision is made [22]. By using IoT utilizing different techniques, computers can learn to make accurate decisions based on health professionals and patients' data and generate appropriately selected feedback.

IoT devices powered by artificial intelligence can operate continuously and monitor people's health. Intelligent robots, intelligent houses, and virtual assistants can provide the necessary support to the elderly and people with disabilities [35]. The use of the IoT in healthcare management can improve the quality of life, especially for the elderly. It is possible to install sensors in the house to monitor the daily life of the residents. In the event of inactivity, the needy people may be informed of the situation [36]. Such a solution is highly desirable in aging societies. IoT in healthcare might be used to connect staff with patients and support them [37], and examples of IOT capabilities used are summarized in Table 1.2.

Thanks to the technology of the patient's health's wireless monitoring system, it is possible to do preliminary, remote diagnosis at home. From the point of view of the healthcare system's operation, it is an economic system for providing health services. Nowadays, it is possible to collect medical data by the sensor placed, for example, in the watch, adhered to the body surface or through the implanted chip [38]. Thanks to using a wireless, remote system for monitoring the patient's vital signs, using medical measuring equipment, and data transmission via the Internet (audio or video), the collected data is transferred to the doctor. The vital signs monitored include blood pressure, heart rate, oxygen saturation, body temperature, expiratory capacity (lung capacity), and blood glucose levels. The use of such an application, effectively

TABLE 1.2
Examples of IoT in healthcare capabilities used

Healthcare Areas of IoT Connections	Examples of Capabilities Used
Urgent and emergency care	• Telecare service to triage alarm calls to the most appropriate responders to reduce emergency service activity. • Teleconsultation between community, ambulance service, and acute care. • Telehealth monitoring of patients not transported to hospital. • Telehealth for pre-operative assessment.
Hospital acute elective	• Text and email appointment reminders. • Telehealth for pre- and post-operative assessment and telecoaching to maintain pre-operative behaviors. • Telecare/telehealth to support earlier discharge.
GP practice	• Self-monitoring kiosks in practices for routine assessments. • Telehealth to assist with self-care and triaging assess to primary care. • Teleconsultation for those hard to reach or having mobility issues. • Telemedicine with specialists to prevent unnecessary outpatients. • Telecare for carer support, medication management, falls/dementia.
Care home	• Education and training apps and web portals to support staff. • Telehealth for care homes including teleconsultations between care home, primary and acute settings. • Teleconsultation between care home, primary and acute settings. • Telecare alarms/sensors, falls monitors, pendant alarms.
Home including re-ablement	• Telecare and telehealth to support rehabilitation. • Telehealth for post-operative recovery assessment. • Digital imaging to inform rehabilitation tailored to home environments. • Internet-based therapeutic interventions and carer support.
Community care	• Telecare to support people with dementia or at risk of falls or at end of life. • Remote audio and video conferencing with care team and patient. • Telecoaching to maintain helpful behaviors and apps to support people to self-care. • Medication management apps to encourage correct use of medication.

integrating the patient's current data into his or her electronic medical records and two-way audio or video communication of the patient with the medical caregiver, can improve healthcare quality and efficiency [39].

Wearable IoT devices in healthcare are intelligent tools providing effective user experiences and services. They are the core of intelligent IoT solutions for healthcare management. These wearable devices, together with the telemedicine, are used for constant reporting of patient's activities. They report by applications and exchange safe data through the IoT. Such wearable devices used to monitor the health signs are tending to be developed with smaller and smaller sizes to better fit the user requirements and to provide them the comfort of wearing them [40]. Another healthcare-related application is HAR, in which IoT serves for reporting the user activities [41]. Detecting and analyzing human activity is a difficult task as it takes significant time together with an expensive equipment. Proper reporting of people activity can help healthcare services improve training guidelines for re- covery or the early indication of medical emergencies encountered in older patients, such as falls and heart failure [42].

It is estimated that more than half of the patients do not take medications at all or take them contrary to the doctor's recommendations. This poses both a medical and an economic problem. Poorly treated patients generate additional treatment costs, especially inpatient treatment. Much research is being done in the health sector management on new technologies in this area. In the context of the current level of technology development, new technologies can be implemented, although, for the time being, there are plans for the future [43]. For example, pharmaceutical com- panies are introducing pilot programs to monitor patient medication intake. The use of silicone microsensors mounted onto tablets allows monitoring of the patient's intake of prescribed medications. The sand-grained chip on each tablet contains small amounts of copper and magnesium. When the chip is swallowed, the metals react with the gastric juice, generating an electrical voltage. This impulse is read by a medical recorder placed on the body's surface (a patch placed on the skin). Thanks to the smartphone, the recorder sends a signal informing about drug intake. If the patient does not take the prescribed medications, the doctor or other au- thorized person—the patient's guardian, will be informed about it. This device has been approved by the United States Food and Drug Administration (FDA) and European Medicines Agency (EMA) for pre-approval clinical trials as medical technology [44].

Smart health devices are also used to report the health of patients with chronic diseases, and they measure many functions: scales, pulse oximeters, blood glucose meters, and cuffs for measuring blood pressure. On the basis of the results, in- formation and alerts are sent to healthcare professionals to diagnose and react or care if necessary. IoT applications in healthcare are beneficial and used to treat chronic diseases related to specific therapy areas [37], and Figure 1.3 presents the classification of such apps by therapy area in 2013.

Diabetes mellitus is a common chronic disease in which blood glucose levels are high for a long time. To deal with this, there is a need for non-invasive glucose sensor. The IoT in healthcare method to deal with is to connect sensors to healthcare pro- viders [45]. Another critical issue is a heart disease. Reporting the heart activity is a necessity. The arrhythmia might be dangerous for the living, so such control prevents the emergency accidents. To prevent this from happening, linking IoT with ECG monitoring makes it possible to remotely offer proper functions and information about

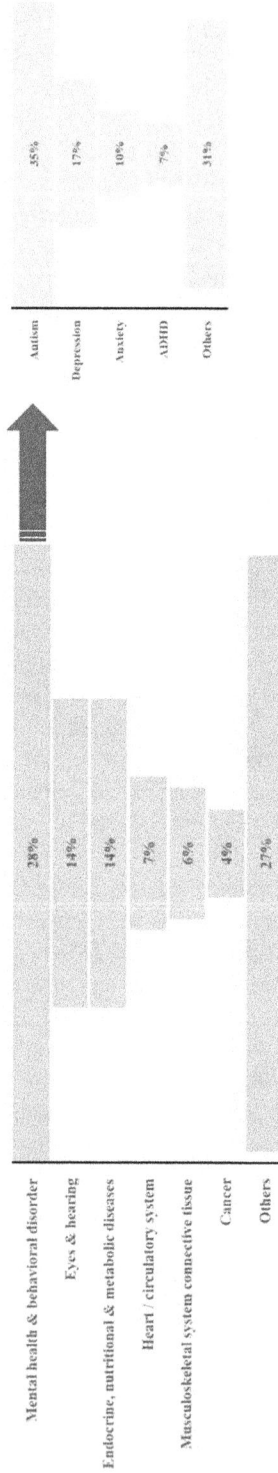

FIGURE 1.3 The classification of IoT healthcare apps by therapy area in 2013.

a patient's symptoms [46]. IoT in healthcare management promises to develop practical solutions for healthcare services, enabling temperature monitoring as it is an essential parameter of the body to monitor body temperature [47].

It is also necessary to ensure that the physician is able to analyze such a vast set of data. A program that detects only abnormal behavior of the patient (no medication) or the state of his or her health that requires intervention may be helpful here. Besides, the medical recorder's sensors can monitor the patient's condition and his or her body's response to a given dose of the drug. Therefore, the doctor has the opportunity to analyze the correlation between the dose of the drug taken by the patient and his or her heart rate, breathing, and level of physical activity. After each data collection, thanks to mobile phones or computers' communication capabilities, they are placed on the server, which allows the doctor to study them. Using such technology, the patient may be instructed to change the drug or its dosage [48].

Another attempt at medical diagnostics using modern technologies involves the implantation of a programmable-bio-nano-chip that can detect heart disease or tumor markers from a sample of the patient's saliva. The implementation of such a chip in the patient's body could provide an early notification system for these diseases long before they discover any symptoms [49]. However, in order for society to be able to adopt all of the above amenities in the medical services sector, it is necessary to solve the problems related to the protection of the privacy of people using them. This type of service provider must clearly state the purpose, frequency, and type of detailed personal information that will be tracked and the circle of entities that have access to this data. Secure transmission of sensitive data between the end user and the service provider must be ensured [50].

When it comes to caring for the elderly, it should be noted that safely supporting older people's independent lives in their place of residence can increase their self-confidence, ensure better autonomy, and provide them with real help. This is the primary goal of ambient assisted living (AAL), an AI-based IoT platform that uses information and communication technologies to achieve this goal. Recognizing activity and understanding behavior are desirable outcomes of using various AAL sensors [51]. It might be done directly with the help of wearable sensors or indirectly with environmental sensors and flux analysis. For example, by tracking a patient's medications, it is possible to track patient consumption.

Virtually everyone can use the IoT in healthcare stages of treatment. It is used in the prevention and diagnosis of disease, observation of patients, as well as at the stage of treatment, including hospital stay. Some hospitals are already part of the IoT. Many of the IoT devices are imperceptible to patients. Hospitals have, among others, devices that, after entering the appropriate parameters, enable communication with each other [52]. After examining the patient's vital signs, they automatically adjust the appropriate doses of drugs and their administration frequency. Another example is endoscopic examinations that do not require the presence of a doctor. The patient swallows a tablet equipped with a camera that takes 36 shots/s, showing an image of the gastrointestinal tract. It is a less stressful and more comfortable test method for the patient [53]. Thanks to the use of intelligent refrigerators, the condition of medical supplies can be monitored in real time [54].

Combining the collected information with an IoT sensor the disease is under control. IoT in healthcare management consists of the essential equipment needed for secure mechanisms and communication technologies, as data and information exchange are a source of solicitude and care the patients, so they are sensitive and must be well protected [55].

1.4   CHALLENGES (ADVANTAGES AND BARRIERS)

The development of modern technologies is rapid and covers all spheres of everyday life. The bases for this development are research and forecasts of the demand for new devices and systems in individual areas of life and economy based on them. One of the dynamically developing sectors in recent years is healthcare. Therefore, technological development is also moving in this direction, creating more and more new challenges. The evolution of digital health technologies is presented in Figure 1.4, in the form of Hype Cycle [56].

The Allied Market Research reports [57] that the global IoT healthcare market will reach $136.8 billion in 2021. More than 3.7 million medical devices are already in use. The development of the healthcare sector in the field of IoT is evidenced by the fact that 60% of healthcare organizations have the IoT. Almost 87% of healthcare providers introduced the IoT services offered in the area, about 40% of the organizations of healthcare in the living biosensors use IoT. About 80% of organizations in the area of healthcare have reported an increase in innovation by implementing IoT, 73% of medical providers were able to reduce costs through the use of IoT. Market segment for smart tablets reached $6.93 billion by 2020. The

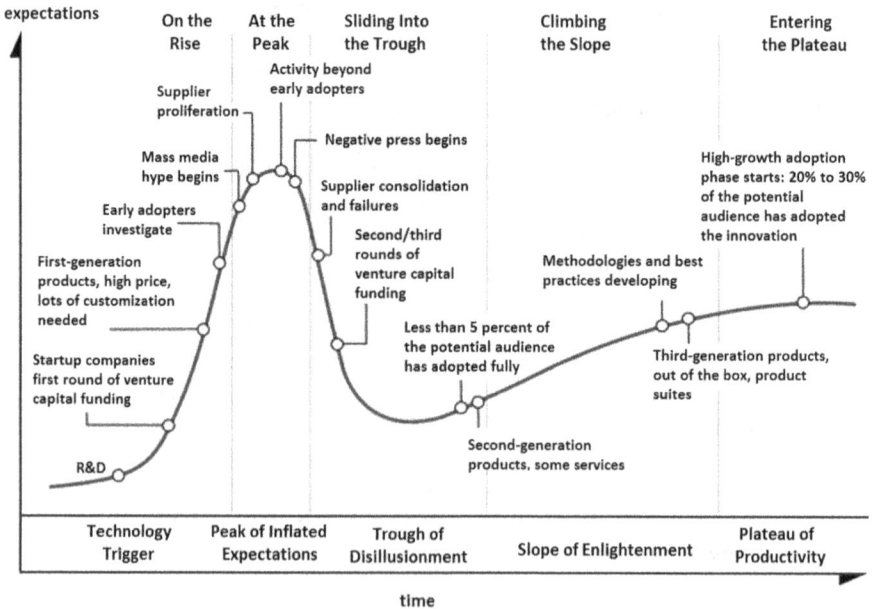

FIGURE 1.4 Evolution of digital health technologies—the Hype Cycle.

most popular IoT solutions in healthcare organizations are used to monitor and keep patients in good condition (73%).

A well-chosen diagnosis with the use of IoT tools and applications allows you to minimize medical costs while increasing the quality standards of service. Therefore, the use of IoT in medicine seems to be an inherent necessity that will allow the free functioning of the healthcare system and avoid injuries, accidents, or sudden deterioration of health. In addition, correctly implemented diagnosis with the use of IoT solutions has the positive impact that is represented by the following data [58]:

- Medical consultations without the need for a personal visit and with the use of electronic communication via IoT and all its tools create a new medical reality and replace the classic approach to patients. This is evidenced by the fact that over 70% of patients, having a choice, would prefer a remote medical visit instead of a traditional one.
- The use of electronic communication tools through IoT medication significantly improves the quality of medical services provided, and additionally allows increasing their number at the same time.
- Telemedicine and IoT tools usage leads to better efficiency of medical services and eliminates the queues, so it makes it possible to the better use of regional medical access points.
- Because of the perspective of costs (direct and indirect) related to civilization diseases (ChS-N and cancer), a huge savings in the healthcare system is possible with the use of IoT solutions to prevent, report, and diagnose such health problems.
- IoT tools enable the better care of people who are under drug therapy, especially through the use of drug dose reminders, guidance on the use of drugs, reconciliation of various types of drug therapies carried out simultaneously, capturing drug interactions.

The data collected thanks to IoT solutions serves to supervise better the companies producing drugs and medical equipment over the use of products. What's more, reporting on drug intake thanks to the use of IoT tools allows you to observe the results of their use and allows you to detect side effects [59]. The implementation of IoT tools for medicine and healthcare management is also associated with the possibility of reporting non-compliance in the operation of these tools. Thanks to this, their producers can make corrections and do the preventive activities, as well as support the lack of response from the device users themselves. On the contrary, the data from IoT tools supplements the information collected from postmarket surveillance of their use [60]. They are utilized to support the determined balance between the positives and negatives of the IoT technology products.

IoT tools increase the everyday life of an aging society, improving and extending the quality of life of patients [61]:

- The data collected by IoT (e.g., certified for medical use wearables) may have an influence on faster diagnose of dementia, and may conduct constant reporting of the health and behavior of an older person.

- The time it takes to perform medical activities is significantly reduced, with the management processes improvement as well.
- IoT tools are able to replace medical assistance in situations where it is possible, for example, reminding about medications, visits, or rehabilitation.

According to a 2015 study, there are more than 165,000 health-related mobile applications on the market. Over the past 2 years, the number of these applications has more than doubled. It is estimated that 90% of downloads are generated by 12% of applications. Most are about nutrition and exercise. The percentage of applications that allow patients to share information safely remains unchanged despite the increasing opportunities resulting from the development of information systems [62]. Nearly two-thirds of the mobile apps focus on lifestyle, diets, stress, and physical activity. In contrast, only 24% of applications concern diseases and their treatment [63], and the usage of health app in US in 2015 is shown in Figure 1.5.

In 2013, over 43,000 health applications on the market had been downloaded more than 660 million times. However, most of them, due to their poor quality, are not very popular. More than half were downloaded by users fewer than 500 times, indicating low interest in most of them. On the contrary, five applications generated 15% of all downloads, which proves their vast popularity. Data from a survey conducted in the USA in 2012 shows that for more than 50% of smartphone users, their phones' primary source of health knowledge is information. Nineteen percent of respondents downloaded a health-related app on their phones. Despite the massive popularity of the application, most of them are not authorized by regulatory bodies such as the FDA in the USA [64].

By using mobile applications, it is easier to promote a healthy lifestyle and preventive care. Lack of motivation for systematic physical activity is a big problem. The solution here is, for example, the competition used by the Endomondo

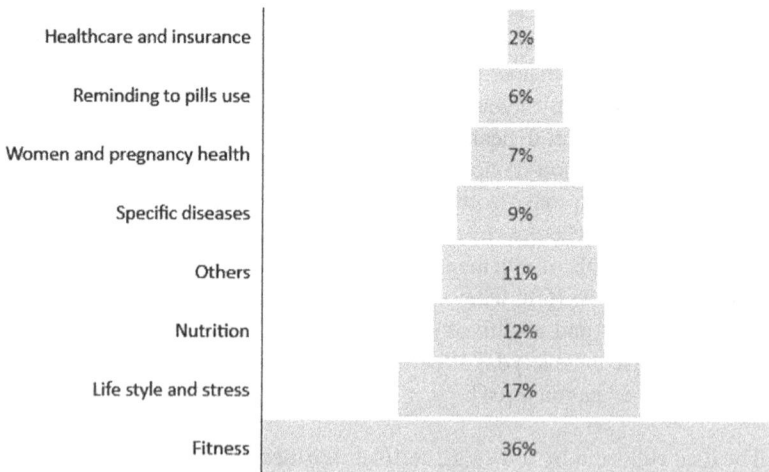

FIGURE 1.5   Breakdown of health app usage in USA in 2015.

application. A considerable number of users compete with each other, for example, who will run more kilometers in a predetermined time [65].

Some mobile applications to function correctly need additional external devices that monitor vital functions, such as pulse, blood pressure, respiratory rate, blood oxygenation. Their data collection is automatic, convenient, and continuous. This way of collecting data reduces the risk of errors. The part of the body for which most devices are produced is the wrist, for which as much as 55% of complementary devices are developed. The chest is in second place with 23% of devices. Other devices are prepared to be placed on the arms, head, clothes, legs. Devices that read vital signs from the ear, where they are unnoticeable, are becoming more popular. It is possible thanks to the progressive miniaturization of these devices [63].

Also, the design of devices and applications for IoT in healthcare takes into account a number of factors and elements that both medics and patients pay attention to. In 2014, a study was carried out to identify users' expectations regarding health applications [66]. These expectations of what patients and carers want from health apps are presented in Table 1.3.

Carried around, wireless and mobile monitoring systems may become the best possible solution for many patients living far from healthcare facilities, whose vital parameters should be monitored on an ongoing basis. Such remote monitoring is a convenient and comfortable solution. It is associated with a reduction in costs and time. Constant monitoring allows for an earlier detection of possible irregularities. It enables immediate medical help in emergency situations, such as immediate drug administration or transport to the hospital. The time needed to make a diagnosis is reduced. It is also crucial that these devices are user-friendly, easy to wear, and intuitive to use. They should be highly acceptable for both the patient and the doctor. They will improve the process of data collection and flow, being the link between the patient and the doctor. Ultimately, however, they will not replace a specialist [67].

The use of IoT in healthcare technology seems to be an extremely beneficial solution for both medicine and patients [68]. Meanwhile, there are not only advantages to using this type of solution, but there are also many barriers, as summarized in Table 1.4.

Thanks to the use of modern technologies, it becomes possible to search vast collections of medical data in search of regularities and anomalies occurring in this data. Automatic search for recurring anomalies allows the finding of unknown dependencies in the development and consequences of diseases [69]. This is, for example, useful for clinical trials thanks to the ability to integrate and share the results of diagnostic tests obtained from patients. Such actions would accelerate the progress of medicine. The companies conduct clinical trials, the results of which are available only in their databases. Generally available medical data on a large number of patients who provide their medical data voluntarily would enable faster and cheaper disease detection and treatment [70]. The researchers emphasize that immediate data sharing will reduce the time needed to collect it when compared to traditional clinical trials. All this is to lead to a better understanding of the causes of disease and improvement in patients' quality of life [71].

TABLE 1.3

Expectations of patients and carers regarding the health apps

Which of the Following Would Convince You to Use Health Apps Regularly		What Is the Single Most Important Service You Think Health Apps Should Provide	
Feature	Indications [in %]	Feature	Indications [in %]
Provide trustworthy, accurate information	69	Give me understandable info on symptoms/medical conditions	23
Is easy to use/simple/well designed	66	Help me communicate with my doctor/nurse	17
Provide guarantees that my personal data is secured	62	Allow me to examine my health records/medical tests online	16
Be free of charge	56	Help me track my medical symptoms	14
Contain no advertisements	51	Help track activities to improve my health or keep me healthy	13
Work effectively and consistently over time	44	Give me understandable info about how to live a healthier life	7
Not expensive to buy, and provide value for money	28	Help me communicate with other people important to me	6
Allow me to network with other people important to me	26	Allow me to comment about, or rate, local healthcare services	3
Be packed with detail (do not mind complex apps)	23		

1. In Poland, the problem is the aging society and the growing number of physically and mentally incapacitated people. The low sense of security of the residents of nursing homes causes a decline in social trust in local governments and foundations. Simultaneously, the amount of time spent on preparing the documentation and the emergency situations are also problematic. There are limited financial resources, staff shortages, and an insufficient number of institutions. This situation makes it necessary to optimize the whole management process.

   The remedy to this problem can be telemedicine bands, namely the SiDLY telecare belt [72], which enables the remote communication, health reporting, fall detection with a call about the need to react. It includes an SOS button to assist in emergencies. Additionally, it reminds to take their medication and allows the user to locate the wristband.

TABLE 1.4

Advantages and barriers of IoT in healthcare

Benefits	Barriers
• Facilitating access to healthcare • Increase in the quality of healthcare • Increase in the quality of life of patients • Increase in the safety of patients and doctors • Time savings for healthcare professionals (including doctors and nurses) and a response to staff shortages • Cost reduction • Modernizing and improving the efficiency of healthcare delivery (by enabling faster information flow and helping to transform healthcare systems from a piecemeal approach that includes prevention, primary care, treatment, and rehabilitation separately, to continuous care where all stages of treatment are closely intertwined (linked) • Improving and increasing the security of transmitting data on patients and their health condition • Accelerating the progress of medicine by facilitating the conduct of clinical trials	• Lack of awareness and trust in e-health solutions among patients, citizens, and healthcare workers • Lack of interoperability between e-health systems • Limited or even lack of evidence describing on a large scale the profitability of using e-health tools and services • Legal uncertainty for the use of mobile health and wellness monitoring applications as well as a lack of transparency regarding the use of data collected by such applications • Lack of sufficient or fragmented legal framework, including no reimbursement system for e-health users • The necessity to incur high costs related to the creation and use of e-health systems • Regional differences in access to ICT services, including limited access to these services in specific areas • Strong fragmentation of the healthcare services market

Thanks to its application, it is possible to notice a number of measurable benefits. Doctors will reduce time spent on documentation by 60%, will have more time for direct patient contact by about 29%, and will consult additional patients. For hospitals, the benefits are reflected in a 35% reduction in hospitalizations, a 53% reduction in emergency room interventions, and a 59% reduction in hospital bed days. While the benefits seen by social policy include improving the implementation of the strategy for the senior care, improving the efficiency of healthcare services, devising more attractive and innovative medical care policies, and enhancing the attractiveness of places of residence for dependent persons, the disabled, senior citizens, who require constant monitoring. SiDLY telecare wristbands allow seniors, people living alone, and people requiring support in everyday life to stay at home [73].

2. In addition to the above case, another problem experienced in Poland is 40,000 cardiac arrests per year. Among people who experience sudden cardiac arrest (SCA) in Poland, only 7% survive, while in the Scandinavian countries, this ratio is 40% (data from the European Resuscitation Council).

The remedy to this problem may be the use of the REANIMATOR application. It is an application that makes it easier to help a person with sudden cardiac arrest (SCA). It consists of two main modules: 1. automated external defibrillator (AED) locator, which will pinpoint the AED localization, and show the shortest way to find it, and 2. 'virtual assistant' that assists the entire situation. This IoT tool may also help in survival, which includes diagnosis of cardiac arrest, calling for professional help, early defibrillation, medical rescue operations conducted by professionals.

The benefits of using this solution include an increase in the survival rate of people with SCA, thus reducing financial losses and deaths of working-age people. The savings might be even at around PLN 400,000. Improving the survival rate by 1% means PLN 160,000,000 of savings [73].

The presented problems and solutions together with the benefits are only two examples illustrating how many benefits can be brought by the appropriate application of IoT in healthcare management.

REFERENCES

[1]. A. M. Rahmani, T. N. Gia, B. Negash, A. Anzanpour, I. Azimi, M. Jiang and P. Liljeberg, Exploiting smart e-Health gateways at the edge of healthcare Internet-of-Things: A fog computing approach. *Future Generation Computer Systems*, 78, 641–658 (2018).

[2]. J. E. W. C. Van Gemert-Pijnen, S. Wynchank, H. D. Covvey and H. C. Ossebaard, Improving the credibility of electronic health technologies. *Bulletin of the World Health Organization*, 90, 323–323A (2012).

[3]. M. M. Dhanvijay and S. C. Patil, Internet of Things: A survey of enabling technologies in healthcare and its applications. *Computer Networks*, 153, 113–131 (2019).

[4]. WHO, *Building Foundations eHealth in Europe. Report of the WHO Global Observatory for eHealth.* Geneva (2008).

[5]. COCIR, COCIR eHealth Toolkit. *Integrated Care: Breaking the Silos*, http://www.cocir.org/fileadmin/4.4__eHealth/15013.COC_2.pdf (2015).

[6]. Communication from the Commission to the European Parliament. The Council, the European economic and social committee and the Committee of the regions, eHealth Action Plan 2012–2020—Innovative healthcare for the 21st century. *COM 736 final*, Brussels (2012).

[7]. T. Lewis, E-health in low- and middle-income countries: Findings from the Center for Health Market Innovations. *Bulletin of the World Health Organization*, 90, 323–340 (2012).

[8]. K. Ashton, That 'internet of things' thing. *RFID Journal*, 22(7), 97–114 (2009).

[9]. A. V. Dastjerdi and R. Buyya, *Internet of things: Principles and paradigms.* Cambridge, MA: Morgan Kaufmann (2016).

[10]. F. Al-Turjman, M. H. Nawaz and U. D. Ulusar, Intelligence in the Internet of Medical Things era: A systematic review of current and future trends. *Computer Communications*, 150, 644–660 (2020).

[11]. A. Botta, W. De Donato, V. Persico and A. Pescapé, Integration of cloud computing and internet of things: A survey. *Future Generation Computer Systems*, 56, 684–700 (2016).

[12]. D. A. Gratton, *The Handbook of Personal Area Networking Technologies and Protocols.* Cambridge: Cambridge University Press (2013).

[13]. J. Pan, S. Ding, D. Wu, S. Yang and J. Yang, Exploring behavioural intentions toward smart healthcare services among medical practitioners: A technology transfer perspective. *International Journal of Production Research*, 57(18), 5801–5820 (2019).

[14]. *Deliotte, Medtech and the Internet of Medical Things. How Connected Medical Devices are Transforming Health Care*. London: Center for Health Solutions (2018).

[15]. N. Dey, A. E. Hassanien, C. Bhatt, A. S. Ashour and S. C. Satapathy, *Internet of Things and Big Data Analytics Toward Next-Generation Intelligence*. Cham: Springer International Publishing (2018).

[16]. J. M. McDonald, C. Gossett, and M. Moore, Moving to the cloud: The state of the art for cloud-based production pipelines. *Journal of Digital Media Management*, 6(3) (2018).

[17]. G. J. Joyia, R. M. Liaqat, A. Farooq and S. Rehman, Internet of Medical Things (IOMT): Applications, benefits and future challenges in healthcare domain. *Journal of Communication*, 12(4), 240–247 (2017).

[18]. W. Raghupathi and V. Raghupathi, Big data analytics in healthcare: Promise and potential. *Health Information Science and Systems*, 2(1), 3 (2014).

[19]. Y. Xiao, Q. Alexander and F. Hu, Telemedicine for Pervasive Healthcare. *Mobile Telemedicine: A Computing and Networking Perspective* (1st ed., 3), 89–404 (2008).

[20]. D. Metcalf, R. Khron and P. Salber, *Health-e Everything: Wearables and the Internet of Things for Health: Part One: Wearables for Healthcare*. Orlando, FL: Moving Knowledge (2016).

[21]. C. A. Figueroa, R. Harrison, A. Chauhan and L. Meyer, Priorities and challenges for health leadership and workforce management globally: a rapid review. *BMC health services research*, 19(1), 1–11 (2019).

[22]. H. Zhu, C. K. Wu, C. H. Koo, Y. T. Tsang, Y. Liu, H. R. Chi and K. F. Tsang, Smart healthcare in the era of internet-of-things. *IEEE Consumer Electronics Magazine*, 8(5), 26–30 (2019).

[23]. A. Gatouillat, Y. Badr, B. Massot and E. Sejdic, Internet of medical things: A review of recent contributions dealing with cyber-physical systems in medicine. *IEEE Internet of Things Journal*, 5, 3810–3822 (2018).

[24]. A. Rajput and T. Brahimi, Characterizing IOMT/Personal Area Networks Landscape. https://arxiv.org/ftp/arxiv/papers/1902/1902.00675.pdf (2017).

[25]. K. Ullah, M. A. Shah and S. Zhang, Effective ways to use Internet of Things in the field of medical and smart health care. *Proceedings of International Conference on Intelligent Systems Engineering (ICISE)*, 372–379 (2016).

[26]. F. Al-Turjman and S. Alturjman, Context-sensitive access in industrial internet of things (IIoT) healthcare applications. *IEEE Transactions on Industrial Informatics*, 14(6), 2736–2744 (2018).

[27]. A. Rajput and T. Brahimi, Characterizing IOMT/personal area networks landscape. *arXiv preprint arXiv*, 1902, 00675 (2019).

[28]. R. Shams, F. Hanif Khan, M. Aamir and F. Saleem, Internet of things in tele-medicine: A discussion regarding to several implementation. *Journal of Computer Science of Newports Institute of Communications and Economics*, 5, 17–26 (2014).

[29]. E. N. Karyagina and R. I. Sitdikova, Telemedicine: The concept and legal regulation in Russia, Europe, and USA. *Journal of History Culture and Art Research*, 8(4), 417–424 (2019).

[30]. E. M. Hayden, K. M. Boggs, J. A. Espinola, C. A. Camargo Jr and K. S. Zachrison, Telemedicine facilitation of transfer coordination from Emergency Departments. *Annals of Emergency Medicine*, 76(5), 602–608 (2020).

[31]. Communication from the Commission to the European Parliament, the Council, the European economic and social committee and the Committee of the regions, eHealth Action Plan 2012–2020, Innovative healthcare for the 21st century. *COM 736 final*, Brussels (2012).

[32]. P. Kotler and J. E. Heppelmann, How smart connected products are transforming competition. *Harvard Business Review*, 11, 4–23 (2014).

[33]. M. Maksimović and V. Vujović, Internet of Things based e-health systems: Ideas, expectations and concerns. *Handbook of large-scale distributed computing in smart healthcare*. Cham: Springer (2017).

[34]. M. Mihai, E. Țițan, D.I. Manea and C. D. Ionescu, Digital Innovation in the Health Sector—a Determinant of Health Status, Records in the EU. *New Trends in Sustainable Business and Consumption*, 2, 579–586 (2020).

[35]. D. Pal, S. Funilkul, N. Charoenkitkarn and P. Kanthamanon, Internet-of-things and smart homes for elderly healthcare: An end user perspective. *IEEE Access*, 6, 10483–10496 (2018).

[36]. V. Jagadeeswari, V. Subramaniyaswamy, R. Logesh and V. Vijayakumar, A study on medical Internet of Things and Big Data in personalized healthcare system. *Health information science and systems*, 6(1), 1–20 (2018).

[37]. Deloitte, Connected health. How digital technology is transforming health and social care, https://www2.deloitte.com/pl/pl/pages/life-sciences-and-healthcare/articles/mobile-health-IP1.html (2015).

[38]. G. Elhayatmy, N. Dey and A. S. Ashour, Internet of Things based wireless body area network in healthcare. In *Internet of Things and Big Data Analytics Toward Next-generation Intelligence*. Cham: Springer (2018).

[39]. M. M. Baig and H. Gholam Hosseini, Wireless remote patient monitoring in older adults, Engineering in Medicine and Biology Society (EMBC), 35th Annual International Conference of the IEEE, 2429 (2013).

[40]. G. Manogaran, R. Varatharajan, D. Lopez, P. M. Kumar, R. Sundarasekar and C. Thota, A new architecture of Internet of Things and big data ecosystem for secured smart healthcare monitoring and alerting system. *Future Generation Computer Systems*, 82, 375–387 (2018).

[41]. S. Nazir, Y. Ali, N. Ullah and I. García-Magariño, Internet of things for healthcare using effects of mobile computing: A systematic literature review. *Wireless Communications and Mobile Computing*, 12(7), 98 (2019).

[42]. Y. Bhatt and C. Bhatt, *Internet of things in healthcare. In Internet of things and big data technologies for next generation HealthCare*. Cham: Springer (2017).

[43]. P. Kaur, R. Kumar and M. Kumar, A healthcare monitoring system using random forest and internet of things (IoT). *Multimedia Tools and Applications*, 78(14), 19905–19916 (2019).

[44]. E. S. Izmailova, J. A. Wagner and E. D. Perakslis, Wearable devices in clinical trials: Hype and hypothesis. *Clinical Pharmacology and Therapeutics*, 104(1), 42–52 (2018).

[45]. K. Guk, G. Han, J. Lim, K. Jeong, T. Kang, E. K. Lim and J. Jung, Evolution of wearable devices with real-time disease monitoring for personalized healthcare. *Nanomaterials*, 9(6), 813 (2019).

[46]. M. W. Condry and X. I. Quan, Digital health innovation, informatics opportunity and challenges. *IEEE Engineering Management Review*, 7, 569 (2021).

[47]. G. Shanmugasundaram and G. Sankarikaarguzhali, An investigation on IoT healthcare analytics. *International Journal of Information Engineering and Electronic Business*, 9(2), 11 (2017).

[48]. M. Chorost, The Networked Pill. *MIT Technology Review*, http://www.technologyreview.com/news/409773/the-networked-pill/ (2008).

[49]. P. Murray, No More Skipping Your Medicine—FDA Approved First Digital Pill. *Forbes*, http://onforb.es/PHcZO8 (2012).

[50]. S. Anderson and A. Bassi, We need a killer business model. Inspiring the Internet of Things, *Internet of Things Initiative*, http://www.alexandra.dk/uk/expertise/publications/documents/iot_comic_book.pdf (2011)

[51]. S. Rosati, G. Balestra and M. Knaflitz, Comparison of different sets of features for human activity recognition by wearable sensors. *Sensors*, 18(12), 4189 (2018).

[52]. J. W. Sharp, The Internet of Things Creeps into Healthcare. http://ehealth. johnwsharp.com/2013/07/19/the-internet-of-things-creeps-into-healthcare/ (2013).

[53]. J. Czechowicz, Raport Internet of Things 2015 (1). http://www.mobiletrends.pl/ raport-internet-of-things-2015-czesc-1/ (2015).

[54]. S. Y. Y. Tun, S. Madanian and F. Mirza, Internet of things (IoT) applications for elderly care: A reflective review. *Aging Clinical and Experimental Research*, 4, 1–13 (2020).

[55]. B.A. Jnr, Use of telemedicine and virtual care for remote treatment in response to COVID-19 pandemic. *Journal of Medical Systems*, 44(7), 1–9 (2020).

[56]. The Digital Health Hype Cycle. https://en.wikipedia.org/wiki/Hype_cycle (2013).

[57]. Allied Market Research report, https://www.alliedmarketresearch.com/iot-healthcare-market (2017).

[58]. K. T. Kadhim, A. M. Alsahlany, S. M. Wadi and H. T. Kadhum, An overview of patient's health status monitoring system based on Internet of Things (IoT). *Wireless Personal Communications*, 114, 2235–2262 (2020).

[59]. A. Dzedzickis, A. Kaklauskas and V. Bucinskas, Human emotion recognition: Review of sensors and methods. *Sensors*, 20(3), 592 (2020).

[60]. A. Jordao, A. C. Nazare Jr, J. Sena and W. R. Schwartz, Human activity recognition based on wearable sensor data: A standardization of the state-of-the-art. *arXiv preprint arXiv*, 1806, 05226 (2018).

[61]. G. Marques and R. Pitarma, mHealth: Indoor environmental quality measuring system for enhanced health and well-being based on internet of things. *Journal of Sensor and Actuator Networks*, 8(3), 43 (2019).

[62]. S. Misra, New report finds more than 165,000 mobile health apps now available, takes close look at characteristics & use, www.imedicalapps.com/2015/09/ims-health-appsreport (2015).

[63]. IMS Institute, Patient Adoption of mHealth. http://www.imshealth.com/fi les/web/ IMSH%20Institute/Reports/Patient%20Adoption%20of%20mHealth/IIHI-Patient-Adoption-mhealth-Exhibits-Full.pdf (2015).

[64]. L. Neubeck, N. Lowres, E. J. Benjamin, S. B. Freedman and G. Coorey, The mobile revolution—using smartphone apps to prevent cardiovascular disease. *Nature Reviews Cardiology*, 12, 85 (2015).

[65]. S. Lomborg and K. Frandsen, Self-tracking as communication. Information, *Communication and Society*, 19(7), 1015–1027 (2016).

[66]. What do patients and carers want from health apps? Results of a global survey of 1,130 people with a long-term condition and their carers. Patient View November 2014; https:// alexwyke.wordpress.com/2014/11/23/what-do-people-want-from-health-apps/ (2014).

[67]. M. M. Baig, H. Gholamhosseini and M. J. Connolly, A comprehensive survey of wearable and wireless ECG monitoring systems for older adults. *Medical and Biological Engineering and Computing*, 51(5), 485–495 (2013).

[68]. J. Qi, P. Yang, G. Min, O. Amft, F. Dong and L. Xu, Advanced internet of things for personalised healthcare systems: A survey. *Pervasive and Mobile Computing*, 41, 132–149 (2017).

[69]. R. Krohn, D. Metcalf and P. Salber, *Connected health improving care, safety, and efficiency with wearables and IoT solution*. Milton: CRC Press (2017).

[70]. C. Bhatt, N. Dey and A. S. Ashour, *Internet of things and big data technologies for next generation healthcare*. Switzerland: Springer (2017).

[71]. J. Wilbanks and S. H. Friend, First, design for data sharing. *Nature Biotechnology*, 34(4), 76 (2016).

[72]. Sidly, http://sidly.eu/pl (2018).

[73]. Polish Ministry of Digitization, IoT in Polish economy report. www.gov.pl/ cyfryzacja (2019).

2 Blending of Internet of Things and Deep Transfer Learning (DTL): Enabling Innovations in Healthcare (COVID-19) and Applications

Atlanta Choudhury and Kandarpa Kumar Sarma

CONTENTS

2.1   INTRODUCTION

Global healthcare systems are currently facing unprecedented hardships while handling the pandemic arising out of this deadly virus. The COVID-19, also called novel corona virus, is responsible for the ongoing pandemic, which causes re-spiratory issues leading even to death. It is transmitted among human beings and starts expanding to all. Contagiousness components in this deadly viruses are very high [1,2], hundreds of millions of people have been contaminated, and huge fatalities have been recorded within months from its outbreak. This deadly disease has been

DOI: 10.1201/9781003171829-2

classified as a pandemic by the World Health Organization (WHO) [3,4]. This is not the only pandemic that has been faced by human beings. Many such outbreaks have occurred in the past, and more may occur in the near future [5,6]. There are no appropriate drugs available in the market, but after clinical trials, vaccination has been started globally. There is no such readymade infrastructure available to deal with such outbreaks, but facilities are being created. To deal with such diseases, building medical and support capacity becomes important [7,8]. Among many support facilities, computation predictive tools are important as these provide a forecast to the emerging scenarios and enable people to visualize probable situations. Many researchers are attempting to develop techniques to obtain solutions for such situations and enable people to face such challenges [9,10]. Artificial intelligence (AI), including data science, is one of the key enabling techniques that are applied in such uncertain situations. Deep learning (DL), a part of AI, is a tool that can be configured to formulate prediction and forecast-based solution so that losses and fatalities could be minimized [11]. Due to deep architectural design and ability to perform feature extraction irrespective of data sources, DL models are the most reliable methods for dealing with medical datasets, particularly in pandemic conditions. Therefore, these techniques could also be applied and customized to handle this type of pandemic situation and help monitor social situation and observe biosafety norms, break the chain of spread, confirm the disease, drug discovery and appropriate use of vaccine, treatment, and many more [12,13]. AI tools are useful for the medical fraternity as these provide predictive analytics. The advantage of such systems is that these tools learn from the surroundings, retain the learning, and use it subsequently. To train such AI-driven techniques, huge datasets and robust computing resources are needed.

For a pandemic situation to be analyzed by AI driven tools, insufficient data and variation in different geographic regions are impeding issues. They seriously influence the performance of AI-aided tools used commonly. Conventional AI tools like the ones based on DL require huge datasets which most of the time might not be available. Further, due to restrictions in mobility in the midst of pandemic situations, it might not be possible to collect sufficient amount of field or real-time data. In such situations, its conventional DL tolls might prove to be ineffective. A solution to such a tricky situation comes from the use of deep transfer learning (DTL). It is an effective tool and works well despite limitations in data volume. DTL takes what it knows from one job and applies it to another after some fine-tuning [14]. In any pandemic scenario, EDs such as the Internet of things (IoT), webcams, drones, intelligent medical equipment, robotic support are beneficial. Concerned organizations should use such facilities to deal with outbreaks because this equipment makes infrastructures sophisticated and automated [15]. As a result, computers are equipped with limited computational resources, which presents a number of challenges. Edge computing (EC) [16] is a method configured for real work situations including medical applications. EC is effective in monitoring, enabling knowledge update with contemporary data, ease of deployment, low cost, user-friendliness, and so on. Further, it can work together with AI tools to generate decision support. Conventional DL tools integrated to EC devices shall also require huge volumes of data, which is a restriction. Therefore, in order to streamline restrictions due to lesser availability of data, DTL can be effectively employed with EC devices. This combination has been discovered to be a viable way to consolidate processing power and allow more systematic EC. Hence, in EDs that use DTL algorithm may be intelligent technique to formulate predictive analytics-based measures to face the devastating nature of COVID-19 pandemic [17]. Here we attempt to report several such issues and challenges with relevant technical backgrounds required to formulate methods for designing AI-driven infrastructure to deal with pandemic-like situations. Further, we also propose possible AI-based architecture as future scope to deploy DTL over EC to assists in efforts of mitigation of such outbreaks. In several countries, the concerned ministries of health have recommended several disease prevention measures for individuals, families, workplaces, schools, childcare centers, and senior citizens [18], many of which are based on AI techniques. These measures include following social distancing norms or increasing physical space between humans and their effective monitoring, autonomous robot for disinfectant spray, support to frontline workers, drug and food delivery, diagnosis, drug discovery and design.

2.2 HISTORICAL BACKGROUND

In Wuhan, Hubei Province, South China, the COVID-19 outbreak was first discovered. On December 31, 2019, local hospitals announced an unidentified pneumonia [19]. This unidentified pneumonia has spread rapidly to almost all countries in the world. These cases were initially linked to the wholesale market, which specially deals with seafood in Huainan. This market is also famous for its wide range of live species. Each of these cases has its own set of clinical characteristics. Many of these cases have common symptoms that are similar to viral pneumonia, such as a dry cough, fever, dyspnea. The imaging findings of lung infiltrates indicated the seriousness of the new outbreak. On January 7, 2020, after examining samples acquired from a throat swab, the Centers for Disease Control and Prevention (CDC) diagnosed the mystery pneumonia as novel corona virus pneumonia (NCP) [20]. It was eventually termed severe acute respiratory syndrome coronavirus 2 (SARS-CoV2) by the International Committee on Virus Taxonomy [21,22]. On February 11, 2020, the WHO called the disease COVID-19 [23]. The corona virus COVID-19 is produced by SARS-CoV-2. There are few indications that the number of contaminated and deceased patient will decrease, and the circumstances will remain volatile.

2.3 TECHNICAL BACKGROUND

Deep learning (DL), also called as hierarchical learning (HL) or deep structured learning (DSL), is a branch of AI that provides tools and methodologies to mimic the abilities of the human brain better than previously known approaches. DL is one of the most recent improvements that have been incorporated in the earlier generation artificial neural network (ANN) systems. Classical machine learning (ML) techniques had been used to make data inferences and predictions in the early 1990s [24]. However, it has a number of disadvantages, such as relying on handcrafted features,

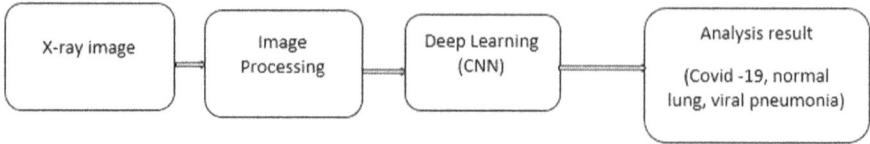

FIGURE 2.1   Proposed schematic diagram of DL-based COVID detection.

data labeling, and being limited by human ability-centric accuracy. The handcrafted function isn't required in DL [25]. With the aid of various innovative algorithms, computational power of modern computers, and the availability of large datasets, DL can make more accurate predictions and classifications.

As already noted DL is a learning algorithm that falls under the AI umbrella, and it is based on ANN but in a much up-scaled level. The back propagation algorithm is used to train these models using the dataset [26]. It is a good optimizer tool for dealing with COVID-19. COVID-19 patients can be detected by checking body temperature (fever) and related symptoms. DL could be used for many other purposes such as patient care as well as detection of systematic social distancing observance and violation. Further, DL methods can be used to formulate robotic systems to handle pandemic-related crisis, provide support to patients, drug and food delivery, decontamination, drug design and discovery, identify and prevent spread of fake news, and create social awareness. The possibilities are enormous. The primary attributes of DL systems that are crucial in this case are their ability to replicate human behavior, provide prediction, and forecast (Figure 2.1).

2.3.1   DEEP TRANSFER LEARNING

After a model has been trained, transfer learning allows it to be employed on a new challenge. In comparison to traditional machine learning methods, a big training data collection is required for DL. As a result, the requirement for a large amount of labeled data is a major impediment to completing some critical domain-specific tasks, especially in the medical domain, where the development of large-scale, high-quality annotated medical data is a major challenge [27]. Although scientists work tirelessly to find ways to reduce the risk and the effects of such constraints [28,29], the basic DL model needs a lot of computing power and the use of specialized hardware like GPU-enabled servers. DTL, a DL-based transfer learning [30], was used to provide a solution to this challenge. DTL greatly minimizes the need for training data and training time for a target domain-specific job by picking a pre-trained model (trained on another large dataset of the same target domain) for a fixed feature extractor or for further fine-tuning [31]. It is now common in DL because it can train deep neural networks (DNN) with a small amount of data (Figure 2.2).

2.3.2   EDGE DEVICES

Edge or IoT devices capture and process data in real time by storing a copy of densely used data from the cloud locally and providing additional functionality to IoT devices. As a result, only the Fog server sends related data from IoT devices to the cloud.

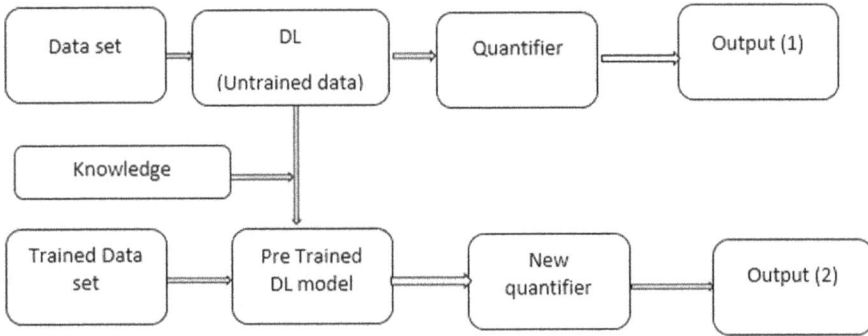

FIGURE 2.2 Schematic diagram of DTL model.

Edge Computing

Data is collected from a variety of IoT devices, then pre-processed before being delivered to the Fog server for analysis and processing, with the Edge providing real-time responses. While the cloud houses the core machine and maintains the whole database, the Fog constantly uploads only the most relevant data or information to the cloud database. Although EC is not a novel concept, it has proven to be extremely useful in the recent development of the IoT.

2.4   LITERATURE SURVEY

Already much work related to application of DL in COVID-19 domains has been reported, DL, which is based on Convolutional Neural Network (CNN) for screening COVID-19 patients using their computed tomography (CT), has been reported with precision, sensitivity, and specificity of 89.5%, 87%, and 88%, respectively [32]. Another study found that chest X-ray images were 83.5% accurate in screening COVID-19 cases [33]. To date, several DTL models have been suggested for application in COVID-19-related domains. Here a few such works are highlighted. In all such works, it is observed that the use of DTL involves the construction of multiple domain-related layers by aligning the joint distribution processes that support a common maximum mean discrepancy. This can be helpful to establish a transfer network. The authors of Ref. [34] suggest that based on the VGG model, a cutting-edge transfer-learning model has been developed. For feature extraction, the researchers used the Image Net [35] dataset, and for fine-tuning, they used handmark construction images. In Ref. [36], authors propose the use of DTL to classify abnormalities in MR images. The researchers used a fine-tuned pre-trained ResNet34 model. However, the global norm diagnostic microbiology laboratory and related research takes time and money, and there are many false-negative results [37]. Around the same time, due to a scarcity of services, studies are rarely performed in community health centers or hospitals. Medical resource management becomes very complex, and the outcome is large numbers of patients are being handled at once. DTL models are thought to be ideal for reducing the difficulties in this type of situation [38,39]. Generative-adversarial-networks (**GANs**) can also be used along with

DTL model. Here, only limited numbers of data are required to run the model. To diagnose COVID-19 disease and analyze, only 307 chest radiographs were taken as a dataset and three pre-trained models, namely Alex net [40], Google Net [41], and Resent [42] have been used. Google Net has reported the highest accuracy among these three pre-trained models.

2.5 DESCRIPTION OF PROPOSED MODEL TO MITIGATE COVID-19

As already highlighted earlier, DTL is effective in building predictive models to deal with COVID-19 situation. DTL does not need much data. There is another technique known as EC that is also useful when computing power is limited. As a result, combining both of these computational approaches or models may be more useful for developing AI-driven methods to deal with COVID. We may assume that DTL on EC (DTLEC) is a special combination to deal with the COVID pandemic. The advantages of both DTL and EC are incorporated to formulate these models. This DTLEC concept is not practically used to mitigate COVID-19 but is evolving [43–69]. It has been observed that such a model could be useful in the healthcare industry, critical care units, quarantine facilities, and other areas where an outbreak could occur. Figure 2.3 shows edge devices or IoT devices implemented on EC and configured to use AI for decision making. Further, the system is designed to trigger an alert system implemented using a cloud-based approach. Later this edge device with a fine-tuning mechanism can be implemented with pre-trained datasets. Further, a DL-based graphical processing unit (GPU) enabled cloud server, which uses a standard dataset for performing feature extraction, is considered. Moreover, a pre-trained data model (DL based) is run over edge devices. With a fine-tuning mechanism, this edge device is considered to be implemented with pre-trained approach and dataset.

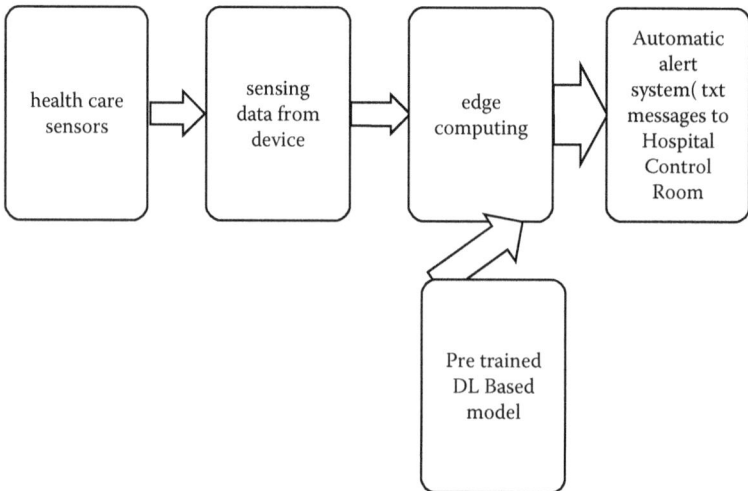

FIGURE 2.3   Proposed model for DTL using EC.

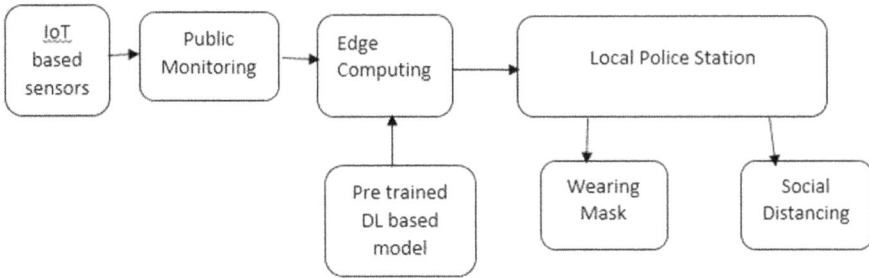

FIGURE 2.4 Proposed IoT-based smart monitoring system.

A typical COVID-19 outbreak scenario is depicted in Figure 2.3, where the proposed model or architecture is visualized for dealing with COVID-19 situations using DTL and EC. This device can monitor if any person is wearing mask in public or not or maintaining social distance. If the model detects any such scenarios, an automated text message with all pertinent information will be sent to the nearest police station as well as pedestrians registered with local mobile networks. Nevertheless, we have not considered a limitation. Children play a major role in spreading the virus. Children are less likely to wear masks on a regular basis because they don't understand the benefits of wearing masks in public areas (Figure 2.4).

2.6 REVIEW OF CERTAIN REPORTED WORKS RELATED TO ML/DL APPROACHES OF COVID-19 DETECTION, PREDICTION, AND OTHER ISSUES

Various research studies have recently reported the application of ML-based approaches for COVID-19 detection, prediction, and monitoring, among other things. Table 2.1 contains a summary of selected works. Some of these works are related to diagnosis [70,71], patient screening [72], observation of COVID-19 from radiographs, scan images, [73–77]; genome sequencing [78], monitoring [79], and prediction [80–82].

Table 2.2 provides a summary of some of the works based on DTL. Here, we see that DTL has been used for prediction [84,85], screening [86], detection, and diagnosis [39,87–91].

There are some works are based on EC (Table 2.3). Here we see that EC has been used for screening [91–93], controlling spreading [13,94], monitoring [95,96].

Table 2.4 includes some recent techniques developed using ML/DL approaches used exclusively for COVID-19 outbreak prediction. The outcomes are found to be accurate.

Table 2.5 shows a few works related to tracking and detection of virus spread. The works use big data and related analysis for tracking and detection of virus spread.

Table 2.6 shows a few works (which use big data from the Kyoto Genes storage) related to diagnosis and treatment of corona virus.

TABLE 2.1
Current DL based works to reduce pandemics

Sl. No.	Work	Specific Objective	Principal Contributions
1	71	Diagnosis using Deep Bayes-Squeeze Nets and X-ray images.	• Using functional DL algorithm for image processing to develop an intelligent recognition system. • A modern COVID-19 decision-making framework that combines traditional and cutting-edge approaches for chest radiographs.
2	72	Screening for corona virus disease pneumonia in 2019.	• Research compared several computational models for classifying different types of pneumonia. • According to CT tests, the accuracy of different cases was 0.996 (95% CI: 0.9891.00), with a sensitivity of 98.2% and specificity of 92.2%.
3	73	Detection and classification of COVID-19 infection from CT images.	• Weakly controlled DL for COVID-19 contamination observation and classification from radiograms. • Reduce the amount of labeling needed for CT pictures.
4	74	Active cases are automatically detected using raw radiograph.	• Different types of pneumonia could be observed by DL-based binary, multi-classification representation. • To ensure good precision, a combination of YOLO and Dark Net models were used as the model's backbone.
5	75	Identification of COVID-19 patterns in radiograms.	• Detection of virus patterns in radiographs. • Datasets from a resource-fullness model giving an accuracy of 91.4%, sensitivity of 90%, and forecasting of 100% were developed [83].
6	76	Distinguishing between novel corona virus and influenza pneumonias.	• An early diagnosis method for distinguishing corona virus pneumonia from standard Influenza with transferability on chest CT images.
7	77	SARSCoV-2 was identified using expanding genomic sequences.	• The interaction of viromics and DL. • A DL-assisted model for developing and future studies.
8	78	Deep learning and CT image analysis are used to automate detection and patient monitoring.	• Clinical awareness model based on 2D- and 3D-DL. • Suggested a continual monitoring method for active patients.

TABLE 2.1 *(Continued)*
Current DL based works to reduce pandemics

Sl. No.	Work	Specific Objective	Principal Contributions
9	79	Predict the COVID-19 outbreak in Iran.	• The information was gathered from the Google Trends website. • Positive COVID-19 cases were estimated using linear regression and LSTM models.
10	80	Using computer-assisted tomography images of the upper body; a fully automated framework to detect COVID-19 has been developed.	• COVNet was developed to detect the presence of this virus using visual features derived from scan. • A large number chest scans of patients were collected from six different hospitals.
11	81	Case detection using an open access chest radiograph image dataset.	• COVID-Net, for detecting active cases from scan images, was proposed as a publicly accessible COVID-Net. • COVIDx is a publicly available chest radiographs dataset.
12	82	A model for pandemic forecasting.	• A forecasting model based on Monte-Carlo approach.
13	83	Applying DL to predict infectious disease with the help of big data.	• Comparison among DL and other models for forecasting possible contamination diseases. • The schematic model aimed to strengthen current monitoring systems in order to spot emerging viral diseases in the future.

Table 2.7 shows a few works related to drug and vaccine development. The research employs molecular docking for drug development, and various peptides have been suggested for the development of a vaccine to combat this deadly virus.

From the above, we may conclude that big data and AI technologies are important in combating the pandemic in different ways. The significant approaches are:

    i. Forecast of outbreak.
    ii. Tracing and detection of spread.
    iii. Detection and therapy.
    iv. Drug and discovery of booster dose.

Learning-based approaches such as DL have also been found to be useful in virus centric modeling, grouping, and approximation. AI supports smart problem-solving tools for projecting successful and secure COVID-19 drug/booster dose design, which would be useful from both a science and a financial standpoint.

TABLE 2.2

Current DTL-based works to reduce pandemics

Sl. No.	Work	Specific Objective	Primary Contributions
1	84	Predicting COVID-19 from radiography.	• To identify COVID-19 disease, radiograms were used to train popular models including ResNet18, ResNet50, Squeeze Net, and DenseNet-121.
2	85	Screening COVID-19 using radiograms.	• Standard, other diseases and Covid-19 are all classified using transfer learning with pre-trained data. • Overall accuracy was 95.3%.
3	86	A case study using a small COVID-19 image dataset.	• On a small COVID-19 image dataset, an analysis of neutrosophic learning models was conducted. • They used pre-trained Alex net, Google Net, and Restnet18 to identify four groups after converting grayscale radiograms into fuzzy images.
4	87	Predicting availability of antiviral drugs using DL model.	• Moving target-DTI model is used to recognize commercially available drugs for corona virus. • This MTDTI model described a list of antiviral drugs, which were proposed.
5	88	Automated Identification of COVID-19.	• ResNet50, InceptionV3, and Inception-ResNetV2 models are used to distinguish between normal viral and COVID infection with the help of radiograms.
6	89	Evaluation of CNN architectures through TL over radiographs.	• DL with radiograms could yield distinct biomarkers related to this disease.
7	90	New crowd source for supporting healthcare deals with pandemic.	• The recognition of cough sound recordings made by handheld devices like mobile phones. Phones may be used as a diagnosis system.
8	91	Detection of COVID-19 using GAN and TL approaches.	• These models are combined to improve testing validity.

In all these applications, ML/DL-based approaches provide a visualization and estimate of the actual situation. In most cases related to COVID-19 infections, uncertainty is a detrimental factor. Where there is uncertainty ML/DL approaches play very crucial roles. In the case of COVID-19 pandemic, if existing infrastructure can have AI attributes, the ability to provide support and execute back-up assistance as a part of COVID-19 crisis handling many of the side effects and limitations arising out of the uncertainties could be minimized. Ability of crisis management teams shall go up considerably.

TABLE 2.3
Edge computing

Sl. No.	Work	Specific Objective	Primary Contributions
1	13	Termination of spreading of corona virus using EC.	• ICU and critical care observing model based on EC. • Computational-based surveillance model is proposed.
2	92	A clinical screening EC system that is open source.	• Detection of fever and cyanosis in the emergency department using detectable cameras. • Here image segmentation is built with open source hardware.
3	93	Energy-efficient smart health care systems.	• Optimizes the transmission of medical record from the edge nodes to the different providers. • Using EC to manage a heterogeneous network in order to furnish rapid emergency reaction.
4	94	In medical healthcare applications, QoS optimization is essential.	• In mobile EC, rate control algorithm is applied for QoS. • Platform for medical applications formed on EC on mobile devices.
5	95	System of intelligent healthcare.	• A smart healthcare mechanism based on edge cognitive computing for dynamic resource utilization in healthcare.
6	96	Healthcare Industry4.0: Efficient approach.	• Evolving of healthcare sector; author proposed body edge architecture applications. • For better health service, a small mobile client module with EC has been created.
7	97	Narrowband-IoT in intelligent hospitals.	• In smart hospitals narrowband IoT architecture is proposed with smart stuffs. • A smart hospital can be developed with less latency by integrating intelligent devices.

2.7 CHALLENGES

For detecting COVID-19, ML and DL methods are useful as these can learn patterns, retain them, and use the learning subsequently. However, in many situations the application of ML and DL systems is confronted with significant challenges, such as data scarcity, the lack of large-scale pre-trained data, large noisy data and false positive labeling, a lack of understanding between medical science and engineering fields, data protection, and regulation, to name a few. A few important terms are highlighted below:

1. **Regulation**—As the pandemic spreads its tentacles to the nooks and corners of the world, the numbers of infected and fatal cases is also increasing. Various measures such as lockdown and social distancing have been proposed

TABLE 2.4
COVID-19 prediction of outbreak

Sl. No.	Work	Specific Objective	Primary Contribution
1	43	Prediction of outbreak.	Using massive data files from Italy, a big data platform suggested estimating the outbreak probability. In Wuhan, it was used to estimate the infected people who will need to be quarantined.
2	44		A big data-based approach for pandemic modeling that interprets the total number of infected and recovered cases. This model will estimate the likelihood of outbreak with a high possibility of pandemic.
3	45		To estimate the pandemic, a system using a large dataset from different parts of countries will adjudge the probability of the outbreak forecasts.
4	46		The analytic approach method allows for the calculation of prediction errors in order to improve estimation accuracy by optimizing the data-modeling model.

TABLE 2.5
COVID-19 tracking and detection

Sl. No	Work	Specific Objective	Primary Contribution
1	50	Tracking and detection of virus spread.	A big data-based unsupervised model that incorporates simple news coverage associated with reported COVID-19 patients to track COVID-19 spread from online data.
2	47		A broad dataset obtained from the China with almost 0.1 million people is being used in a big data-based analytic approach for monitoring the COVID-19 distribution. The analytic findings reveal a strong connection between active cases and inhabitant size.
3	48		For virus spread monitoring, a big data-based analytic model was developed using datasets collected from different countries. The highest number of affected human beings in a given area can be estimated using this model.
4	49		For corona virus monitoring, a temperature-based model was proposed to determine the relationship between the number of infected cases and the average temperature in different countries.

to combat the pandemic. The outcomes of such measures are analyzed beforehand using ML and DL systems.

2. **Scarcity of data**—Mostly, AI-based DL techniques depend on large-scale trained model and data for such situations, which also include medical images like X-ray, CT scan, and different data related to environment. However, due

TABLE 2.6
COVID-19 detection and therapy

Sl. No.	Work	Specific Objective	Primary Contribution
1	51	Detection and therapy.	To diagnose this, a stable, responsive, precise, and quantitative solution based on numerous polymerase pattern responses is proposed. The proposed method for diagnosing *Plasmodium falciparum* infections has been shown to be effective and low-cost.
2	52		The use of 6,381 proteins in cells infected with this virus is suggested as a tool. This project aims to examine data from Kyoto Genes to aid COVID-19 diagnosis.
3	53		The large dataset has been used to conduct a variety of clinical studies, ranging from normal and a typical radiogram or scan manifestations to hematology examinations and pathogen recognition in the inhaling tract.

TABLE 2.7
State-of-art on applications (drug and vaccine) of big data for COVID-19

Sl. No.	Work	Specific Objective	Primary Contribution
1	54	Drug and vaccine development.	The spike proteins of various other earlier human corona virus strains are investigated using a method proposed. It allows for crucial screening of the SARS CoV-2 spike sequence and structure for vaccine production.
2	55		Different peptides have been suggested for creating a new COVID-19 vaccine.
3	56		Molecular docking-based approach is suggested for drug and booster dose discovery involving over a large numbers of small molecules, with the aim of repositioning it against COVID-19.

to COVID-19's rapid spread, it is observed that there is little growth in the number of databases available for training of DL systems.

3. **Large noisy data**—There are a large number of audio information and fake reports about COVID-19. Due to unreliability and imprecise verification of the source and content, such data cannot be used for training of ML/DL systems.

4. **Rumors**—There are many online data available for training process, which might not be reliable. Therefore, while taking data from such sources we should be very careful.

5. **Limited awareness and association between medical science and engineering fields**—Most ML/ DL researchers have a background in engineering, such as computer science or electronics, but finding a proper way

to combat COVID-19 involves strong specialization in medical imaging, virology, and many other fields. Only with an adequate knowledge of the background, proper systems involving the use of ML/DL systems can be designed.

6. **Data security**—Governments require a variety of personal details, such as an ID number, a phone number, a date of birth, and other related personal information, as well as medical information like COVID-19 status, travel and infection history, vaccination. Here the problem arises about the security of such data and how effectively the ML/DL based systems can use such repositories and never compromise on personal information.

2.8 FUTURE RESEARCH DIRECTION

AI-based DL and ML are already playing significant roles to combat COVID-19. The benefits of these models and graphical representation aid the automatic detection of the virus. Different types of pneumonia have already become standard methods adopted by the medical community. Extensive developments in this domain shall enable the medical professionals to correctly employ such tools to reduce probable faulty diagnosis while using scanning and detection medical instrument (X-ray machine, CT scan machine) to detect which one is simple pneumonia and which one is due to COVID-19. Primarily, both diagnosis and treatment of COVID-19 are important. However, finding a cure for COVID-19 is critical, which is critically related to the application of ML/DL tools for drug discovery and design. Smart robots are being used for sanitization of public arenas, delivery of products and drugs to COVID patients. This measure is helpful to stop the spread of COVID-19. ML/DL methods can monitor and track the behavior and social interaction characteristics of people and warn about impending danger due to their proximity to patients with COVID-19 if any. These approaches can help to create social networks, and spread the awareness about avoiding all forms of proximity with COVID-19 cases and effectively decelerate the potential spread of the disease. These standard machine-learning algorithms can be applied to recognize false information, then remove false news, data, or audio from the online portals so that scientific information about COVID-19 only is circulated. The possibility of use of ML/DL methods for combating COVID-19 is limitless.

2.9 CONCLUSION

Globally people are carrying out extensive research to find ways and means to combat COVID-19. This involves the use of ML/DL tools to monitor crowd behavior with regard to biosafety norms, build social networks to spread awareness, prevent circulation of fake news and information, assist in diagnosis between normal pneumonia and COVID-19 using images and scans, etc. The widespread COVID-19 has a major influence on many people's lives around the world, and the number of individuals who have died because of this virus continues to climb. As a result, it is critical to examine various forecasting and prediction methods that will be useful in this pandemic situation in order to support the government and healthcare sectors. Though AI has made inroads into our daily lives with a slew of victories, a significant number of systems are enlisting AI's support in the battle against COVID-19. Here we have included a detailed overview of ongoing work associated with the application of these techniques for predicting COVID-19 infection and suggest intelligence-based measure with which humanity can prevent the damages of this deadly disease.

REFERENCES

[1]. H. A. Rothan and S. N. Byrareddy, The epidemiology and pathogenesis of coronavirus disease (COVID-19) outbreak, *Journal of Autoimmunity*, 102433, 1–4 (2020).

[2]. Y. Jin, H. Yang, W. Ji, W. Wu, S. Chen, W. Zhang and G. Duan, Virology, epidemiology, pathogenesis, and control of COVID-19, Viruses, 12 (4), 1–17 (2020).

[3]. W. H. Organization, et al., Coronavirus disease 2019 (COVID-19): Situation report (2020).

[4]. C. Sohrabi, Z. Alsafi, N. ONeill, M. Khan, A. Kerwan, A. Al-Jabir, C. Iosifidis and R. Agha, World health organization declares global emergency: A review of the 2019 novel coronavirus (COVID-19). *International Journal of Surgery*, 76, 71–76 (April 2020). doi: 10.1016/j.ijsu.2020.02.034

[5]. E. D. Kilbourne, Influenza pandemics of the 20th century, *Emerging Infectious Diseases* 12 (1), 9 (2006).

[6]. Y. C. Hsieh, T.-Z. Wu, D.-P. Liu, P.-L. Shao, L.-Y. Chang, C.-Y. Lu, C.-Y. Lee, F.-Y. Huang and L.-M. Huang, Influenza pandemics: Past, present and future, *Journal of the Formosan Medical Association* 105 (1) (2006) 1–6.

[7]. W. H. Organization, et al., Rational use of personal protective equipment for coronavirus disease (COVID-19) and considerations during severe shortages: Interim guidance, 6 April 2020, Tech. rep., World Health Organization (2020).

[8]. P. Daszak, K. J. Olival and H. Li, A strategy to prevent future pandemics similar to the 2019-ncov outbreak (2020).

[9]. A. S. Fauci, H. C. Lane and R. R. Redfield, COVID-19 navigating the uncharted (2020).

[10]. D. Fanelli and F. Piazza, Analysis and forecast of COVID-19 spreading in China, Italy and France. *Chaos, Solitons & Fractals,*134, 109761 (2020).

[11]. Y. LeCun, Y. Bengio and G. Hinton, Deep learning, *Nature* 521 (7553), 436–444 (2015).

[12]. F. Shi, J. Wang, J. Shi, Z. Wu, Q. Wang, Z. Tang, K. He, Y. Shi and D. Shen, Review of artificial intelligence techniques in imaging data acquisition, segmentation and diagnosis for COVID-19, *arXiv preprint arXiv* 2004, 02731, DOI: 10.11 09/RBME.2020.2987975 (2020, April).

[13]. A. Sufian, D. S. Jat and A. Banerjee, Insights of artificial intelligence to stop spread of COVID-19, in: Big Data Analytics and Artificial Intelligence against COVID-19: Innovative vision and approach. *Nature Public Health Emergency Collection*, doi: 10.1007/978-3-030-55258-9_11 (2020, July).

[14]. C. Tan, F. Sun, T. Kong, W. Zhang, C. Yang and C. Liu, A survey on deep transfer learning, in: International conference on artificial neural networks. Springer, pp. 270–279 (2019).

[15]. D.S.W. Ting, L. Carin, V. Dzau and T.Y. Wong, Digital technology and COVID-19. *Nature Medicine, 26* (2020) 13.

[16]. W. Z. Khan, E. Ahmed, S. Hakak, I. Yaqoob and A. Ahmed, Edge computing: A survey, *Future Generation Computer Systems* 97, 219–235 (2019).

[17]. X. Wang, Y. Han, V. C. Leung, D. Niyato, X. Yan and X. Chen, Convergence of edge computing and deep learning: A comprehensive survey, *IEEE Communications Surveys & Tutorials,* 22 (2), 869–904 (2019).

[18]. Ministry of Health, Malaysia (MOHM) official portal, COVID-19 GUIDELINESS [ONLINE]. Available at https://www.moh.gov.my/index.php/pages/view/2019-ncov-wuhan-guidelines (Accessed 8th May 2020).

[19]. S. Peter, K. Madelon and P. John. Reassessing the global mortality burden of the 1918 influenza pandemic. *American Journal of Epidemiology,* 187(12), 2561–2567 (2017).

[20]. Z. Gensheng, et al. A review of breast tissue classification in mammograms. In: Proceedings of the 2011 ACM Symposium on Research in Applied Computation (2011).

[21]. B. Christopher, M. Pattern recognition and machine learning. Springer (2006).

[22]. P. M. Kumar and S. Karthikeyan, Performance analysis of time series forecasting of Ebola casualties using machine learning algorithm. Proceedings ITISE 2011: 201 (2011).

[23]. H. George and A. David, Next-generation phenotyping of electronic health records. *Journal of the American Medical Informatics Association,* 20(1), 117–121 (2013).

[24]. L. Nanni, S. Ghidoni and S. Brahnam, Handcrafted vs. non-handcrafted features for computer vision classification. *Pattern Recognition,* 71, 158–172 (2017).

[25]. I. Goodfellow and Y. Bengio, A. Courville, Deep Learning. MIT Press, 2016.

[26]. D. E. Rumelhart, G. E. Hinton and R. J. Williams, Learning internal representations by error propagation. Tech. rep., California Univ San Diego La Jolla Inst for Cognitive Science (1985).

[27]. R. Altman, Artificial intelligence (AI) systems for interpreting complex medical datasets. *Clinical Pharmacology & Therapeutics,* 101 (5), 585–586 (2017).

[28]. Y. LeCun, Deep learning hardware: Past, present, and future. in: 2019 IEEE International Solid-State Circuits Conference—(ISSCC), pp. 12–19 (2019).

[29]. S. Mittal and S. Vaishay, A survey of techniques for optimizing deep learning on gpus. *Journal of Systems Architecture,* 99, 101635. doi:https://doi.org/10. 1016/j.sysarc.2019.101635 (2019).

[30]. M. Long, H. Zhu, J. Wang and M. I. Jordan, Deep transfer learning with joint adaptation networks, in: Proceedings of the 34th International Conference on Machine Learning. Vol. 70, JMLR. Org, pp. 2208–2217 (2017).

[31]. S. Koitka and C. M. Friedrich, Traditional feature engineering and deep learning approaches at medical classification task of image. *clef2016.In: CLEF (Working Notes),* 304–317 (2016).

[32]. K. He, X. Zhang, S. Ren and J. Sun, Deep residual learning for image recognition. in: Proceedings of the IEEE conference on computer vision and pattern recognition, pp. 770–778 (2016).

[33]. L. Wang and A. Wong, Covid-net: A tailored deep convolutional neural network design for detection of COVID-19 cases from chest radiography images. *arXiv preprint arXiv*: 2003, 09871 (2019).

[34]. Y. Gao and K. M. Mosalam, Deep transfer learning for image-based structural damage recognition. *Computer-Aided Civil and Infrastructure Engineering,* 33 (9), 748–768 (2018).

[35]. J. Deng, W. Dong, R. Socher, L. Li, K. Li and L. Fei-Fei, Image net: A large-scale hierarchical image database. in: 2009 IEEE Conference on Computer Vision and Pattern Recognition, pp. 248–255, (2009).

[36]. M. Talo, U. B. Baloglu, O. Yıldırım and U. R. Acharya, Application of deep transfer learning for automated brain abnormality classification using MRI images. *Cognitive Systems Research,* 54, 176–188 (2019).

[37]. T. S. Santosh, R. Parmar, H. Anand, K. Srikanth and M. Saritha, A review of salivary diagnostics and its potential implication in detection of COVID-19 Cures. DOI: 10.7759/cureus.7708, 12 (4) (2020).

[38]. M. Loey, F. Smarandache and N. E. M. Khalifa, Within the lack of COVID-19 benchmark dataset: A novel gan with deep transfer learning for corona-virus detection in chest X-ray images, 12 (4), 651; 10.3390/sym12040651 (2020).

[39]. I. D. Apostolopoulos and T. A. Mpesiana, COVID-19: Automatic detection from X-ray images utilizing transfer learning with convolutional neural networks. *Physical and Engineering Sciences in Medicine* (2020) 1.

[40]. I. S. A. Abdelaziz, M. Ammar and H. Hesham. An enhanced deep teaching approach for brain cancer MRI images classification using residual networks. *Artificial Intelligence in Medicine*, 102, 101779 (2020).

[41]. H.I. Rizwan and N. Jeremiah. Deep learning approaches to biomedical image segmentation. *Informatics in Medicine Unlocked: 100297*, 81, 1–12 (2020).

[42]. A. K. Jaiswal, et al. Identifying pneumonia in chest X-rays: A deep learning approach. *Measurement*, 145, 511–518 (2019).

[43]. G. Giordano, F. Blanchini, R. Bruno, P. Colaneri, A. Di Filippo, A. Di Matteo and M. Colaneri, Modeling the COVID-19 epidemic and implementation of population-wide interventions in Italy. *Nature Medicine*, 1–6 (2020).

[44]. L. Peng, W. Yang, D. Zhang, C. Zhuge and L. Hong, Epidemic analysis of COVID-19 in China by dynamical modeling. *arXiv preprint arXiv,* 2002, 06563 (2020).

[45]. D. Tátrai and Z. Várallyay, COVID-19 epidemic outcome predictions based on logistic fitting and estimation of its reliability. *arXiv preprint arXiv,* 2003, 4160 (2020).

[46]. S. Heroy, Metropolitan-scale COVID-19 outbreaks: How similar are they? *arXiv preprint arXiv,* 2004, 01248 (2020).

[47]. X. Zhao, X. Liu and X. Li, Tracking the spread of novel coronavirus (2019-ncov) based on big data. *medRxiv* (2020).

[48]. P. Castorina, A. Iorio and D. Lanteri, Data analysis on coronavirus spreading by macroscopic growth laws. *arXiv preprint arXiv,* 2003, 00507 (2020).

[49]. A. Notari, Temperature dependence of COVID-19 transmission. *arXiv preprint arXiv*, 2003, 12417 (2020).

[50]. V. Lampos, S. Moura, E. Yom-Tov, I. J. Cox, R. McKendry and M. Edelstein, Tracking COVID-19 using online search. *arXiv preprint arXiv*, 2003, 08086 (2020).

[51]. C. Li, D. N. Debruyne, J. Spencer, V. Kapoor, L. Y. Liu, B. Zhou, L. Lee, R. Feigelman, G. Burdon and J. Liu, High sensitivity detection of coronavirus SARS-CoV-2 using multiplex PCR and a multiplex-PCRbased met genomic method. *bioRxiv* (2020).

[52]. I. Ortea and J.-O. Bock, Re-analysis of SARS-CoV-2 infected host cell proteomics time-course data by impact pathway analysis and network analysis a potential link with inflammatory response. *BioRxiv* 2020).

[53]. Y. H. Jin, L. Cai, Z. S. Cheng, H. Cheng, T. Deng, Y. P. Fan, C. Fang, D. Huang, L. Q. Huang and Q. Huang, A rapid advice guideline for the diagnosis and treatment of 2019 novel coronavirus (2019-ncov) infected pneumonia (standard version), *Military Medical Research*, 7 (1), 4 (2020).

[54]. A. Banerjee, D. Santra and S. Maiti, Energetics based epitope screening in SARS CoV-2 (COVID 19) spike glycoprotein by immuno-informatic analysis aiming to a suitable vaccine development. *bioRxiv* (2020).

[55]. M. I. Abdelmageed, A. H. Abdelmoneim, M. I. Mustafa, N. M. Elfadol, N. S. Murshed, S. W. Shantier and A. M. Makhawi, Design of a multiepitope-based peptide vaccine against the E PROTEIN OF HUMan COVID-19: An immunoinformatics approach. *BioMed Research International*, 2020, 1–17 (2020).

[56]. Z. Li, X. Li, Y.-Y. Huang, Y. Wu, L. Zhou, R. Liu, D. Wu, L. Zhang, H. Liu and X. Xu, FEP-based screening prompts drug repositioning against COVID-19. *bioRxiv*, 2020.

[57]. Centers for Disease Control and Prevention. Principles of epidemiology in public health practice: An introduction to applied epidemiology and biostatics (2006).

[58]. M. Stephen, S. Factors in the emergence of infectious diseases. In: Plagues and politics. London: Palgrave Macmillan; 2001. pp. 8–26.

[59]. H. D. Ainslie *Small pox: The death of a disease*. Amherst, NY: Prometheus Books (2009).

[59]. J. B. Peter, J. J. Lars and B. Soren. Mining electronic health records: Towards better research applications and clinical care. *Nature Reviews Genetics*, 13 (6) 395–405. (2012)

[60]. L. Jake, Big data application in biomedical research and health care: A literature review. *Biomedical Informatics Insights*, 8, BII-S31559 (2016).

[61]. T. Muhammed, Application of deep transfer learning for automated brain abnormality classification using MR images. *Cognitive Systems Research*, 54, 176–188 (2019).

[62]. K. N. Eldeen, Artificial Intelligence Technique for gene expression by tumor RNA-seq data: A novel optimized deep learning approach. *IEEE Access*, 8, 22874–22883 (2020).

[63]. Ho Chi-Sing, Rapid identification of pathogenic bacteria using Raman spectroscopy and deep learning. *Nature Communications*, 10 (1), 1–8 (2019).

[64]. F. A. Martínez, Corona virus optimization algorithm: A bio inspired met heuristic based on the COVID-19 propagation model. *arXiv preprint arXiv*, 2003, 13633 (2020).

[65]. N. Zhu, et al. A novel coronavirus from patients with pneumonia in China, 2019. *New England Journal of Medicine* (2020). doi: 10.1056/NEJMoa2001017.

[66]. H. Swapnarekha, H. S. Behera, J. Nayak, B. Naik, Role of intelligent computing in COVID-19 prognosis: A state-of-the-art review. Elsevier, 29 May 2020.

[67]. T. T. Nguyen, Artificial Intelligence in the Battle against Coronavirus (COVID-19): A Survey and future Research Directions. 30th July, 2020.

[68]. Orbann Carolyn, Defining epidemics in computer simulation models: How do definitions influence conclusions? *Epidemics* 19, 24–32 (2017).

[69]. https://worldhealthorg.shinyapps.io/covid.

[70]. F. Ucar and D. Korkmaz, Covidiagnosis-net: Deep bayes-squeezenet based diagnostic of the coronavirus disease 2019 (COVID-19) from X-ray images. *Medical Hypotheses*, 109761 (2020).

[71]. S. Hu, Y. Gao, Z. Niu, Y. Jiang, L. Li, X. Xiao, M. Wang, E. F. Fang, W. MenpesSmith and J. Xia, Weakly supervised deep learning for COVID-19 infection detection and classification from CT images. *arXiv preprint arXiv*, 2004, 06689 (2020).

[72]. C. Butt, J. Gill, D. Chun and B. A. Babu, Deep learning system to screen coronavirus disease 2019 pneumonia. *Applied Intelligence,* 8(3), (2020) 1.

[73]. T. Ozturk, M. Talo, E. A. Yildirim, U. Baloglu, O. Yildirim and U. R. Acharya, Automated detection of COVID-19 cases using deep neural networks with X-ray images. *Computers in Biology and Medicine*, 11, June (2020).

[74]. E. Luz, P. L. Silva, R. Silva and G. Moreira, Towards an efficient deep learning model for COVID-19 patterns detection in X-ray images. *arXiv preprint arXiv*, 2004, 05717 (2020).

[75]. M. Zhou, Y. Chen, D. Wang, Y. Xu, W. Yao, J. Huang, X. Jin, Z. Pan, J. Tan and L. Wang, Improved deep learning model for differentiating novel coronavirus pneumonia and influenza pneumonia. *medRxiv* (2020).

[76]. L. Li, L. Qin, Z. Xu, Y. Yin, X. Wang, B. Kong, J. Bai, Y. Lu, Z. Fang and Q. Song, Artificial intelligence distinguishes COVID-19 from community acquired pneumonia on chest CT Radiology. 200905 (2020).

[77]. L. Wang and A. Wong, Covid-net: A tailored deep convolutional neural network design for detection of COVID-19 cases from chest radiography images. *arXiv preprint arXiv*, 09871, 1–12 (2003).

[78]. A. Lopez-Rincon, A. Tonda, L. Mendoza-Maldonado, E. Claassen, J. Garssen and A. D. Kraneveld, Accurate identification of sars-cov-2 from viral genome sequences using deep learning. *bioRxiv*.

[79]. O. Gozes, M. Frid-Adar, H. Greenspan, P. D. Browning, H. Zhang, W. Ji, A. Bernheim and E. Siegel, Rapid AI development cycle for the coronavirus (COVID-19) pandemic: Initial results for automated detection & patient monitoring using deep learning CT image analysis. *arXiv preprint arXiv*, 2003, 05037 (2020).

[80]. S. M. Ayyoubzadeh, S. M. Ayyoubzadeh, H. Zahedi, M. Ahmadi and S. R. N. Kalhori, Predicting COVID-19 incidence through analysis of google trends data in Iran: Data mining and deep learning pilot study. *JMIR Public Health and Surveillance*, 6 (2), e18828 (2020).

[81]. S. J. Fong, G. Li, N. Dey, R. G. Crespo and E. Herrera-Viedma, Composite montecarlo decision making under high uncertainty of novel coronavirus epidemic using hybridized deep learning and fuzzy rule induction. *Applied Soft Computing*, 106282, 1–14 (2020).

[82]. S. Chae, S. Kwon and D. Lee, Predicting infectious disease using deep learning and big data. *International Journal of Environmental Research and Public Health*, 15 (8) 1596 (2018).

[83]. J. P. Cohen, P. Morrison and L. Dao, COVID-19 image data collection. *arXiv preprint arXiv*, 2003, 11597, March(2020).

[84]. S. Minaee, R. Kafieh, M. Sonka, S. Yazdani and G. J. Soufi, Deep-covid: Predicting COVID-19 from chest X-ray images using deep transfer learning. *arXiv preprint arXiv*, 09363. (2004).

[85]. B. R. Beck, B. Shin, Y. Choi, S. Park and K. Kang, Predicting commercially available antiviral drugs that may act on the novel coronavirus (sars-cov-2) through a drug target interaction deep learning model. *Computational and Structural Biotechnology Journal* (2020).

[86]. S. Basu and S. Mitra, Deep learning for screening COVID-19 using chest X-ray images. *arXiv preprint arXiv*, 2004, 10507 (2020).

[87]. N. E. M. Khalifa, F. Smarandache and M. Loey, A study of the neutrosophic set significance on deep transfer learning models: An experimental case on a limited COVID-19 chest X-ray dataset. *Symmetry, 65*, 1–10, (2020).

[88]. A. Narin, C. Kaya and Z. Pamuk, Automatic detection of coronavirus disease (COVID19) using X-ray images and deep convolutional neural networks. *arXiv preprint arXiv*, 2003, 10849 (2020).

[89]. B. Subirana, F. Hueto, P. Rajasekaran, J. Laguarta, S. Puig, J. Malvehy, O. Mitja, A. Trilla, C. I. Moreno and J. F. M. Valle, Hi sigma, do I have the coronavirus?: Call for a new artificial intelligence approach to support health care professionals dealing with the COVID-19 pandemic. *arXiv preprint arXiv*, 2004, 06510 (2020).

[90]. N. E. M. Khalifa, M. H. N. Taha, A. E. Hassanien and S. Elghamrawy, Detection of coronavirus (COVID-19) associated pneumonia based on generative adversarial networks and a fine-tuned deep transfer learning model using chest X-ray dataset. *arXiv preprint arXiv*, 2004, 01184 (2020).

[91]. C. Hegde, P. B. Suresha, J. Zelko, Z. Jiang, R. Kamaleswaran, M. A. Reyna and G. D. Clifford, Autotriage-an open source edge computing raspberry pi-based clinical screening system. *medRxiv*, doi: https://doi.org/10.1101/2020.04.09.20059840 (2020).

[92]. A. A. Abdellatif, A. Mohamed, C. F. Chiasserini, A. Erbad and M. Guizani, Edge computing for energy-efficient smart health systems: Data and application-specific approaches. in: Energy Efficiency of Medical Devices and Healthcare Applications. Elsevier, pp. 53–67 (2020).

[93]. A. H. Sodhro, Z. Luo, A. K. Sangaiah and S. W. Baik, Mobile edge computing based qos optimization in medical healthcare applications. *International Journal of Information Management*, 45, 308–318 (2019).

[94]. M. Chen, W. Li, Y. Hao, Y. Qian and I. Humar, Edge cognitive computing based smart healthcare system. *Future Generation Computer Systems*, 86, 403–411 (2018).

[95]. P. Pace, G. Aloi, R. Gravina, G. Caliciuri, G. Fortino and A. Liotta, An edge-based architecture to support efficient applications for healthcare industry 4.0. *IEEE Transactions on Industrial Informatics*, 15 (1), 481–489 (2019).

[96]. H. Zhang, J. Li, B. Wen, Y. Xun and J. Liu, Connecting intelligent things in smart hospitals using nb-iot. *IEEE Internet of Things Journal*, 5 (3), 1550–1560 (2018).

3 Potential Applications and Challenges of Internet of Things in Healthcare

Neha Sharma and Chander Prabha

CONTENTS

3.1 INTRODUCTION

An important aspect of life is healthcare. Unfortunately, the growing senior citizens and the resulting increase in lifelong disorders put enormous pressure on current healthcare services, and the demand for assets from clinic wards toward nurses and physicians is high [1]. Today, healthcare uses information technology to provide intelligent networks that improve medical evaluation and also provide reliable and efficient treatment. Intelligent clinical screening mechanisms and automatic medical diagnostic technologies offer services in diverse contexts and situations, including clinics, offices, and households, and travel enables to significantly decrease the cost of clinic visits and improve the overall healthcare outcomes [2]. Wearable sensors, data transmission technologies, wireless sensor networks (WSN), wireless body area network (WBAN), and human bond interactions (HBI) will be an embryonic field of research worldwide in the future. A body sensor network (BSN) is another name for a body area network (BAN). It is a handheld computing system with a wireless network, and it is similar to other wireless network technologies. This includes the individual body with either a collection of native sensors or gadgets, for instance, observing the individual's vital signs, fitness data, heart monitoring for medical purposes. Using a wearable fixed position technique, the BAN could be integrated into the human body as a device in various situations, wallets, and clothes. As a data hub or information gateway in a BAN application, these small smart gadgets play an important and effective role [3]. IoT healthcare system is shown in Figure 3.1.

3.1.1 HEALTHCARE AND INTERNET OF THINGS

The IoT is a relatively new field of study, and its potential use in healthcare is only in its early stages. The IoT is discussed in this chapter, and its appropriateness for healthcare is illustrated. Several innovative attempts to develop IoT in healthcare are discussed.

IoT—It is emerging into an ubiquitous digital computer network where something and all can be connected to the Internet as a result of continual technological advancements and future advancements [4]. IoT consist of six-layered architecture described as follows [5,6]:

   i. **LAYER 1**—It is known as a coding layer, and it is the backbone of the IoT that determines the objects of interests. Every object is given a unique ID in this layer that makes it easy to distinguish the objects [5].
   ii. **LAYER 2**—Second layer is the perception layer that interacts via smart devices and physical devices including RFID, sensors, actuators. Its key

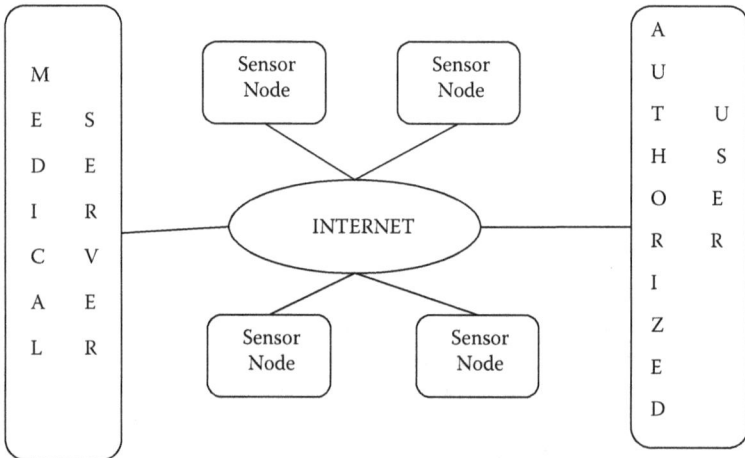

FIGURE 3.1   IoT healthcare system [3].

goals are to link things to the IoT network and, via deployed smart devices, to calculate, capture, and transfer state information associated with all of these things, transmitting the information to the upper layer via layer interfaces [5,6].

iii. **LAYER 3**—The objective of network layer is to extract relevant data from the second layer in the form of digital signals and transfer it to the middleware layer processing systems using transmission media, such as Bluetooth, WiFi, Zigbee, WiMaX,GSM, and 3 G through protocols, such as IPv4, IPv6, DDS, and MQTT [5,6].

iv. **LAYER 4**—The information collected from the wireless devices is handled by middleware layer. It involves technology like cloud storage and cloud connectivity that deposits immediate access to the database to supply all the acquired information. The information is examined using secure intelligent computing gadgets, and a fully automatic activity is captured based on data-refined results [5].

v. **LAYER 5**—Application layer realizes IoT frameworks, based on the processed data, for all types of industry. Since IoT growth is promoted by apps, it is valuable in the extensive growth of the IoT system. Smart houses, smart transportation, smart world could be IoT-related applications [5,6].

vi. **LAYER 6**—Business layer handles Internet of Things program, and the abilities are accountable for every IoT-related studies. For productive market strategies, it produces numerous business models [5] (Figure 3.2).

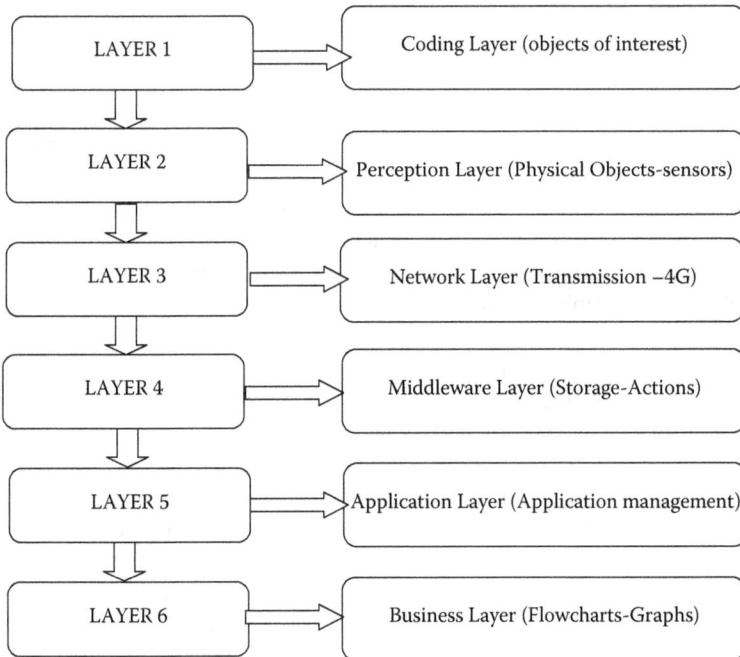

FIGURE 3.2 IoT architecture [5].

3.1.2   IoT HEALTHCARE

Due to a sizeable population, conventional healthcare does not satisfy the demands of everyone. Health facilities are not available or open to all, considering the excellent infrastructure and modern technology. One of the wise aims of healthcare is to inform individuals about their health and tell them about their health. Smart healthcare requires any of their crises to be handled by users. The focus is on enhancing patient interface and reliability. It helps to remotely track patients and to reduce the cost of healthcare. It also allows doctors without regional boundaries to extend their facilities. As the movement toward smart cities continues to expand, an efficient smart healthcare system would offer healthy life to citizens [7]. An IoT has the capacity to detect individuals, appliances, specimens, materials, or even service animals reliably and examine the collected data. Problems could be more easily detected, greater standard of care provided, and services used more accurately by patient's link to the detectors to monitor pulse rate, and other biometric data [8].

3.1.3   IoT HEALTHCARE APPLICATIONS

The below are only a few examples of IoT healthcare technology frameworks:

   a. Sensors in the patient's room and in a clinic or home healthcare facility could detect a raised pulse rate, heart rate, or even the appearance of vomit in a bulimia (eating disorder) patient. Sensors could be used to monitor exercise aggression, such as extended aerobic workout or rapid walking movement, in comparison to walking at a standard pace [1].
   b. For monitoring cardiac activity, which is controlled by a microcontroller, an ECG sensor is used. This detail will be delivered to the patient's gadgets via Bluetooth, by which the ECG information is again refined and displayed into the individual application. The deployment of software for heart disease prediction, according to the authors, would improve the method. Further enhancement can be done by assessing the pulse rate, which is considered to help in the detection of cardiac attack [1].
   c. Imagine the Alzheimer's disease (AD) patient. Here, to avoid roaming or other undesirable movement habits, an IoT may use Geolocation. Comorbidities of other conditions like high blood pressure (BP), mental retardation, or diabetes mellitus are also observed in people with AD. Relevant integrated instruments may then collect data to monitor the specific signs and effects of certain conditions [8].
   d. Forgetting the dosage of the medicine is common among many patients, particularly among elderly patients who take multiple medicines. A medical care alternative for patients was suggested in this research report. The smart pill box is designed for use in hospitals as well as nursing homes. This medicine pill box is customizable to take pills as the pill number and timing. The pill box will remind the patients to take pills [9].
   e. As a personal home healthcare approach, ultrasound-based technologies now used in hospitals can be deployed to identify and monitor the movement of a

senior citizen and predict slips. Emergency services are treated by a cost-effective, sensor device that is simple to implement and needs only a wide-area communications channel [10].

3.2 LITERATURE SURVEY

In homes, engineering, community, and vehicles, technology has improved. Healthcare is one of the areas where emerging technologies often require attention and development. By applying various approaches and technology, different scholars have made different analyses on healthcare challenges and their monitoring methods.

Stephanie et al. [1] presented a specific paradigm for potential work in this chapter. Healthcare programs based on IoT can be extended to all general structures and processes that track specific situation. Authors then provided a concise and structured description. State-of-the-art works owe to each aspect of the suggested model. Numerous portable, non-intrusive detectors, especially those measuring blood pressure, heart rate, and oxygen levels, were studied and discussed. Mrinai et al. [3] provides information on research studies and disease monitoring, exercise management, pediatric, private health, and elderly care management. The IoT medical field is resourceful, and safety, protection, accessibility, resource allocation are the most critical elements.

Pace et al. [11] proposed INTER-Health framework aims to impose an inter-active IoT framework for the decentralized smartphone tracking of the lifestyle of people to prevent health problems emerging from nutrition and physical activity disorders. This screening process can be delegated from the health center to the homes of the tracked individuals, and assisted by the use of on-body physical activity sensors during mobility.

Inderpreet et al. [12] presented the structure of the sensors to easily demonstrate how the sensors perform in the healthcare sector. The cloud server receives the information, and then the information is transmitted to the web servers, then interconnected with a gateway with the support of WiFi or modem, and then transfers data to the single SoC platform with the support of the sensor nodes. Further, transmitting the information to the 6LoWPAN server then transferring information to the star-based 6LoWPAN health sensor and connecting this entire device or architecture to the Internet browser with the help of smartphone, phone, computer, one can quickly download the information and see all the information one needs.

Further, Adarsh et al. [13] introduced a strategy that makes use of Healthcare 4.0 to secure central authority from disease and implemented a decentralized technique, device and data protection, capacity enhancement, simple data maintenance, and offered comprehensive healthcare monitoring functionality. To improve the quality of the entire system and subsystems, a simulation optimization technique is implemented. Through experimentation and execution, the suggested solution is evaluated, checked, and verified.

Deepak et al. [14] developed IoT-based intelligent medical care to avoid the isolation of a patient to an observation area. A patient can get a therapy plan tailor-made for his bodily needs in this method. The purpose of this technique is the removal of human oversight in the monitoring process and the automation of the whole monitoring process. The context principle of the framework proposed is to provide a one-stop response to all observation needs.

Mohamed et al. [15] suggested a security paradigm for healthcare to protect the transfer of medical information in IoT systems. The suggested framework consists of the following processes: first, the sensitive information of the patient is encoded using a proposed encryption method built from the both AES and RSA encryption. Second, the encrypted information is stored in a cover picture and creates a stego-image, the third step is the retrieval of embedded data, and the fourth step is the decryption of processed data to recover the actual information.

The authors presented an analysis of current work along with research topics on the 5 G and IoT networking component of smart healthcare. First they presented a framework for 5 G smart healthcare and the critical strategies for allowing 5 G smart healthcares, Network Feature Virtualization (NFV). Second, they discussed the 5 G smart healthcare definition, and analyzed the current 5 G smart healthcare criteria and targets. Finally, they performed a comprehensive overview of network layer technologies applicable to IoT-based 5 G smart healthcare, involving timing, scheduling, and congestion management, addressing both current work and future development opportunities [16].

Anar et al. [17] introduced the concept of an EHMS test bed in which a patient's body was connected to multiple small sensors. A practical healthcare database was collected by the author with more than 16,000 records of usual and MITM attack packets. In order to construct an effective IDS, the author recommended the integration of the network flow statistics with the biometrics of the patient as functions to increase device performance; four distinct ML approaches, RF, KNN, SVM, and ANN, are used.

3.3 HEALTHCARE SERVICES AND APPLICATIONS IN IOT

A number of areas may be extended to IoT-based healthcare organizations, including caring for adolescent and aged patients, chronic illness supervision, and private health management and exercise administration, among others. The IoT will intend to allow a variety of treatments in which a range of healthcare options are offered by each provider. Various kinds of IoT healthcare services and the applications are included in the following sections (Figure 3.3).

3.3.1 IoT HEALTHCARE SERVICES

Services are used to create applications, and they are user-centric and specifically used by consumers and patients. Distinct services provided by IoT are shown below:

a. **Ambient assistant living (AAL)**—In general, it is inevitable that neither a smart device nor a traditional IoT-based healthcare services can provide specialized services to elderly people, that is, mandatory for a definite IoT action. Ambient assisted living is an IoT process pushed by artificial

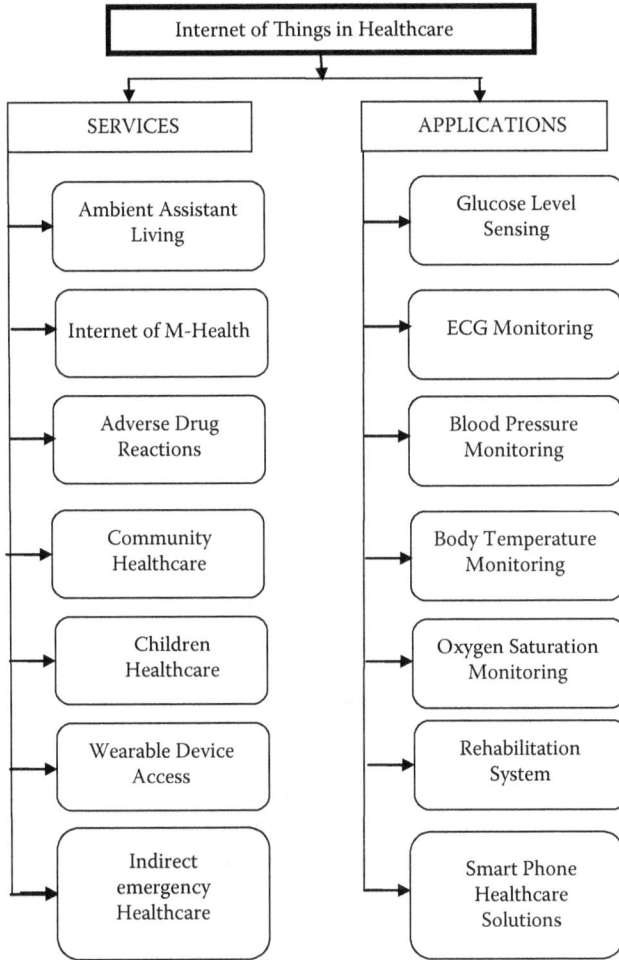

```
┌─────────────────────────────────────┐
│      Internet of Things in Healthcare │
└─────────────────────────────────────┘
```

SERVICES	APPLICATIONS
Ambient Assistant Living	Glucose Level Sensing
Internet of M-Health	ECG Monitoring
Adverse Drug Reactions	Blood Pressure Monitoring
Community Healthcare	Body Temperature Monitoring
Children Healthcare	Oxygen Saturation Monitoring
Wearable Device Access	Rehabilitation System
Indirect emergency Healthcare	Smart Phone Healthcare Solutions

FIGURE 3.3 Services and applications of IoT healthcare [18].

intelligence that can accommodate the medical treatment of older people and people with disabilities. Its main objective is to maintain and promote the autonomy of those individuals and, therefore, to enhance the security of their lifestyle as well as their family environment. The need for these applications stems from the demographic shift in industrialized nations where lifespan is increasing and the rate of birth is decreasing. Such situations require imaginative and cost-effective ways to keep medical costs under the boundaries of economic opportunity. In order to improve the quality of life, well-being and security of older people, AAL applications provide services, goods, and ideas [19,20]. In AAL implementations, the areas of need for senior citizens are healthcare, safety, peace of mind, social interaction, and mobility.

b. **Internet of M-health (IoMH)**—Digital health is a health technology framework made up of mobile devices and the IoT, and it involves the use of a smart phone's basic functionality, GPRS, 4 G systems, location services, and wireless technologies. It makes decisions, and gives the information, which is obtained through detectors in IoT environment. Heart rate recordings and body behavior during a variety of physical exercises are used in the M-health dataset. To monitor the patient's breathing, these sensors may be placed at various body positions, such as the right hand, abdomen, and left ankle [21].

c. **Adverse drug reactions (ADR)**—A consequence of consuming a drug is known as an adverse drug reaction (ADR). Due to a combination of two or more drugs or a single dose or prolonged injection of a drug this can occur. Since the ADR is essentially generic, that is, not relevant to a single disease drug, certain appropriate quantitative problems and their solutions need to be separately formulated (called ADR services). Along with putting an added pressure on healthcare system, it may have lethal effects on patients. It is one of the world's fastest-growing risks of sickness and mortality, and they will become a major health issue for the care of multiple diseases in an elderly population [22].

d. **Community healthcare (CH)**—It is a program that serves in a selected limited area. This structure of community hospitals is often the same as that of a 'digital health center'. It's an IoT-based network that monitors rural neighborhoods and the housing areas that surround them [21].

e. **Children healthcare (CH)**—The children's healthcare system (CHS) is a forum for toddlers to improve their quality of life with their eating habits while they are not with their family and eating outside of their residences. Toddlers who use a mobile food monitoring device receive notification from their physicians, care workers, or guardians. Through the increased application, customers can access information about food. To provide guidance to the children, the healthcare professional uses the stored data and send a note to guardians. This helps parents talk to their kids about food to help them develop healthy eating habits [21].

f. **Wearable device access (WDA)**—For a broad range of health applications, especially for WSN-based medical care, different non-intrusive sensors are available. Such detectors have the potential to provide the same services through the IoT. The incorporation of the mentioned sensors through wearable devices is apparent [18,23].

g. **Indirect emergency healthcare (IEH)**—There are a number of emergency conditions in which medical care is deeply engaged, including bad weather, transportation (aircraft, airplane, train, and car) collisions, and earthen field disaster. In such instances, a centralized platform called indirect urgent medical care can provide a range of solutions like accessibility of information, notification of changes, post-accident intervention, and records management [18].

3.3.2 IoT Healthcare Applications

It is important to remember that services are used to build applications, but clients and patients access apps directly. As a result, services are developer-focused, while apps are user-focused.

a. **Glucose level sensing (GLS)**—An individual with diabetes is primarily concerned with regulating the blood sugar levels to prevent glucose boundary abnormalities. Non-invasive, minimally invasive, and invasive approaches for controlling these levels are divided into three groups [24].

    i. The invasive group contains often-used approaches because, due to the direct contact with the blood of the patient, it has the greatest consistency in outcomes.

    ii. One of the methods under review concerns the minimally invasive group. This method makes use of small pores caused through laser radiation, which are tiny holes in the skin. When the holes are open, a system uses a steady vacuum to remove a small quantity of transdermal body fluid. An enzyme-based electrode processes and tests glucose rate with the sample collected.

    iii. Non-invasive category are non-invasive glucometers that have the goal of replacing a blood component with another from which external access is achieved. The procedure involves putting a sensor on a specific area of the body to receive a glucose measurement.

b. **ECG monitoring (ECGM)**—The best tool for detecting heart irregularities is known to be an ECG. The ECGs differ between single and 12-lead ECG recording equipment. On the one side, ECG acquisition instruments in hospitals are typically large in size and facilitate high-precision, and long-term surveillance. They, however, restrict the movements and participation of the patients. Wearable health-monitoring devices offer continuous actual monitoring of patients by installing sensors. The data collection process, the lifecycle procedure of ECGM devices, includes the selection of the following processes [23]:

    i. The categories of sensors (e.g., wireless or wired),

    ii. The location of the sensors,

    iii. The numbers of sensors, and

    iv. The hardware needed to capture, store, and transmit data.

c. **Blood pressure monitoring (BPM)**—One of the most significant parameters for detecting cardiovascular disorders is BP. The patient's BP should be tested on a regular basis, based on his or her age and overall health. Several instruments for monitoring BP outside of the hospital are available to achieve this goal. These instruments are supplemental hardware that the patients must bring with them at all times and are frequently inaccessible in the event of a medical emergency. In today's world, the current research is made to have knowledgeable, internet-connected measurement tools that the patient can always have with them. The new monitoring framework, including such instruments, allows the Internet of Medical Things (IoMT) paradigm to be applied [25].

d. **Body temperature monitoring (BTM)**—Hypothermia, fever, normothermia, hyperthermia, hyperpyrexia, euthermia, or natural are the various forms of human body temperature, according to medical science. The first step in a complete clinical test is to take an individual's temperature. Medical thermometers come in a range of shapes and sizes and can be used in different body parts: in the mouth, in the bladder, in the ear, in the vagina, under arm, and over the temporal artery on the membrane of the forehead. The safe and convenient method of calculating temperature of the body is the auxiliary temperature calculation. The temperature below the arm is approximately 36.4 deg C. Aside from mercury thermometers, digital temperature sensors, such as thermocouple, thermistor, and IC (integrated circuit) temperature sensors, are even used. In medical diagnosis, electronic thermometers with thermocouple sensors are commonly used. The calculation is often influenced by the ambient temperature in the auxiliary measurement [18,26].

e. **An oxygen saturation monitoring (OSM)**—BP is ideal for continuous, non-invasive oxygen saturation monitoring. For innovation medical healthcare applications, the combination of IoT with BP is helpful. The promise of IoT-based pulse oximeter is explored in a survey of CoAP-located healthcare facilities. Connectivity based on a pro-le wireless healthcare system comes with this system, and the detector directly connects to the Monere network. An IoT-optimized moderate pulse oximeter for remote patient monitoring has been proposed. This software could be useful over such an IoT network to constantly monitor the health of patients [18].

f. **Rehabilitation system (RS)**—Smart recovery technologies focused on IoT are becoming a safer way to minimize issues related to elderly population and shortages of healthcare workers. While it has come into being, there are still critical problems in automating the design and reconfiguration of such a device so that it can adapt quickly to the needs of the patient. This model successfully demonstrates that the IoT can be an efficient model for enabling all the tools required to deliver interactions with actual information. To help successful remote consultation in extensive recovery, IoT-based innovations will shape a valuable framework. An innovative prison proposed system, a smart community hospital RS, hemiplegic patient rehabilitation training, and a childhood autism language immersion system are among the IoT-based treatment programs [18,27].

g. **Smartphone healthcare solutions (SHS)**—The advent of digital equipment with a mobile phone sensor has been observed in recent years, which illustrates the growth of smartphones as an IoT engine. Smartphones can now be used as a flexible healthcare system thanks to a range of hardwired and software devices. To access diagnosis and treatment information, diagnostic applications are used. Drug reference applications usually contain drug names, signs, dosages, prices, and distinguishing characteristics. Literature search applications make it easier to locate specific medical knowledge and medical literature repositories. Usually, medical education applications deal with videos, instruction, advanced treatment presentations, color images of various pictures, and medical journals. Calculator apps include a variety of medical formulas and equations that can be used to determine different parameter values. Medical contact applications make it easier for physicians and nurses to interact inside a hospital [18].

3.3.3 Techniques for Promoting Services

IoT-based medical services can be facilitated by cloud computing (CC), big data, grid computing (GC), and other innovations [28].

Load balancing, high availability, and high performance are all problems that CC presents. Additionally, it could be expanded through data centers to the mobile phone end-user, and as a cloud hosting provider, it allows for edge mobile connectivity. The introduction of CC into IoT-based medical care technology can allow services access to shared information from anywhere. In this way, services can be requested over the system, and services for various needs can be carried out.

CC is said to be built on the base of GC. The inadequate computing functionality of medical sensor nodes is resolved by incorporating GC into the healthcare network.

As the next move in computing, big data presents multiple obstacles to the science society, and necessitates a shared view, and discussion of a number of fields, like healthcare. It contains a vast volume of medical data obtained from sensor devices. There are also techniques for enhancing the quality of health-related diagnosis, and also tracking methods and shops.

Which network style is best for IoT-based healthcare is a hot topic. Data, service, and patient-service models are the three basic ways of designing. The healthcare system is divided into items in the data-centric scheme depending on the health data collected. In a service-centric system, the healthcare framework is assigned depending on the characteristics that it would have. Finally, the patient-centric approach divides hospital systems based on the number of patients they accept for treatment.

3.4 IOT HEALTHCARE SECURITY ISSUES AND CHALLENGES

3.4.1 Security Issues

Since hackers or attackers can easily identify sensor information, protection has become a big issue in the IoT, and therefore the investigation of the most current security approaches in IoT is crucial. Holding various IoT vulnerabilities in consideration, security deployment and defense design typically has three stages.

Health data could be an attractive and appealing target for a deceptive doer due to a lack of appropriate security measures. Mobile devices with cameras and other wearable technologies are also being used to gather computerized data from patients. In most cases, these are linked to applications that process and analyze information and indications. The functionality of these applications is often expanded by sending information to the server, and this phenomenon necessitates the use of sophisticated algorithms. Confidentiality, genuine use of intelligence, and legal concerns are the three essential elements in this area of protection.

In addition, there are three points of security flaw: data transfer, devices, and data storage. It's worth noting that data stealing from smartphones isn't as common as it once was. However, using ransom ware would not eliminate the risk of data leakage from computers. Physical computers are often at risk of being hacked or misplaced. In addition, safety does not imply the use of wearable sensors. But, users will configure their mobile devices. During the transfer of information, though, data can be compromised using various malwares. To prevent data hacking, an effective encryption technique and authentication system is needed. However, there are several issues of encryption and authentication that must be addressed.

These include a decrease in data transmission rate, difficulties in implementing in a practical manner, and strong energy usage. Finally, the information is encrypted in a CC architecture archive. However, this service is provided by a variety of third-party providers, and thus there are more opportunities for assaults. Furthermore, these databases are connected to the Internet network, allowing data to be retrieved by users. It increases the likelihood of attacks even more. Multidimensional authenticity, certain access managing procedure, and a complex code are needed to overcome these problems, making the device more difficult to use [27] (Table 3.1).

As shown in Figure 3.4, there are many factors that lead to safety concerns.

3.4.2 IoT Healthcare Challenges

IoT has been incorporated into a number of systems to benefit the healthcare sector, including patient management and a mobile home system for diabetic patients. Main challenges that exist in the healthcare sector are listed below [29,30]:

i. To guarantee the confidentiality of the patient's private information, data sharing in IoT systems should be encrypted. It will help to prevent unwanted access to a patient's records, as well as attacker snooping on the details.

ii. Powerful credentials and authentication mechanisms can be used to secure IoT web portals. To the IoT devices and data, role-based connectivity should be planned so that only approved individuals have access to

TABLE 3.1
IoT healthcare security issues [27]

	IoT Layer	Issues	Description
1	Perception layer	Device security	It is a device-level security that relies on the privacy of smartphones, smartphone applications, and web applications. At this stage, the IoT protection risk is a physical threat that threatens physical equipment.
2	Network and transport layer	Communication securities	Used to secure networks and information channels.
3	Application layer	Cloud security	Cloud platforms that are especially sensitive to vulnerabilities, such as SQL injection bugs, would almost definitely be the first to be attacked. Cloud encryption guarantees data security and avoid privacy breaches.

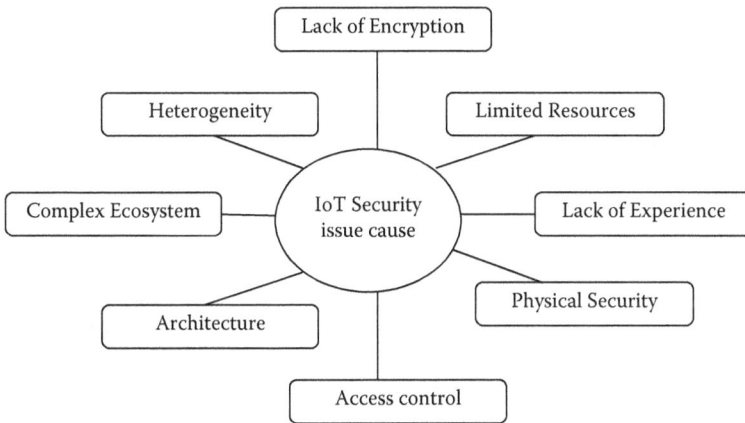

FIGURE 3.4 Reasons of security issues in IoT [29].

confidential medical information, such as the practicing physician panel, which is authorized for the patient's diagnosis, treatment, and supervision.

iii. By ensuring the physical security of the device, various threats like tampering of the device, data theft through USB, or stealing of the storage media can be prevented. Middleware connects the applications to the things/sensors, and it should be secured.

iv. IoT allows for more convenience, for example, if a patient needs continuous treatment, he or she will remain at home rather than in a hospital and can be supervised on an as-needed basis using IoT technology. Any wearable gadgets, such as cameras, are harmful to the patient's body.

v. The information transferred from the sensor to the control system and then to the monitoring center would be affected by noise, lowering the data quality. A better infrastructure aids in the transmission of data without compromising its integrity. The use of a noise-reduction technique will also help to improve the data signal.

vi. When the number of wearable sensors grows, the amount of energy used to process them grows, resulting in increased power leakage and energy usage. Power consumption is an optimization technique that can be used.

vii. In the IoT, tracking a huge number of devices necessitates further storage and computer system, which can be avoided by encrypting information in the cloud. The IoT combined with the cloud, on the other hand, adds to the difficulty.

viii. Another significant issue with the IoT is secrecy, as computers are more susceptible to attack. These devices have little resources, making encryption methods impossible to implement.

ix. The majority of ECG testing methods currently in use include a supervised signal analysis. This increases the cost, and it can result in a detection error. Machine learning can be used to evaluate the signal, resulting in increased performance and lower costs.

3.5   IoT Wearable Sensors

Smart sensors that can be used as external attachments, inserted in clothes and dresses, inserted in the body, or even adhered to or covered in tattoos on the skin are all examples of IoT-enabled wearable devices. These devices can connect to the network in order to store, transmit, and retrieve data which can be used to make informed decisions. Wearable devices are becoming a bigger part of IoT, and they're evolving from basic gadgets to more advanced and realistic applications. For communication and computing, smart wearables may communicate with a variety of other gadgets, such as smartphones.

The wearable IoT system for health is mostly used for remote healthcare control, and in certain cases of recovery. Until uploading the user/health patient's information over the Internet for further study, the devices capture health-related data, and the system can conduct limited computing. Data can also be received by the system, allowing the individual to create additional decisions. In several implementations, wearable sensors are linked to devices to monitor the data gathered and then transfer it to a CC system like Microsoft Azure or Amazon Web Services (AWS) for storage, processing, and analysis.

Mobile wellness apps can be used to visualize examined data and offer information about a person's or patient's wellness. Furthermore, the examined data may be used to transmit special instructions to the wearable devices, like heating the body or delivering a shock, in treatment processes [31,32] (Figure 3.5).

Vital sign monitoring—Body temperature, respiratory oximetry, and oxygen saturation are the key vital signs that medical practitioners and healthcare services track on a regular basis.

Non-vital monitoring—Non-invasive evaluation is what non-vital symptoms surveillance entails.

The following parameters, such as respiration rate and sugar levels, may be tracked.

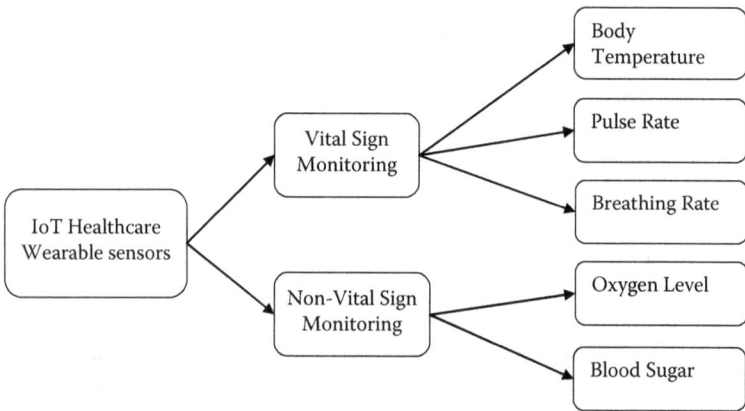

FIGURE 3.5   IoT healthcare wearable sensors [31].

3.5.1 HEALTH MONITORING WEARABLE SYSTEMS

The health tracking system differs based on the type of sensors used. There are four main types of wearable devices [31]:

1. **Bio-potential sensors**—Electrocardiography (ECG), electroencephalography (EEG), photoplesmography (PPG), and electromyography (EMG) are examples of bio-potential sensors.
2. **Motion sensors**—The examples of the motion sensors are gyroscope and accelerometer.
3. **Environmental sensors**—The examples of the environmental sensors are ultrasound, temperature, and pressure.
4. **Biochemical sensors**—Analyzing the above signs provides a wealth of information about the patient's or user's well-being.

3.6 CONCLUSION AND FUTURE SCOPE

New technologies and applications of cloud-based IoT in healthcare have emerged as a result of the exponential growth of the IoT and CC. The challenge is that how cloud-based IoT can be integrated into the next-generation medical system. This chapter discuss the various healthcare applications and services provided by IoT. The study has been carried out with an outline drawn on various IoT healthcare challenges and the security issues. Further, the concepts of wearable sensors in IoT healthcare are also discussed. Increased security, versatility, and power usage will all help to increase IoT in healthcare.

REFERENCES

[1]. Stephanie, B., Wei, X. and Ian, A. Internet of things for smart healthcare: Technologies, challenges, and opportunities. *IEEE*, 5, 26521–26544 (2017).
[2]. Syed, U. and M.H. Shamim. Edge intelligence and internet of things in healthcare: A survey. *Special Section on Edge Intelligence for Internet of Things IEEE*, 9, 45–59 (2021).
[3]. Mrinai, M. and Shailaja, C. Internet of things: A survey of enabling technologies in healthcare and its applications. *Computer Networks*, 153, 113–131 (2019).
[4]. Mahdi, H., Maaruf, A., Peter, S. and Rich, P. A review on Internet of Things (IoT), Internet of Everything (IoE) and Internet of Nano Things (IoNT). *IEEE Xplore*, 219–224 (2015).
[5]. M.U., F., Muhammad, W., Sadia, M., Anjum, K. and Talha, K. A review on Internet of Things (IoT). *International Journal Of Computer Applications*, 113(1), 1–7 (2015).
[6]. Jie Lin, L., Wei, Y., Nan, Z., Xinyu, Y., Hanlin, Z. and Wei, Z. A survey on Internet of Things: Architecture, enabling technologies, security and privacy and application. *IEEE Internet Of Things Journal*, 4, 1–16 (2017).
[7]. Zahra, N., Amir, M. and Mehdi, H. The role of the Internet of Things in healthcare: Future trends and challenges. *Computer Methods And Programs In Biomedicine*, 199, 1–64 (2020).
[8]. Phillip, A. and Nancy, L. The Internet of Things in healthcare potential applications and challenges. *US National Institute Of Standards And Technology IEEE*, 1–4 (2016).

[9]. Madushan and Rashmika Gamage, G. A review on applications of internet of things (IOT) in healthcare. *Journal of the American Society for Information Science and Technology* (2021).

[10]. Alok, K. and Sampada, S. Healthcare applications of the Internet of Things: A review. *(IJCSIT) International Journal Of Computer Science And Information Technologies, 5* (5), 6229–6232 (2014).

[11]. P.P., G.A., A.C. and R.G. INTER-health: An interoperable IoT solution for active and assisted living healthcare services. *IEEE 5Th World Forum on Internet of Things (WF-Iot)*, 81–86 (2019).

[12]. Inderpreet, S. and Deepak, K. Improving IOT based architecture of healthcare system. *4th International Conference on Information Systems and Computer Networks (ISCON)*, 113–117 (2019).

[13]. Adarsh, k., Rajalakshmi, K., Anand, N. and Kriti, S. A novel smart healthcare design, simulation, and implementation using Healthcare 4.0 processes. *Special Section on Blockchain Technology: Principles and Applications, IEEE, 8,* 118433–118471 (2020).

[14]. Deepak, K. and hi va m, C. IoT based healthcare services for monitoring post injury. *Proceedings* of the *International Conference on Intelligent Computing and Control Systems (ICICCS 2019) IEEE Xplore*, 293–296 (2019).

[15]. Mohamed, A., Gunasekaran, M., Mai, M. and Ehab, R. Internet of things in smart education environment: Supportive framework in the decision-making process. *Wiley*, pp. 1–12 (2018).

[16]. Abdul, A., Mohammad, T. and Kok-Lim, A. 5G-based smart healthcare network: Architecture, taxonomy, challenges and future research directions. *IEEE, 7,* 100747–100762 (2019).

[17]. Anar, A., Ali, G., Tara, S. and Devrim, U. Intrusion detection system for healthcare systems using medical and network data: A comparison study, *IEEE, 8,* 106576–106584 (2020).

[18]. S.M.R., Daehan, K., Md., H., Mahmud, H. and Kyung-Sup, K. The internet of things for health care: A comprehensive survey. *IEEE, 3,* 678–708 (2015).

[19]. A. Dohr, R. Modre-Opsrian, M. Drobics, D. Hayn and G. Schreier, "The Internet of Things for Ambient Assisted Living," Seventh International Conference on Information Technology: New Generations, 2010, pp. 804-809 (2010).

[20]. Dragorad, M. and Zoran, B. Cloud-based IoT healthcare applications: Requirements and recommendations. *International Journal of Internet of Things and Web Services, 2,* 60–65 (2017).

[21]. Shah, N., Yasir, A., Naeem, U. and Ivan Garc, ı. (2019). Internet of things for healthcare using effects of mobile computing: A systematic literature review. *Wireless Communications And Mobile Computing,* 1–20.

[22]. H.K. and C.H. Adverse drug reactions in primary care: A scoping review. *Khalil And Huang BMC Health Services Research,* 20(5), 1–13 (2020).

[23]. Mohamed, A., Hadeel, T., Heba, I. and Alramzana, N. ECG monitoring systems: Review, architecture, processes, and key challenges. *Sensors,* 20, 1–40 (2020).

[24]. Francisco, V., Armando, G., Erica, R., Mabel, V. and Joaquín, C. An IoT-BASED GLUCOSE MONITORING ALGORITHM TO PREVENT DIABETES COMPLICATIONS. *Applied Science,* 10, 1–12 (2020).

[25]. Francesco, L. and Domenico, L. An overview on internet of medical things in blood pressure monitoring. *IEEE,* 1–6 (2019).

[26]. H.R.F., M.R.I., B.S.H. and I.P.S. Body temperature monitoring based on telemedicine. *The 1St International Conference on Engineering and Applied Science,* 1–9 (2019).

[27]. Pranjal, P., Ubhash, C. and Upendra, K. Security issues of internet of things in health-care sector: An analytical approach. *Research Gate*, 2, 307–329 (2019).

[28]. Dragorad, M. and zoran, B. Cloud-based IoT healthcare applications: Requirements and recommendations. *International Journal Of Internet Of Things And Web Services*, 2, 60–65 (2017)

[29]. Sweta, A. and Anil Kumar, G. Challenges of IoT in healthcare. *Research Gate*, 1–15 (2020).

[30]. Sureshkumar, S. and Suresh, S. Challenges and opportunities in IoT healthcare systems: A systematic review. *SN Applied Sciences*, 1–8 (2019).

[31]. F. John D. and R., V. (2021). Wearables and the internet of things (IoT), applications, opportunities, and challenges: A survey. *IEEE Access*, 1–12.

[32]. C. F. Pasluosta, H. Gassner, J. Winkler, J. Klucken and B. M. Eskofier, An emerging era in the management of Parkinson's disease: Wearable technologies and the internet of things. *Biomedical and Health Informatics*, 19, 1873–1881 (2015).

4 IoT and Smart Health Management

M. Starostka-Patyk and P. Bajdor

CONTENTS

4.1 INTRODUCTION

The modern environment shows an increased need to transform natural world objects into virtually intelligent objects. Intelligent systems, assemblies of interconnecting intelligence hoists, have integrated into the integrity surrounding us for good. Prof. John McCarthy (1929–2011) in the mid-1950s defined artificial intelligence (AI) as the science and engineering of creating intelligent machines, brilliant computers, to use humans' intelligence. Nevertheless, AI is not limited to biologically observable methods. McCarthy defined intelligence as the computational part of achieving goals in the world [1].

The phenomenon of AI described in this way remains unchanged to the present day, and on its basis, new concepts, methods, and IT tools are created that enable full or partial support of human-implemented processes. Among them, the following can be distinguished [2]:

- **Data mining**—Methods of data mining involving the discovery of new, potentially useful patterns from large datasets and the use of algorithms to extract hidden information [3].
- **Machine learning**—Learning systems in which changes in the value of their parameters occur autonomously and based on experience and lead to the improvement in the quality of their operation [4].
- **Decision support systems** [5].
- **Natural-language processing (NLP)**—Computer methods of understanding and deriving information from natural human language, i.e., that is used in everyday life by people [6].

DOI: 10.1201/9781003171829-4

- **Expert systems**—Expert systems that can collect and process enormous resources of knowledge and carry out inference processes that enable the formulation of answers to the questions asked [7].

The Internet of Things (IoT) is also a response to this challenge of modern information technologies and AI. Its goal is to unify all fundamental elements and place them in a shared infrastructure, which will allow not only to control the environment, keep informed about the state of affairs but also have a huge impact on management [8]. Due to the dynamic development of devices with access to the Internet, the idea of the IoT has become not only natural but is also even indicated as one of the key growth drivers of the future global economy and management. The scale of IoT solutions' application is enormous: from clothing, intelligent home appliances, building automation, and smart cities to management, defense systems, and health.

4.2   DEFINING THE IOT

The name IoT was first used in the 90s of the last century. British entrepreneur Kevin Ashton first used this concept in 1999. He described this phenomenon as a mutual cooperation of devices gathering, processing, and transmitting data between each other [9]. This cooperation in communication takes place without human intervention, which allows for systematic automation of processes and autonomous decision-making. He emphasized that the information powering computers and the Internet comes entirely from humans, and from the very beginning, all the data describing things and phenomena on the web was created and recorded by humans. The problem, however, is that man has limited time, attention, and precision, which is why he is not the best at collecting data about objects of the surrounding world.

Meanwhile, it is on these objects (things), not on ideas, that the economy, society, and generally understood existence are based. Therefore, it is necessary to use computers to observe, identify, and understand the world without the limitations of human imperfection [10]. Communication devices without the human factor differ from the typical industrial systems because it is the idea of generally available and common network connected more and more new things, in suitably equipped and functional stand-alone sensors.

The IoT became an increasingly well-known concept globally that concerns ordinary everyday human life in society and has countless application possibilities. The development of the IoT was initially based on the needs of large corporations that wanted to get the most significant benefit from the management and predictability provided by the ability to track all objects in the chains of cooperation in which these companies were involved [11]. Object coding and tracking capabilities have enabled enterprises to increase their productivity, improve their management, accelerate processes, reduce errors, prevent theft, and implement a comprehensive and flexible system organization using the IoT [12]. The IoT is, therefore, a technological revolution that represents the future of information technology and communication and that is developed depending on the dynamics of technological innovation in a diverse environment, because regardless of the area in which it is applied, it allows each object to be marked for identification, automation, monitoring, and control.

The available literature in information technologies does not indicate a clear and consistent definition of the term IoT. However, based on the existing literature, it can be indicated that the IoT is a kind of ecosystem in which objects equipped with sensors communicate with computers [13]. Additionally, in this ecosystem, objects can communicate with or without human involvement [14].

The IoT enables objects/things to take an active part in human environment, for example, by making information available to other users or members of the network wirelessly, using the same IP protocol that connects the Internet. In this way, objects/things can independently recognize events and changes taking place in their environment and autonomously take appropriate action or reaction without human intervention [15].

Speaking of the development of the IoT, we are talking about a wave of innovations using a network of intelligent objects (objects equipped with the ability to process data and cooperate), the essence of which is not only to meet the needs known today. As was the case with the first 'Internet revolution', we are also dealing with creating new application areas, unexpected consumer behavior, and new management models [16]. This is undoubtedly an area of great opportunities and significant risk inherent in mass waves of innovation. When defining the IoT, one should consider the prospects of its use and its structure and functionality.

The definitions of the IoT from the perspective of use in services, interoperability, and technology with different approaches are presented by many authors in the literature [17], and they are summarized in Table 4.1.

However, considering the aspects of construction and functionality, the IoT can be defined from a technological and architectural perspective.

TABLE 4.1
Definitions of the IoT from different perspectives and approaches

Perspective	Approach	Definition
Services	IoT as a business ecosystem	A set of services using objects capable of collecting and processing information (interacting), networked, ensuring interoperability and synergy of applications.
Interoperability	Internet of everything	Consumer devices and products are connected to the Internet and equipped with extensive digital functionalities. The concept assumes that technology's future is the cooperation of devices, objects, and applications in the global network.
Technology	IoT	A network of physical objects containing built-in technology allows for communication, observation of phenomena, manipulating the internal state of objects, and influencing their surroundings.

In terms of technology, IoT is a network that connects devices with a wired or wireless connection, characterized by autonomy (not requiring human involvement) to obtain, share, process data, or interact with the environment under the influence of these data. It is a concept of building telecommunications networks and highly dispersed information systems that can be used, among others, to create intelligent control and measurement systems, analytical or control systems, practically in every area of life, economy, management, or science [18].

The architectural approach defines the IoT as a concept of IT architecture that enables cooperation (interoperability) of various ICT systems supporting various domain applications and is based on the following layers [19]:

- **Equipment**—Devices (or items equipped with them), in particular sensors, actuators, controllers, smartphones, tablets, laptops, or computers, can communicate and process data without human involvement or limited interaction.
- **Communication**—Telecommunications infrastructure and telecommunications network (wired or wireless), operating based on any data transmission standards with any range (here the Internet).
- **Software**—IT systems of IoT devices and software for data exchange, processing, system management, and security.
- **Integration**—sets of defined IT services ensuring software interoperability at all architecture levels.

According to the business and management definition, the IoT is an ecosystem of business and management services, using objects capable of collecting and processing information (interacting), connected in a network, ensuring interoperability and synergy of applications [20]. Combining IoT products/services allows us to understand better the consumer, environment, products, and processes identify critical events; and react to optimize immediately or, more precisely, personalize.

The problem of standardizing nomenclature and definitions was also dealt with by the European Commission. In the study entitled IoT. Position Paper on Standardization for IoT technologies from January 2015, prepared by the European Research Cluster on the IoT, IoT is defined as a dynamic global network infrastructure with self-configuring capabilities, based on standard and interoperable communication protocols in which physical and virtual 'things' have an identity, physical characteristics, and a virtual personality, use intelligent interfaces, and are seamlessly integrated into the information network [15].

According to the Cisco Internet Business Solutions Group (IBSG), the IoT concept describes four main elements that interact with each other in a network: people, data, processes, and things [21]. The basic architecture of IoT is presented in Figure 4.1.

All elements of the IoT are connected via the Internet and provide direct communication [22]:

- People to people (P2P).
- Machines to people (M2P).
- Machines to machines (M2M).

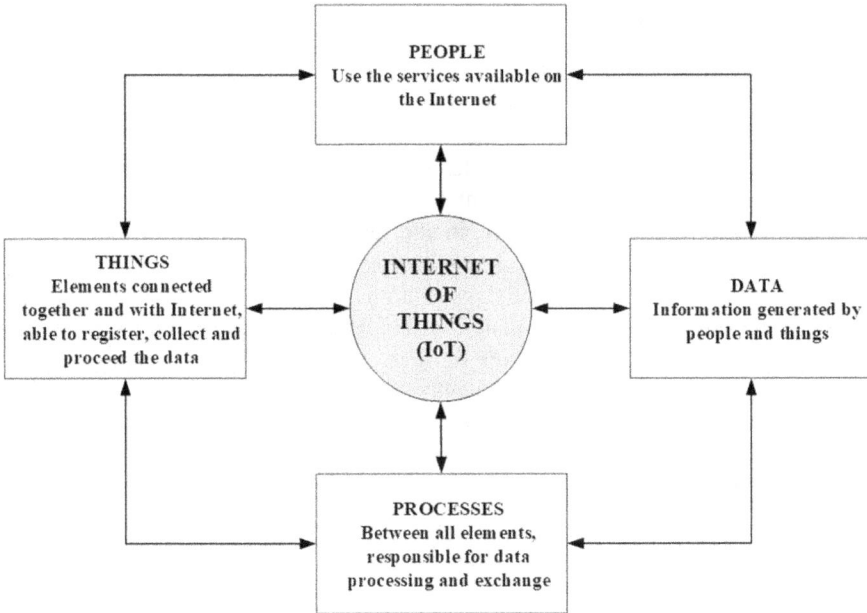

FIGURE 4.1 Basic architecture of IoT.

Simultaneously, the IBSG believes that the IoT represents a specific point in time, at which point the number of things or objects connected to the Internet has exceeded the total population. Cisco defined this moment in the period between 2008 and 2009 [23], and the moment of the emergence of the IoT is shown in Table 4.2.

In conclusion, it should be considered that the Internet owes its origins and development to the growing number of intelligent, interconnected devices and now wide possibilities that they can present [24].

TABLE 4.2
Emergence of the IoT

The population of the world [in billion]	6.3	6.8	7.2	7.6
Number of connected devices [in billion]	0.5	12.5	25	50
Number of connected devices per person	0.08	1.84	3.47	6.58
	2003	2010	2015	2020

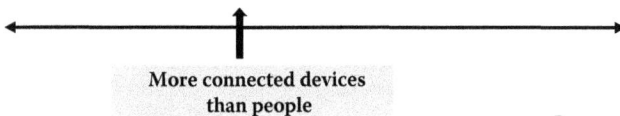

**More connected devices
than people**

4.3   THE ARCHITECTURE OF THE IOT

The critical element of the IoT is the global Internet network as an open communication channel. This is not without reason, because the last decades of the development of the Internet network have allowed for the creation and launch of entirely new services and functionalities of the Internet, which at the same time directly translates into the development of individual sectors of the economy.

Using the IoT requires a change in the approach to building and applying mathematical models. IoT means that it is necessary to depart from the existing practices, where the predictive model was built based on the collected data and then used operationally as long as it maintained the required quality parameters. In the world of permanently communicating devices, where the stream of data available for analysis is vast and changes dynamically, the use of the classic approach will not give a sufficient opportunity to discount its hidden values [25]. Effective models must be built on data whose storage is economically unjustified. Their quick update has become a necessity, and analytical-supported decisions should be made immediately. Thus, the architecture of the tools that make up the IoT solutions, in the simplest terms, is based on:

- Objects that can communicate or receive commands or transmit information, that is, objects equipped with sensors, sensors (temperature, vibration, humidity, motion, etc.) and transmitters enabling communication, receiving commands, and collecting and transmitting information.
- Teleinformatic network meditating in dialogue, that is, infrastructure that enables communication, that is, data transfer between objects (examples and the most popular solutions include WiFi, Bluetooth, NFC wireless network, and also, mainly used in home automation systems, the Z-Wave system).
- IT systems and solutions for processing collected data and transferring information to devices, that is, systems and IT solutions that are receivers of data collected and transferred by objects and places for their processing and decision-making (e.g., laptops, tablets, smartphones, and home cloud computing).

Therefore, the idea of the IoT solutions' functioning (Figure 4.2) is based on using a computer network connected to the Internet, which connects all the cooperating elements [26].

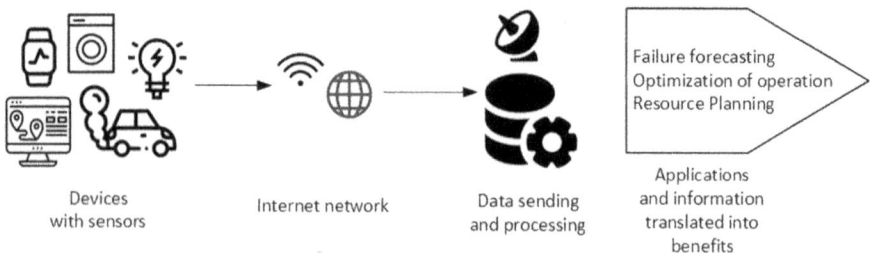

Devices with sensors   Internet network   Data sending and processing   Failure forecasting / Optimization of operation / Resource Planning — Applications and information translated into benefits

FIGURE 4.2   Idea of the IoT solutions' functioning.

Figure 4.2 shows the complexity of technologies, standards, and subsequent revolutionary solutions included in the IoT environment, divided into layers based on the ISO-OSI (Open System Interconnection) model, starting from a physical device equipped with sensors enabling data acquisition, through communication systems, data collection, and processing systems, up to specific business models and applications [27].

The Internet network was initially intended to connect computer units located in different locations for mutual information exchange. However, the further development of the Internet, including using a standardized language for communication with the TCP/IP protocol stack, allowed its global users to use e-mail and publish and search for information on websites. Over time, the use of network technologies has become more and more intensive, which made it possible to use them in e-commerce and create connected supply chains, in which cooperating enterprises work together on one product. Further the development of network technology made it possible for more efficient use of data and video and audio streams. Simultaneously, wireless access technologies started to develop, which enabled the launch of service mobility. As a result, social media, streaming services, and cloud services on a mass scale and in conjunction with mobile technologies began to be used. Today, the Internet is a global network connecting millions of private, public, business, academic, and government users, operating locally to international levels, connected by a wide range of electronic, wireless, and optical devices [28].

Therefore, the natural effect of the further development of this technology is the connection to the Internet of more and more new things which, thanks to the possibility of data exchange, are characterized by completely new functionalities, thus becoming an integral part of the IoT. However, things can be all kinds of objects or people from the real world. What is more, everyday objects do not only mean electronic devices or technologically advanced products; they can be all things, even those in no way associated with electronics, such as food, clothes, furniture, raw materials, parts, art, culture, health. [29].

Understanding the IoT as an ecosystem where objects can communicate with each other, with or without human intervention, is important. For information to be exchanged there are four necessary elements for the IoT functioning, presented in Figure 4.3, and three conditions must be met between two 'things' [30]:

1. First of all a device equipped with a sensor that can collect certain information from the environment and then pass it on is needed. These can be objects equipped with various sensors: temperature, vibration, humidity, motion, GPS. The role of the transmitter can also be played by a smartphone

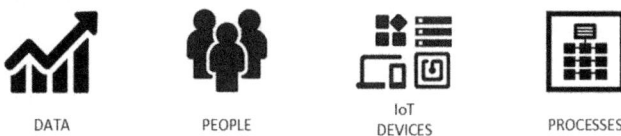

DATA   PEOPLE   IoT DEVICES   PROCESSES

FIGURE 4.3 Elements of the IoT functioning.

from which commands are issued. The only difference is that the data is not downloaded automatically but through an action triggered by the user (e.g., clicking, voice command). Examples include a smart band wristband that monitors the heart rate, a sheet equipped with a motion sensor, or a beacon that detects human movement.

2. Second a device that will receive the transmitted signal, process it, and trigger if a specific reaction occurs is needed. It can be a smartphone, tablet, or computer on which specific information will be displayed, but also another item that will automatically perform a specific action, for example, developing roller shutters integrated with the home-automation system, traffic lights adapted to the traffic volume, or a library book displaying a reminder about the return date.

3. The last element that makes up this ecosystem is the means of communication, that is, the way of sending data. Currently, several technologies on the market enable the transfer of information between two objects, ranging from the most popular ones, such as WiFi or Bluetooth, to NFC or Z-WAVE (used, e.g., in building automation systems).

4.4   APPLICATION OF THE IOT

In the developed world of the IoT, thousands of information exchange processes take place every second, and communication between devices, in many cases, will be multi-path—using a more significant number of transmitters and receivers. All this to display one message—the most important from the user's point of view—at the very end (e.g., on a smartphone screen). It is not difficult to imagine, for example, sensors located throughout the city, thanks to which, after analyzing many variables, the user will receive information about the optimal time to leave home in order to avoid traffic jams on the way to work.

Direct management benefits, including financial ones, resulting from the wide use of the IoT are manifested on three levels [31]:

1. Data to discovery, where, based on new data and with the use of analytics, it is possible to find and identify phenomena whose existence was previously unknown. These can be, for example, new patterns of the course of the disease found thanks to detailed data from telemedicine devices.

2. Data to decisions, where an action can be taken based on the acquired knowledge, often even autonomously. An example may be sending a welcome message and product recommendations to a returning customer, but also an emergency shutdown of a power turbine in the event of a failure.

3. Data to dollars—dividends, where a real financial benefit for the organization or a new business development opportunity emerges from the combination of two previous skills. This level should also include innovative services and products that could not exist without the application of the idea of the IoT (e.g., the new smart home market).

The IoT creates excellent opportunities for the economy, business, and management, influencing, among other things, the design process and service and human

resource management. The benefits of IoT solutions include, among others, reduction of costs, increased productivity and safety of employees, better allocation of
capital, and improvement in customer relations or management processes [32]. The
IoT is also a challenge—it changes the mechanisms of competition, customer expectations, and the products themselves, and offers innovative functionalities, thus
satisfying new consumer needs.

Application of IoT technology is powerful and so far unlimited. Its solutions can
be found both in the private sector in industries such as [33]:

• Telecommunications and media.
• Finances.
• Logistics and production.
• The retail trade.
• Automotive.
• Energy and media.
• Agriculture.

And in the public sector, healthcare management, and households.

Based on the analysis of surveys and reports, scientists from IERC have published an extensive list of IoT applications, which confirms its strategic dimension
among the technological trends in the coming years. The most important among
them are [34]:

1. **Smart Life**—Innovative, state-of-the-art technology aims to make life simpler and safer for consumers. Smart life includes management of:
   • Healthcare—A patient-centered and tailored business approach. Smart
     health covers a wide range of applications used in monitoring health con-
     ditions and physical activity (e.g., older people), vitality (e.g., people ac-
     tively practicing sports), patient safety (both in hospital and at home).
     Thanks to the IoT, it is possible, for example, to control sleep (intelligent
     mattresses) or teeth (using smart brushes). Applications at the industrial
     level include monitoring of hygiene (e.g., informing about the need to wash
     hands in plants), the condition of goods (e.g., monitoring medical re-
     frigerators) and safety (e.g., UV levels or radiation in nuclear power plants).
   • Banking—New banking and personal finance models.
   • Insurance—Moving from statistics to individual policies based on facts.
   • Public services—Improving efficiency and convenience for both admin-
     istrations and managers and citizens.

2. **Smart mobility**—Real-time route management and solutions to make travel
   more enjoyable and transport more reliable. Connecting vehicles to the
   Internet creates many new possibilities and applications that facilitate mo-
   bility and keep users safe. Smart Mobility includes:
   • Autonomous vehicle driving and all connected car services.
   • Mobility in the city—intelligent traffic management.
   • Intercity mobility—connecting communication systems.

- Fee management and payment solutions.
- Distribution and logistics.
- Vehicle fleet management.
- Direct communication between vehicles and the vehicle concerning the infrastructure.
- Identification and monitoring of critical system components.

3. **Smart city**—Innovations aimed at improving the quality of life in cities, including safety and energy efficiency issues. Smart City includes:
   - Intelligent management of city infrastructure, using data analysis tools specific to big data.
   - Cooperation of various administrative bodies, using cloud technologies.
   - Real-time data collection and processing using mobile technologies, enabling immediate response.
   - Increasing the sense of security by improving law enforcement and more effective response to crises.
   - Sustainable city planning—improved schemas and management of spatial planning projects.
   - 'Connected utilities'—intelligent metering devices and management of the gas, water, networks.
   - Construction development—greater automation, better management, and security.

4. **Smart manufacturing**—Manufacturing and logistics solutions specifically designed to optimize processes, management, control, and quality. The omnipresence of communication, the development of micro-robotics, adaptation to individual needs are possible thanks to software that significantly changes the world of production. Intelligent production includes:
   - Machine learning—intelligent, automated decision makings.
   - Networking—network control and management of production devices.
   - Optimized processes—rapid prototyping and production, improved processes, and more efficient supply chain operations.
   - Proactive equipment management—through preventive diagnostics and maintenance.
   - Smooth integration of infrastructure—overcoming the problem of interface standards.

5. **Intelligent energy and grid (smart energy, smart grid)**—technologies that revolutionize the way of producing and transmitting energy to the end user, characterized by a high level of security and applicable in both concentrated and distributed installations. Intelligent Energy and Grid include:
   - Energy savings through the use of more reliable and intelligent sensors and actuators.
   - Scalability of the safety functions.

6. **Smart home, smart buildings, and infrastructure**—Use of the growing role of wireless Internet access (WiFi) in home automation, which is primarily due to the network nature of the electronics used in new electronics/

household appliances, which are beginning to be part of the home IP network, as well as the number of mobile computing devices (smartphones, tablets, etc.) connected to home networks. These technologies include:

- integration of intelligent devices and equipment for buildings or apartments with, for example, entertainment systems.
- Healthcare monitoring.
- Wireless monitoring of energy consumption in the context of a house or building.
- Intelligent building management systems.

IoT technology is horizontal. This means that it can be used in many different industries and business solutions. Additionally, within each industry, IoT systems may appear at different stages of the supply chain, creating ecosystems of solutions that permeate individual market segments. Nevertheless, some industries will be much more dependent on IoT systems, and activities supporting the IoT market's development should focus on them. Therefore, Figure 4.4 summarizes the global spending on IoT 2015–2020 [35], by industry sector in billion U.S. dollars.

Based on the trends described earlier, the most critical industries in terms of the volume of benefits resulting from using IoT [36] are pointed out in Figure 4.5.

The importance and growing possibilities of IoT technology applications will result in the continuation of the development of new digital devices, replacing

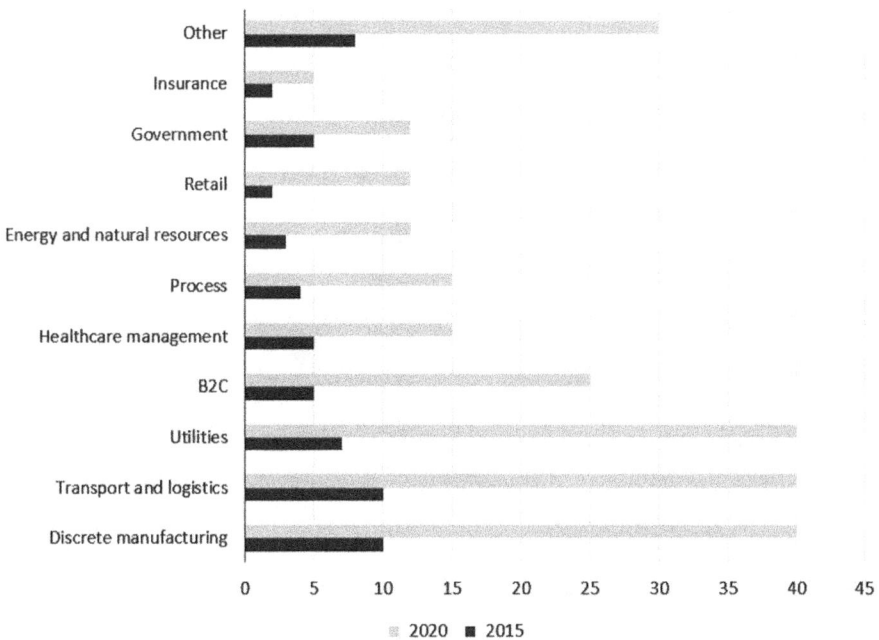

FIGURE 4.4 Global spending on IoT by industry sector in billion U.S. dollars in 2015–2020.

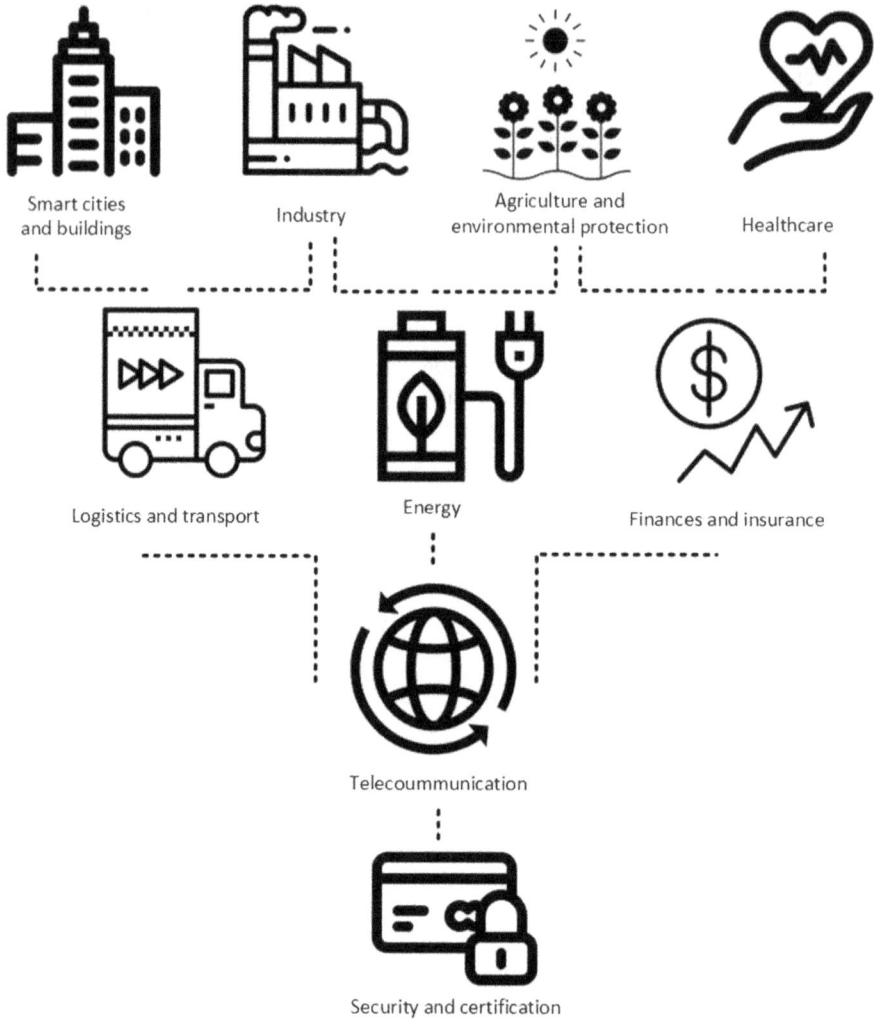

FIGURE 4.5 Industries with the best benefits of IoT usage.

primarily non-digital objects, creating new Internet-X classifications, an example of which is the Internet of Everything, considered to be the next important step in the digital industrial revolution and of which the IoT is only a constituent part.

4.5 THE IOT IN POLAND—A CASE STUDY

Although the potential of IoT in Poland is tremendous, its further direction and development will depend on adaptation at producers' and service providers' levels. A big challenge—especially for RTV/household appliances producers—will increase competitiveness and create added value for users. Smart home services and products show the most significant growth potential.

To determine the development prospects of IoT and the degree of adaptation to this ecosystem among Polish Internet users, IAB Polska, in cooperation with the media and science representatives, carried out a dedicated research project [37]. The study covered the following issues related to the IoT:

- Awareness of the phenomenon and readiness to adapt.
- Degree of adaptation and purchasing potential.
- Barriers and benefits.

As part of the study, 1,121 interviews with Polish Internet users aged over 14 were conducted. The sample was representative in terms of sex, age, and frequency of use of the network, and the participation of the websites in the survey ensured coverage at the level exceeding 90%. The measurement was carried out using the CAWI method between May 6–31, 2015. The maximum estimation error at the 95% confidence level was 2.84%.

The study decided to determine the readiness to use IoT solutions, understood as the degree of use of three types of devices with Internet access: home WiFi, mobile devices, and a car. Access to the first two channels was confirmed by all of the respondents, and every sixth of them declared that their car could connect to the Internet (e.g., playing music, navigation). In total, the vast majority of Internet users (86%) have access to wireless devices that support the network. It should be emphasized that it is mainly dependent on the age of network users—in the youngest group of respondents, it slightly exceeds the general level, then gradually increases to reach the maximum (93%), from the marketing perspective, in the target group of people of mobile working age (35–44 years old), then decreases among people over 44 years old.

The study also verified Internet users' level of knowledge about the term 'IoT'. It shows that only 11% of Internet users have come across the term IoT. It is essential to note that although the level of knowledge is independent of age, significantly more men than women declared knowledge of this term. This knowledge is also correlated with the degree of digitization—people who use smart devices (smartphone, tablet) more often encountered this term. However, rarely a technological or industry language is understandable to average users, even if they use a given technology solution. It should therefore not be surprising that—according to the 'IoT' study—despite such a low technical knowledge of the concept, currently about 40% of Polish Internet users have equipment that can function in the IoT ecosystem, and another 50% would use such devices if they had such a possibility.

As of today, IoT solutions in the smart home category are characterized by the lowest degree of use (only a few percentage of respondents declare having such solutions), but this is an area with the most significant development potential among consumer applications of the IoT (Figure 4.6). This is evidenced by several indicators determined in the study [38]. First, Internet users' households are characterized by a high degree of wireless data transmission—77% use their home WiFi (Figure 4.7). Moreover, this technology is widely used as 86% of its users use a wireless link to operate more than one device [38].

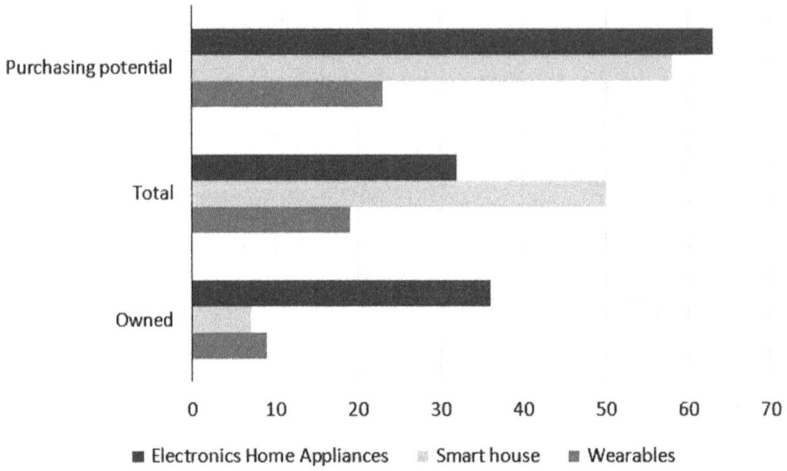

FIGURE 4.6   Potential among consumer applications of the IoT.

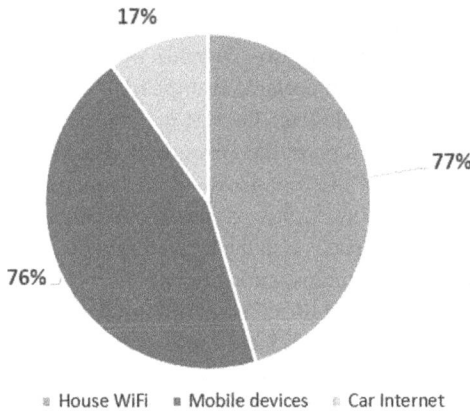

FIGURE 4.7   Characteristics of Internet users' households.

Second, taking into account the desire to use the various IoT through the Internet, the most significant increase in the number of potential users was recorded precisely in this category, which can translate into the penetration of services in smart house among Polish Internet users at a level exceeding 50%. Finally, among the expected benefits associated with IoT, most often it applies to smart homes—saving energy (44%). It should also be emphasized that—taking into account the currently low penetration of this type of device—further directions and pace of development of this category will largely depend on the degree of adaptation of the IoT at the level of producers and service providers.

Personal belongings, clothing items, and IoT accessories are as lowly popular as building automation—they are owned by only a few percentage of respondents. However, they are characterized by a much smaller, moderate development potential.

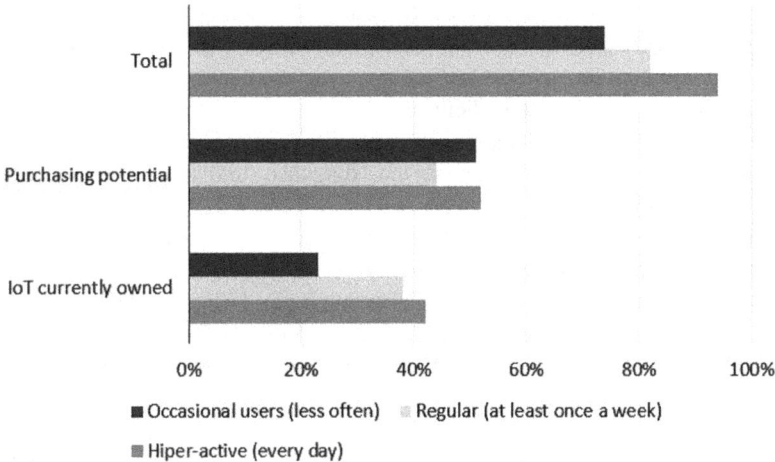

FIGURE 4.8 Potential of IoT devices with Internet usage.

Considering people who consider using this type of device in the future, the growth index in the number of potential users is slightly above 200%. However, in this category, special attention should be paid to health protection equipment, which enjoyed the most significant interest among the wearables accessories presented.

Above, the focus was on the most typical consumer solutions, but the portfolio of products and services associated with the IoT is vast [38]. It should also be noted that the potential of IoT devices depends on the intensity of Internet use (Figure 4.8).

An example may be the use of IoT in the automotive industry, sport, and tourism, as well as culture and art (museums, cinemas) and many public places (hotels, airports, shops, etc.). The results of the study indicate that Polish Internet users are primarily prepared for this—76% use WiFi on mobile devices at least from time to time (e.g., phone, smartphone, tablet), 49% being in a museum or gallery would like to receive information and interesting facts about the exhibitions on the phone, and 41% being in the store get information about the products, discounts, and promotions. The IoT opens up great opportunities for the entire economy, innovation, and creativity.

4.6 SMART HEALTH MANAGEMENT—INTERPRETATION OF THE PHENOMENON

Regardless of the individual or social approach, human health is the most crucial good that should be constantly looked after. Along with the development of civilization, healthcare improves its activities from year to year. Modern technological achievements also help in this development. Smart health management (SHM) is defined as using information and communication technologies to support activities related to health protection [39].

SHM is the name used to describe tools or solutions that include products, systems, processes, and services for health authorities and professionals, and tailored health systems for patients and citizens, such as health information networks, electronic health books, telemedicine services, personal portable communication systems, health portals, and many other tools based on information and communication technologies, helping to prevent, diagnose, and treat diseases, monitor health, lead an appropriate lifestyle.

Besides, this term covers many other terms such as telemedicine, telehealth, remote medical care, telematics in healthcare, medical IT, health information management, information, and communication technologies [40]. In addition to computer applications, smart health management includes cognitive information processing and communication tasks for medical practice, education, and research [41]. The essence of SHM is that it should support the transformation of healthcare processes to benefit patients and the healthcare system.

At the same time, SHM aims to support patients by educating them about their health condition and prevention. It also allows patients to deal with crises on their own. It provides its users with services of a high-quality standard, supported by experienced health professionals, and also enables the maximum use of the potential of knowledge from available online sources. Thanks to this, using SHM, it is possible to monitor patients and reduce costs related to their treatment remotely, and eliminate geographical barriers in providing medical care [42].

Despite the effective use of SHM in practice and its wide use by physicians and society it is possible to identify several success factors as well as some determined barriers. Additionally, some of the factors may exist in certain circumstances and, depending on them, may be considered severe (as a best practice) and less often as threats due to the lack of an appropriate implementation approach [43]. Success and failure factors in implementing smart health are collected in Table 4.3.

The broad classification of the SHM is based on the services, medical devices, technologies used, applications, system management, and end users [44]. Classification of smart healthcare is presented in Figure 4.9.

Connectivity technologies that are used play a vital role in expanding the applications for which the healthcare system is designed. The efficient integration of small devices through wireless technologies can help in implementing remote health monitoring through the IoT [45].

The healthcare sector is transforming as a result of the digital revolution. New technologies are creating a new world of online healthcare, from robotic surgery to hyper-precise treatment. The IoT technology accelerates the change in healthcare management by enabling doctors to use data collected by medical devices. In this way, reactive healthcare becomes proactive care, helping to improve early diagnosis. In addition to facilitating remote healthcare, IoT technology can help health organizations become more efficient by tracking resources such as hospital beds [46].

Data from the IoT help drive smart hospitals' management and development, but it also helps to track the person's health. IoT devices enable patients to be more active in controlling their health, which is especially important for the elderly and patients suffering from chronic diseases. Using IoT devices can also help to get out of the hospital faster and even prevent hospital stays [47].

TABLE 4.3

Success and failure factors in implementing smart health

Success Factors	Implementation Barriers
• A medical need and strong patient orientation • Political and social support • Long-term view of projects • Predefined investment goals • Involvement of all key actors • A multidisciplinary approach involving politicians, specialists, researchers, and business • Public-private partnership • Selection of the right technology, continuous technical support • Interoperability and open standards	• Inability to adapt the strategy to the changing environment • Reorganization of healthcare processes in the process of establishing new technologies • Isolation from organizations and potential users • Resistance to change • Lack of political support • Lack of a long-term perspective. • Lack of understanding of healthcare processes and changes in medical environments • Lack of market analysis, comparing the solution to the existing ones • Lack of existing information systems (e.g., clinical information systems) • Bad communication of technical problems in the project

Opportunities (or Threats)

• Involvement at all levels and user participation
• Projects based on actual needs and clear goals
• Contacts and interpersonal communication within the project
• Compliance, as far as possible, with technical standards for interoperability
• Long-term approach, endurance, and development stability.

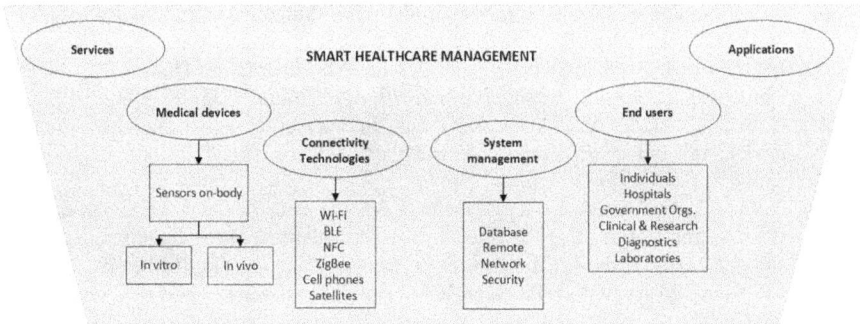

FIGURE 4.9 Classification of smart healthcare.

To sum up, SHM is healthcare based on the latest technology and information achievements. As a result, both the providers of medical services and their recipients obtain highly qualified support, improving its management processes and significantly facilitating healthcare's daily functioning.

REFERENCES

[1]. J. McCarthy, What is artificial intelligence. http://www-formal.stanford.edu/jmc/whatisai.pdf (2007).

[2]. W. Shi, J. Cao, Q. Zhang, Y. Li and L. Xu, Edge computing: Vision and challenges. *IEEE Internet of Things Journal*, 3 (5), 637–646 (2016).

[3]. F. Chen, P. Deng, J. Wan, D. Zhang, A.V. Vasilakos and X. Rong, Data mining for the Internet of things: Literature review and challenges. *International Journal of Distributed Sensor Networks*, 1, 17 (2015).

[4]. E. Alpaydin, *Introduction to machine learning*. Cambridge: MIT press (2020).

[5]. S. Reddy, J. Fox and M. Purohit, Artificial intelligence-enabled healthcare delivery. *Journal of the Royal Society of Medicine*, 112 (1), 22–28 (2019).

[6]. J.T. Wu, F. Dernoncourt, S. Gehrmann, P.D. Tyler, E.T. Moseley, E.T. Carlson and L. Celi, Behind the scenes: A medical natural language processing project. *International Journal of Medical Informatics*, 112, 68–73 (2018).

[7]. J. Liebowitz, *The handbook of applied expert systems*. Boca Raton: CRC Press (2019).

[8]. R. Shah and A. Chircu, IOT and ai in healthcare: A systematic literature review. *Issues in Information Systems*, 19 (3), 49 (2018).

[9]. K. Ashton, That 'Internet of Things' thing, http://www.rfidjournal.com/articles/view? 4986 (2011).

[10]. N. Gershenfeld, R. Krikorian and D. Cohen, The Internet of Things. *Scientific American*, 291, 76–81 (2004).

[11]. M. Lianos and M. Douglas, Dangerization and the End of Deviance: The Institutional Environment. *British Journal of Criminology*, 40, 261–278 (2000).

[12]. T. Ferguson, Have your objects call my object. *Harvard Business Review*, 6, 1–7 (2002).

[13]. R. Lombreglia, *The Internet of Things*. Boston: Boston Globe (2010).

[14]. G. Jayavardhana, B. Rajkumar, S. Marusic and M. Palaniswami, Internet of Things: A vision, architectural elements, and future directions. *Future Generation* (2013).

[15]. IERC, IERC—European Research Cluster on the Internet of Things, *Internet of Things. Position Paper on Standardization for IoT Technologies*, 1645–1660 (2015).

[16]. E. Bertino and N. Islam, Botnets and internet of things security. *Computer*, 50 (2), 76–79 (2017).

[17]. J.H. Nord, A. Koohang and J. Paliszkiewicz, The Internet of Things: Review and theoretical framework. *Expert Systems with Applications*, 133, 97–108 (2019).

[18]. G. Singh, L. Gaur and R. Ramakrishnan, Internet of Things-technology adoption model in India. *Pertanika Journal of Science & Technology*, 25 (3), 835–846 (2017).

[19]. I. Yaqoob, E. Ahmed, I.A.T. Hashem, A.I.A. Ahmed, A. Gani, M. Imran and M. Guizani, Internet of things architecture: Recent advances, taxonomy, requirements, and open challenges. *IEEE Wireless Communications*, 24 (3), 10–16 (2017).

[20]. J.P. Shim, M. Avital, A.R. Denniś, M. Rossi, C. Sørensen and A. French, The transformative effect of the internet of things on business and society. *Communications of the Association for Information Systems*, 44 (1), 5 (2019).

[21]. Cisco, The Internet of Things: How the Next Evolution of the Internet Is Changing Everything. Cisco Internet Business Solutions Group (IBSG), http://www.woodsidecap.com/wp-content/uploads/2015/02/WCP-IOT-M_and_A-REPORT-2015-21.pdf (2011).

[22]. S. Li, L. Da Xu and S. Zhao, 5G Internet of Things: A survey. *Journal of Industrial Information Integration*, 10, 1–9 (2018).

[23]. D. Evans, The IoT—How the next evolution of the Internet is changing everything. *CISCO Internet Business Solution Group (IBSG)*, https://www.cisco.com/c/dam/en_us/about/ac79/docs/innov/IoT_IBSG_0411FINAL.pdf (2011).

[24]. M.E. Porter and J.E. Heppelmann, How smart, connected product are transforming competition. *Harvard Business Review*, 11, 64–89 (2014).

[25]. J. Lin, W. Yu, N. Zhang, X. Yang, H. Zhang and W. Zhao, A survey on internet of things: Architecture, enabling technologies, security and privacy, and applications. *IEEE Internet of Things Journal*, 4 (5), 1125–1142 (2017).

[26]. S. Al Hinai and A.V. Singh, Internet of things: Architecture, security challenges and solutions. 2017 International Conference on Infocom Technologies and Unmanned Systems (Trends and Future Directions ICTUS) IEEE, 1–4 (2017).

[27]. A. Passemard, The Internet of Things Protocol stack—from sensors to business value. https://entrepreneurshiptalk.wordpress.com/2014/01/29/the-internet-of-thing-protocol-stack-from-sensors-to-business-value/ (2014).

[28]. B. Yang, Y. Lu, K. Zhu, Y. Zhang and J. Liu, Evolution of the Internet and its measures. 2017 First International Conference on Electronics Instrumentation & Information Systems (EIIS) IEEE, 1–4 (2017).

[29]. E.A. Kosmatos, N.D. Tselikas and A.C. Boucouvalas, Integrating RFIDs and Smart Objects into a Unified In-ternet of Things Architecture. *Advances in Internet of Things: Scientific Research*, 1, 5–12 (2011).

[30]. V. Krotov, The Internet of Things and new business opportunities. *Business Horizons*, 60 (6), 831–841 (2017).

[31]. K. Borne, Big data—what is it good for? https://mapr.com/blog/big-data-what-it-good/ (2014).

[32]. H.F. Atlam, A. Alenezi, M.O. Alassafi and G. Wills, Blockchain with internet of things: Benefits, challenges, and future directions. *International Journal of Intelligent Systems and Applications*, 10 (6), 40–48 (2018).

[33]. G. Lampropoulos, K. Siakas and T. Anastasiadis, Internet of things in the context of industry 4.0: An overview. *International Journal of Entrepreneurial Knowledge*, 7 (1), 4–19 (2019).

[34]. G.N. Satish and P.S. Varma, Internet Of Things—Opportunities, applications and challenges in the prospective smart world. *International Journal of Computer Science and Information Technologies*, 4 (3), 8–16 (2017).

[35]. L. Shanhong, Global spending on IoT by industry sector. https://www.statista.com/statistics/1095375/global-spending-on-iot-by-industry-sector/ (2021).

[36]. Q. Guo and Q. Xu, The economic benefits of agglomeration of the internet of things industry based on 5 G network and markov chain. *Microprocessors and Microsystems*, 103438 (2020).

[37]. M. Grodner, W. Kokot, P. Kolenda, K. Krejtz, A. Legoń, P. Rytel and R. Wierzbiński, *Internet Rzeczy w Polsce*. Warsaw: IAB Polska (2015).

[38]. IAB Polska, Internet Rzeczy Report (2015).

[39]. M.I. Pramanik, R.Y. Lau, H. Demirkan and M.A.K. Azad, Smart health: Big data enabled health paradigm within smart cities. *Expert Systems with Applications*, 87, 370–383 (2017).

[40]. M.K. Al-Azzam and M.B. Alazzam, Smart city and smart-health framework, challenges and opportunities. *International Journal of Advanced Computer Science and Applications*, 10 (2), 171–176 (2019).

[41]. H. Hamidi, An approach to develop the smart health using Internet of Things and authentication based on biometric technology. *Future Generation Computer Systems*, 91, 434–449 (2019).

[42]. S.P. Mohanty, U. Choppali and E. Kougianos, Everything you wanted to know about smart cities: The Internet of Things is the back-bone. *IEEE Consumer Electronics Magazine*, 5 (3),60–70 (2016).

[43]. A. Solanas, C. Patsakis, M. Conti, I. Vlachos, V. Ramos, F. Falcone, O. Postolache, P.A. Pérez-Martínez, R. Di Petro, D.N. Perrea and A.M. Ballesté, Smart health: A context-aware health paradigm within smart cities. *IEEE Communication Magazine*, 52 (8), 74–81 (2014).

[44]. P. Sundaravadivel, E. Kougianos, S.P. Mohanty and M.K. Ganapathiraju, Everything You Wanted to Know about Smart Health Care: Evaluating the Different Technologies and Components of the Internet of Things for Better Health. *IEEE Consumer Electronics Magazine*, 7 (1), 18–28 (2018).

[45]. K. Ullah, M.A. Shah and S. Zhang, Effective ways to use Internet of Things in the field of medical and smart health care. Proceedia of International Conference on Intelligent Systems Engineering (ICISE), 372–379 (2016).

[46]. M. Díaz, G. Juan, O. Lucas and A. Ryuga, Big data on the Internet of Things: An example for the e-health. Proceedings of 6th International Conference on Innovative Mobile and Internet Services in Ubiquitous Computing, 898–900 (2012).

[47]. J. Wang, L. Li, L. Wang and W. Zhao, The Internet of Things for resident health information service platform research. Proceedia of IET International Conference on Communication Technology and Application, 631–635 (2011).

5 Current Status of Alzheimer's Disease in India: Prevalence, Stigma, and Myths

Surekha Manhas, Zaved Ahmed Khan, and Meenu Gupta

CONTENTS

DOI: 10.1201/9781003171829-5

5.1   BACKGROUND

In 1906, Dr. Alois Alzheimer was the first person who illustrated this potent disastrous Alzheimer's through the observation of shrinkage in the nerve cells of the brain in her patient who suffered from memory loss and psychological changes. It is estimated that more than 4 million people in India suffer from Alzheimer's disease (AD), yet many people, especially rural people, are not aware of this disease because they usually consider the loss of memory as a sign of inexorable part of aging rather than the sign of any kind of neurodegenerative disease. AD keeps on increasing at a faster rate and thus there is increase in burden of Alzheimer's in India. After China and USA, India has the third-highest caseloads in the world. But still there are no effective drugs and treatments available to cure this disease. More research is needed in this field to treat AD.

5.2   INTRODUCTION

AD is one of the heterogeneous disastrous neurodegenerative diseases that cause progressive relentless loss in relation to cognitive functions including thinking, language and behavior associated with the accumulation of amyloid-ß (Aß) peptides and tau proteins that ultimately result in the formation of senile plaques in the hippocampal region of the brain. Dementia usually affects the elder population, and is caused by AD, which is the most common form of dementing illness, showing a huge impact on family, personal, and societal life. The early typical symptoms that usually appear after the age of 60 are the loss of recent memories, language problems, mild coordination problems, and psychological issues. There are reports related to coronal T1-weighted magnetic resonance imaging (MRI) scan studies in a patient who suffered from moderate AD. The study shows that disease progression in the hippocampus area leads to hippocampal atrophy [1].

5.3 CHANGES OCCUR IN BRAIN DURING AD

In central nervous system, neurons are the basic potent cells that help transmit information from one nerve to another. A normal healthy adult brain has over a billion neurons, each having long branching extensions, with an axon and several dendrites. Neurons communicate with each other by establishing a connection between them, called synapses, which are usually over trillions in number. The flow of information is usually carried out in the form of tiny chemicals like neurotransmitters which are released by single specific neuron and detected by other specific receiving neuron through the brain's neuronal circuit which develops thoughts, emotions, movements, and cellular basis of memories.

The two main changes in the brain associated with AD are accumulation of ß-amyloid (protein fragment), a peptide made up of 36–43 amino acids outside neurons, and accumulation of tau protein in the defective form inside neurons that no longer stabilize the properties of microtubules. Accumulation of ß-amyloid (beta-amyloid plaques) is believed to be responsible for the cell death because they restrict the transmission of information within the neurons at synapses, while tau protein (tau tangles) blocks nutrients exchange within the neurons. When the concentration of ß-amlyoid starts increasing in the neurons, the point is reached at which defective tau protein spreads all over the brain. Inflammation and atrophy are the conditions that have been detected during AD. High concentration of toxic ß-amyloid and abnormal form of tau protein results in the activation of immune cells in the brain called microglia, which are the defense cells present in the central nervous system by acting as macrophages to remove plaques, cell debris, and dead neurons through the process of phagocytosis. Due to loss of cells in the brain, it gets shrunk, which is the main cause of atrophy. The loss of cells results in the decrease in the capacity of the brain to metabolize the glucose (fuel source), causing slow cognitive function and loss of memory [2].

According to research, several changes that occur in brain related with Alzheimer's start showing symptoms at the age of 20 before the symptoms are visible. After developing early changes, the brain tries to recover it in order to perform the functions properly. When the disease gets worse, the brain is not able to recover instantly and then the person starts showing symptoms like the loss of cognitive functions [3].

5.4 MILD COGNITIVE IMPAIRMENT

Mild cognitive impairment (MCI) is a state in which individuals show benign but noticeable changes that are easily perceptible to the family others. Despite this condition, individuals are able to perform daily activities. MCI affects 20% of the individuals under the age of 65. The people who are suffering from MCI are more likely to develop Alzheimer's rather than those without MCI [3].

5.5 NEURAL MECHANISM

During AD, numerous brain cells get affected and the numbers vary with respect to different regions by the expression of neuropeptides and neurotransmitters, including claustrum, substantia nigra, striatum, thalamus, locus ceruleus. Due to degenerative process, usually cells come under this process and thus loss of neuronal cells as a result of cellular atrophy. The pathobiology of this subtle disease also has potential to affect the non-neuronal cells like microglia, astrocytes, oligodendroglia, blood vessels, choroid plexus. The AD models of transgenic mice showed that the presence of amyloid plaques in the brain tissues has a great potential to disturb the normal brain functioning due to the loss of dendrite spines or synaptic dysfunction. Postmortem studies of brain tissues illustrated that individuals who suffer from this deadly disease usually have a strong decline in dendritic spines and density of synapses in the hippocampus region of the brain relative to normal brain tissues. Loss of dendritic spines is directly co-related with the worsening mental status and also acts as an indicator of disease [4].

5.6 PATHOBIOGENESIS

For the detailed explanation of AD, different hypotheses have been given: (a) Aß amyloid hypothesis, (b) lysosome hypothesis, (c) calcium dysregulation hypothesis, (d) A-ß amyloid oligomer hypothesis, (e) the tau hypothesis. Among all of these, amyloid hypothesis is the best studied one, on the basis of multiple reports that explain the weak interrelationship between A-ß deposition in the brain, loss of neuron (neuronal atrophy), and cognitive impairments. In 1984, two scientists, George Glenner and Caine Wong, discovered the basic mechanism of Alzheimer's by isolating multiple forms of meninvascular Aß by proteolytic cleavage from protein amyloid precursor protein (APP). Thus, Alzheimer's pathobiology is directly associated with the presence of Aß peptide that results in spine instability and functional deficit in neuronal structures [3]. Toxic protein formation (amyloid and tau protein) and involvement of other non-neuronal cells like microglia cells act as macrophages to remove unwanted material from the brain to maintain normal functioning of brain [5].

5.7 IMPAIRMENT IN MITOCHONDRIA LEADS TO PRODUCTION OF REACTIVE OXYGEN SPECIES

Due to high metabolic activities in the brain, neurons require enormous energy for performing normal functions of the brain that are specifically carried out in the presence of mitochondria in the brain tissues through oxidative phosphorylation, during which reactive oxygen species (ROS) are generated in tremendous quantity, and then increased level is conventionally offset by the normal process of homeostasis in mitochondria. Aß is a potent solitary molecule that has a great tendency to develop huge numbers of small clusters having potential to move freely in the brain and then ultimately form plaques which are indications (hallmark) of AD. Aß molecules have the ability to penetrate the plasma membrane and come into contact with defective internal proteins of mitochondria, which causes the decline in the activities of electron transport chain and increased ROS production. Increased Aß concentration is responsible for cellular toxicity. ROS is also a hallmark of AD [6].

5.8 GENES LINKED WITH ALZHEIMER DISEASE

Several numbers of different genes, including *PSEN-1*, *APP*, and *PSEN-2*, play a potent role in the progression of this devastating disease. Mutation in these genes results in the generation of amyloid plaques whose accumulation outside the neurons causes hindrance in cell signaling pathways (Tables 5.1 and 5.2).

TABLE 5.1

Different genes involved in the genetics of Alzheimer's disease with their description and their ID [7]

S. No.	Gene Symbol	Gene ID	Description
1.	*APP*	GC21M027252	Beta-amyloid (A4) precursor protein: AD risk factor: found on chromosome 21
2.	*BPTF*	GC17P065821	Bromodomain PHD finger transcription factor
3.	*PSEN1*	GC14P073603	Presenilin 1: found on chromosome17: ß-secretase activity determination results in the proteolysis
4.	*COL25A1*	GC04M109731	Collagen, type XXV, alpha 1
5.	*APBB1*	GC11M006414	Beta-amyloid (A4) precursor protein-binding, member 1 (Fe65), family B
6.	*PSEN2*	GC01P227058	Presenilin 2: beta-secretase activity responsible for proteolysis
7.	*GSK3B*	GC03M119540	Glycogen synthase kinase 3 ß
8.	*PSENEN*	GC19P036236	Presenilin enhancer gamma-secretase subunit
9.	*CHAT*	GC10P050817	Choline *O*-acetyltransferase
10.	*MAPT*	GC17P043971	Microtubule-associated protein tau: location: chromosome no.17: neurofibrillary tangles formation: AD risk hallmark
11.	*APBA1*	GC09M072042	Amyloid-beta (A4) precursor protein-binding, family A, member 1
12.	*CDK5R1*	GC17P030813	Regulatory subunit 1 (p35), cyclin-dependent kinase 5
13.	*CASP2*	GC07P142985	Apoptosis-related cysteine peptidase, caspase 2
14.	*LRP1*	GC12P057497	Low-density lipoprotein receptor-related protein 1
15.	*APOE*	GC19P045408	Apolipoprotein E: neuronal protection: lipid haemostasis
16.	*APBA2*	GC15P029213	Beta-amyloid (A4) precursor protein-binding, member 2, family A
17.	*NCSTN*	GC01P160313	Nicastrin
18.	*CLSTN1*	GC01M009789	Calsyntenin 1
19.	*APBB1*	GC11M006414	Beta-amyloid (A4) precursor protein-binding, family B, member 1 (Fe65)
20.	*GSK3A*	GC19M042734	Glycogen synthase kinase 3 alpha

TABLE 5.2

Three specifically mutated genes that are observed under the case study of Alzheimer's disease with their location and their molecular effects [7]

S.No.	Protein	Mutations	Gene	Location	Pathogenic Effects at Molecular Level
1.	Presenilin 2	14	*PSEN-2*	14q24	Ratio of Aß42:Aß40 increases
2.	ß-Amyloid precursor protein	32	*APP*	21q21	ß-Amyloid production increases/ ratio of Aß42:Aß40 increases
3.	Presenilin 1	182	*PSEN-1*	14q24	Rise in the ratio of Aß42:Aß40

5.8.1 AMYLOID PRECURSOR PROTEIN

The specific gene for amyloid precursor protein (APP) is located on chromosome 21 in humans that comprises 19 exons, and in DNA, it spans approximately 240 kbp that plays a vital role in cell synaptic development, neuronal injury, iron export, and repair mechanism [8–12]. Mutation in *APP* gene causes proteolysis of this gene product and results in the formation of amyloid plaques [13–15]. APP and Aß are the two potent indicators of AD, which are normal products of neuronal protein generated by the sequential process of proteolysis through the enzymes beta and gamma secretase that cut specifically at beta and gamma sites of APP. Patients who are generally suffering from Down syndrome usually have a high risk of AD because both the diseases occur due to changes in chromosome 21. APP undergoes certain post-translational modifications like tyrosine sulfation, glycosylation, sialyation, and other proteolytic processes to generate peptide fragments [16]. It has been found that the translation of APP mRNA can be disrupted by changing a single nucleotide in the 5'UTR region of APP (single nucleotide polymorphism) [17].

5.8.2 *PSEN-1* AND *PSEN-2* GENES

Gene for Presenilin-1 and Presenilin-2 is located on chromosome 14 which determines the activity of ß-secretase that is responsible for proteolysis that usually takes place in the APP and other NOTCH receptor-related proteins [18–20]. These genes are protagonist in structure, having 13 exons in which 10 exons consist of a coding sequence, whereas on the 4 different exons, the 5' UTR region is present [21–24]. The *PSEN-1* gene contains CAAT box, STAT elements, and TAAT box in its promoter region that is responsible for the activation of transcription process that depends on signal transduction [24]. The proteins encoded by these both genes display 67% similarities to each other [25–27]. In the case of *PSEN-1*, intronic polymorphism has been observed between exonS 8 and 9 that display a remarkable affiliation with late-onset disease [28]. However, several different dataset studies display different reports to confirm the association, but there are other reports too that give no description about association [29–35].

5.8.3 *Tau* Gene

Tau is a protein (phosphoprotein) that plays a potent role in the stabilization of neuronal structure and maintains the microtubule stability [36,37]. The gene that controls the production of protein tau is located on chromosome 17, which when gets mutated results in the development of neurofibrillary tangles inside the neurons, which in turn interfere the flow of information among the cells. Alternative splicing of a microtubule-associated protein tau (*MAPT*) gene results in the formation of tau proteins [38,39]. The changes in the post-transcriptional modification processes thus result in the excessive phosphorylation of tau into an abnormal form called neurofibrillary tangles [40]. In AD, phosphorylation usually occurs in 19 amino acids at serine position 119, 202, 409, 396 and threonine at 231 [41,42].

5.8.4 *APOE* Gene

Apolipoprotein E consists of 299 amino acids that play a major role in neuronal protection and also in the lipid haemostasis [43–45]. There are three different major alleles found in the brain, e2, e3, and e4, according to their respective positions 112 and 158. The positions of wild-type e3, e2, and e4 are Cys 112 and Arg 158, Cys 112 and Arg158, and Cys 112Arg and Arg158 [46–48]. The most frequent allele is e3 that is found in most old adults, whereas e4 is observed mostly in AD patients [49–51]. Allele e4 is recognized as a genetically risk factor of AD [52]. The expression frequency of allele e4 has been observed highest in the study of Nigerian population with less prevalence of AD among them, which may be associated with low levels of cholesterol [53–56]. In a number of studies, it has been observed that e2 allele plays a protective role in AD [57,58] (Figure 5.1).

5.9 BLOOD–BRAIN BARRIERS

For the effective drug delivery to the target site, drugs should have potential to cross the blood–brain barriers (BBB) so that it could reach the target site, but BBB

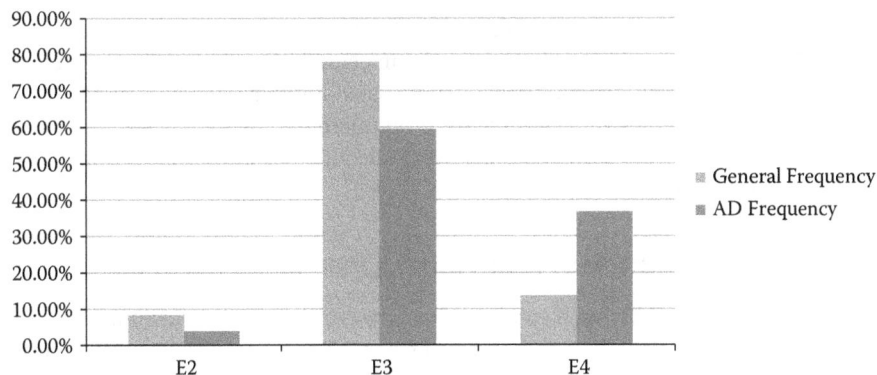

FIGURE 5.1 Estimated allelic frequencies related to the *APOE* gene in humans in case studies associated with Caucasian population [58].

doesn't allow the paracellular passive diffusion, which creates a hindrance during drug delivery. This hindrance can be overcome by using advanced nanotechnology. BBB consists of a number of capillaries of endothelial cells in the central nervous system attached together with the strong tight junctions that allow only nutrients or ions which provide neuronal protection to enter the brain part in order to maintain haemostasis to restrict the access of toxic substances or drug. The other additional barrier that inhibits the movement of certain molecules or drug entry is blood-CSF whose main role is the separation of blood from cerebrospinal fluid that is located at the choroid plexus and covers the subarachnoid space by enclosing the brain. There is some part of central nervous system where BBB is not present, but despite that, that particular regions contain micro vessels which are analogous to periphery, called as circumventricular organs, and consist of median eminence, choroid plexus. The free solute movement within interstitial fluid and blood is carried out by the capillaries which are present in the circumventricular organ. The presence of membrane transporters (influx and efflux transporters) acts as a barrier which permits the entry and exit of xenobiotics or drugs. Hindrance and degradation of drugs during drug delivery occur due to the presence of different potent enzymes in the brain which generate their effects to block the entry of drugs. To easily cross BBB by the process of passive diffusion, the drugs should be lipid molecules having the molecular weight of about less than 500 kDa with partition coefficient of 0.5 and 6.0 and pH should be neutral [59]. Certain different approaches have been used thus to overcome the problem that occurs during drug delivery to pass BBB that include biomimetics, intracranial infusion, diuretic agents, and convectional enhanced delivery [60–63]. With issues associated with safety, specificity which poses a problem to effective drug delivery to the target site [64,65]. In order to check the effectiveness of a wide range of drugs, animal models are used and are treated with the focused ultrasound that delivers a specific drug to the target site, including stem cells, viruses, antibodies, herceptin, nanoparticles, and chemotherapy [66–73].

5.10 ACTIVATION OF MICROGLIA TO GENERATE RESPONSE TO INJURY

During neurodegeneration, microglia gets activated and transformed into phagocytes which act as an antigen-presenting cells in central nervous system to generate response to remove cell debris. T-cells get activated through the receptors like Fcγ, MHC-class I&II, and B7 that are expressed by microglia. Microglia gets activated during death of neurons, and when there is no death of neuronal cells, they return back to their resting phase [74].

5.11 EARLY SYMPTOMS FOR DIAGNOSIS OF ALZHEIMER'S

Dr. Parveen Gupta, HOD of Neurology Department from Fortis Institute, has explained certain Alzheimer's-related symptoms:

- Decline in the cognitive activities like thinking, learning, and other mental processes.

- Changes in the behavioral pattern like forget the way to communicate with others.
- Memory loss.
- Problems related to language (aphasia) like difficulty in speaking the words.
- Inability recognize faces and objects.
- Inability to reading text.
- Facing difficulties to solve problems by analyzing it [75].

5.12   MAGNETIC RESONANCE IMAGING

Magnetic resonance imaging (MRI) is the common medical-based brain diagnostic technique in which the anatomy of brain is characterized non-invasively through the estimation of energy liberated by protons within different components of tissues including cerebrospinal fluid, gray matter, and white matter under the influence of high magnetic field and high-frequency radio waves. It is mainly used for the detection of the level of blood–oxygen within the various regions of brain and its related activities [76] (Figure 5.2).

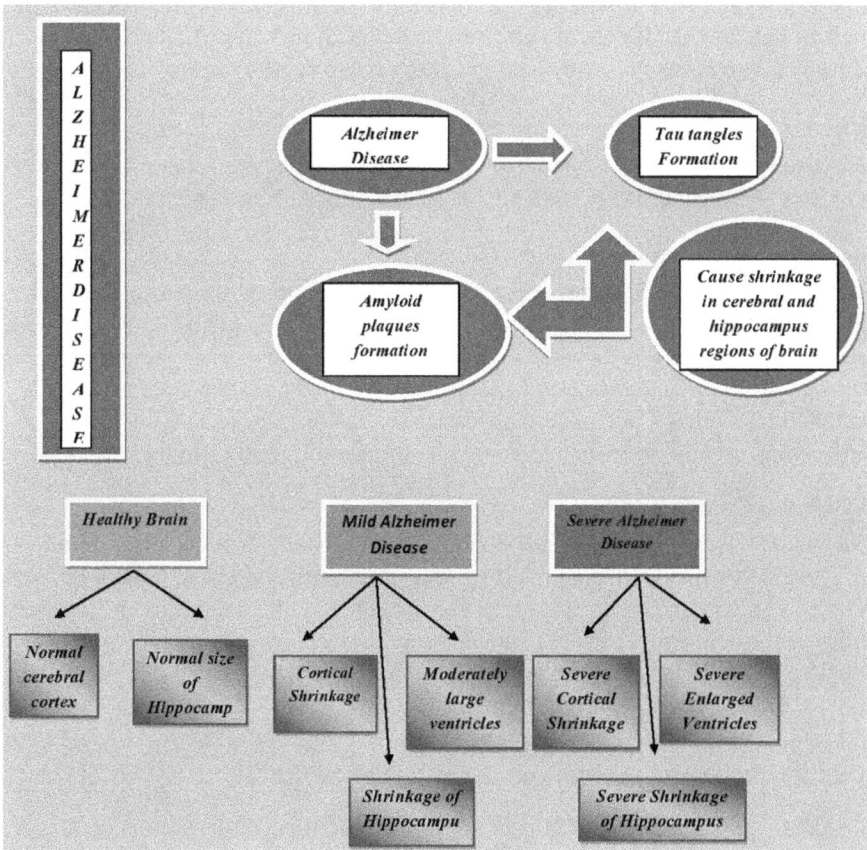

FIGURE 5.2   Differences observed between normal and Alzheimer's patient brain during MRI.

5.13 MEDICATIONS FOR ALZHEIMER'S

5.13.1 Inhibitors of Cholinesterase

Cholinesterase inhibitors are potent drugs available in the market in order to control the progression of deadly AD by inhibiting the action of cholinesterase enzyme that breaks down the neurotransmitters like acetylcholine, and thus there is a deficit in the amount of neurotransmitters that result in the delay or stoppage in the cell signaling transmission.

The common drugs that are used for the cholinesterase inhibition are discussed here.

5.13.1.1 Tacrine

Tetra-hidro-aminoacridine (THA) acts as a vigorous reversible anti-cholinesterase drug metabolized in the liver having the half-life period of about 2–4 hours.

Side effects associated with tacrine are ataxia, anorexia, vomiting, mialgias, nausea, bradicardia, and increase in the concentration of transaminase glutamic-oxalacetic acid (found in 40% cases) which is a hepatic enzyme. The concentration of hepatic enzyme increases during the initial 12 weeks of treatment, but after the treatment the level of hepatic enzyme reverts to the normal state. There are a number of tacrine derivatives under research: methoxitacrine, velnacrine, and suronacrine.

5.13.1.2 Donepezil

It is also a potent reversible inhibitor of cholinesterase having certain side effects: bradicardia, bronchospasm, anorexia, nausea, diarrhoea, syncope, vomitting.

5.13.1.3 Rivastigmine

Rivastigmine is a pseudo reversible cholinesterase inhibitor used as a formidable drug against carbonate acetylcholintrease and has a half-life period of about 1 hour and has the potential to remain active for 10 hours because when the enzyme and acetylcholine combine together in the acetate site, hydrolization occurs so quickly and the enzyme has a potential to appear again within microseconds. The common side effects usually observed are nausea, diarrhoea, dizziness, fatigue, insomnia.

5.13.1.4 Galantamine

Galantamine is a potent reversible cholinesterase inhibitor with the half-life period of about 7 hours and is metabolized by glucuronidation and cytochrome P-450; its action is associated with allosteric modulation on the receptors of nicotine. Presynaptic activation leads to the increase in the concentration of glutamate, GABA, acetylcholine, and mono-amines. The common side effects include vomiting, nausea, and shaking.

5.13.2 Neuronal Protection

5.13.2.1 Estrogen

Through a number of studies, it has been found that AD usually mostly affects women after menopause than men because of a strong deficit in the concentration of estrogen in the female body. The risk of this disease can be reduced to a certain level by the regular intake of estrogen. The effectiveness of estrogen is carried out by several mechanisms including activation of cholinergic neurons, reduction in *APOE* in the plasma, increased neuronal uptake of glucose.

5.13.2.2   Vitamin E

It is a powerful antioxidant and plays a vital role to inhibit the oxidative degradation of lipids to cure a number of diseases like Alzheimer's in which it delays the symptoms of that disease. The side effects usually observed are syncope and cataract, and the deficiency of vitamin E increases the risk of hemorrhage. Other antioxidants that have a huge impact on this disease are selegiline, ginkgo biloba, idebenone.

5.13.2.3   Anti-inflammatory Drugs

Certain anti-inflammatory drugs, including indomethacin, ibuprofen, prednisone, aspirin, have been identified to delay the regular progression of Alzheimer's [62].

5.14   CSF AND PLASMA PROTEIN DEPENDENT BIOMARKERS

Various different biomarkers are being developed for the proper diagnosis of AD. The blood from patient is taken in order to check the concentration of certain proteins or ions whose increased or decreased level in the blood helps diagnose the disease. It has been found that in AD the level of Aß-42 decreases with the simultaneously raised level of tau phosphorylated peptide protein [76].

5.15   STIGMA

Public stigma toward the people suffering from mental illness is a worldwide issue that shows the marked negative impacts on the individual's personal life. The public point of view toward stigmatised group totally relies on several elements: First, they usually have pessimistic beliefs toward the stigmatized group and consider them as a stereotype. Second, they show emotional side towards stigmatized individuals. Third, they start discriminating these people. General public consider stigmatized groups as a sign of danger and start maintaining distance from them that results in social isolation [77]. According to the report of NCRB 2016, more than 13,200 individuals under the age of 65 were unable to find out their homes and then lost (Figure 5.3).

5.16   CARE GIVING IN INDIA

AD mostly affects the individual under the age of 65. In India, 1.25 billion people comes under the age of 35, and 80% Indians will cross the age of 65 in the upcoming years due to age shifting period. It means that more new cases would rise related to Alzheimer's in India in the near future. In rural areas where the elder individuals live alone and earn for their living, they forget their homes and then start sleeping on roads or other places. It shows the ugly face of that disease because it

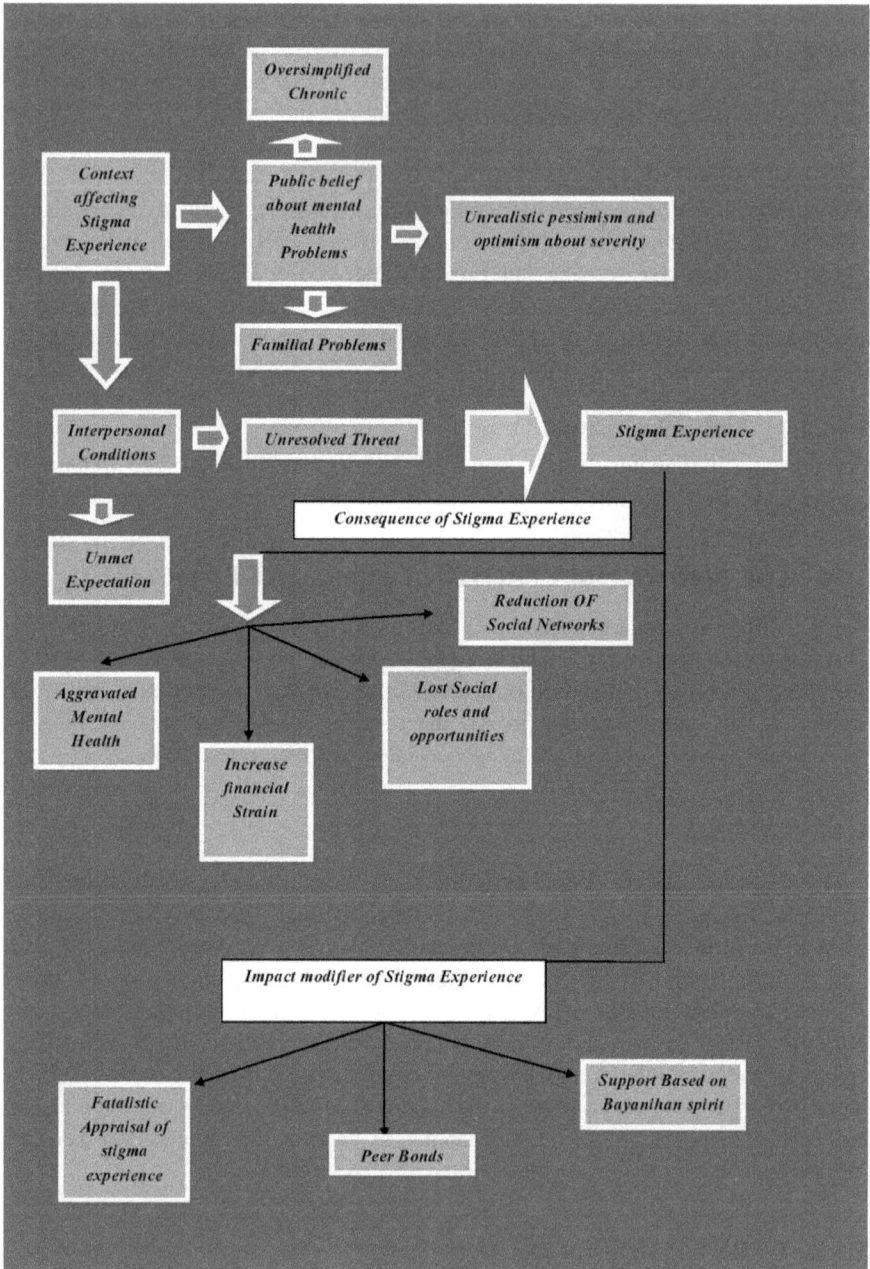

FIGURE 5.3 Mentally retarded people or individuals who have mental health issues experienced stigma [78].

makes the people homeless. Several ashrams are there for the old-aged people, specifically people who suffer from AD or homeless people; they are provided with accommodation and other home facilities in addition to treatment to the

Alzheimer's patients, for example, Guru Vishram Vridh Ashram, an old-age home in Delhi, specifically for the people who are facing this insidious disease [77].

5.17 NON-GOVERNMENTAL ORGANIZATIONS PROVIDING SHELTER TO THE DEMENTIA PATIENTS [60]

Some non-governmental organizations (NGOs) provide a warm care to the dementia patient:

- Silver Innings
- Help Age India
- ARDSI

5.18 NO AWARENESS IN INDIA

India, having a population around 133.92 crores, is growing at a faster rate, out of whom more than 1.6 million people are suffering from this subtle disease, and this number is estimated to triple at the end of 2050. Alzheimer Day is celebrated on September 21 to create awareness among people about this neurodegenerative disease and its dreadful impacts on our daily lives.

The president of ISCR, Dr. Chirag Trivedi, explains certain impacts of Alzheimer disease: In India, population keeps increasing, especially the elder population, so the burden of this disease is increasing. More women than men are more affected because of lower life expectancies of men. According to a *Lancet* study in 2016 on healthy life expectancy, women have a higher life expectancy than men and indeed women spend their lives in disabled conditions facing lots of problems. For the proper cure of this disease, clinical research should be modified at an extent level [74].

5.19 MYTHS ASSOCIATED WITH AD

People have a number of myths related to Alzheimer's.

5.19.1 MYTH 1

Alzheimer and dementia both are the same disease: Dementia is a mental illness that results in the reduction in the brain functions, including problems associated with memory, language, and reasoning, whereas AD commonly affects the people between the age of 60 and 80, that is recognized as a common form of dementia. The common symptoms associated with Alzheimer's are loss of memory, which mostly affects individual's daily life.

5.19.2 MYTH 2

Alzheimer's affects only elder population: AD generally affects the individuals under the age of 65, but a number of cases have been identified in which people under the age 40 s and 50 s also come in contact with this disease, the situation of early-onset AD. Sometimes, symptoms that appear during AD are similar to symptoms associated with aging that can be distinguished from each other.

5.19.3 MYTH 3

Alzheimer is a gene associated disorder: Many genes when mutated result in the development of Alzheimer's. *APOE* e4's presence increases the chances of Alzheimer's, usually inherited from parents. Not only genetic factors lead to the development of this particular disease, but there are also certain environmental factors and daily lifestyle activities responsible for that. The disease affects not only those individuals who have *APOE e4* genes, but also those who don't have *APOE e4* genes.

5.19.4 MYTH 4

No preventions for Alzheimer's: There are no specified methods or techniques or drugs available in the market for the prevention of Alzheimer's. But a number of studies have shown that a regular intake of omega-3, vitamins E, B, and C along with herbal remedies, selenium and folate and regular exercise can reduce the effects of this disease to a certain level.

5.19.5 MYTH 5

Alzheimer's is not lethal: Alzheimer's destroys the nerve cells and then creates lots of problems in cell signaling pathways specifically associated with the normal brain functions that result in the loss of memory and changes in the behavioral pattern that can easily be predicted by family members.

5.19.6 MYTH 6

Memory loss is a sign of Alzheimer: Alzheimer's is responsible for the distorted activities that occur due to degeneration of nerve cells, including forgetting their names, their way to reach home, their close friends, and the way to communicate with the people.

5.19.7 MYTH 7

Suffered from Alzheimer doesn't indicate a specific sign which associated with the death of Alzheimer patient inspite of that Alzheimer patient could survive for certain period of times with this disease. Alzheimer does not directly lead to death of individuals but inspite of that AD patients could survive upto many more years after disease diagnosis. A number of different drugs are available in the market that slows down the progression of this disease to a certain extent [60].

5.20 INDIAN ATTITUDE TOWARD MENTAL ILLNESS

The survey related to attitude toward mental illness encompasses the four main different broad themes:

- Mental illness associated with fear
- Awareness among people related to mental illness
- Attitude of community toward people with mental illness
- Recognizable causes associated with mental disorder

The following statements have been selected on which the survey has been done: Mostly 60% of the people agreed with the statement that described about the mental illness related to lack of will power and self-confidence. About 60% admitted that mentally unhealthy people should live in a group at a separate place to avoid danger for healthy people. Nearly 46% of the respondents thought that they should maintain distance from the mentally depressed individual. About 41% agreed to the statement that they should sit with the mentally retarded people and talk to them. About 40% respondents did not imagine living with mentally ill individuals. Rest of 68% agreed to the statement that they should give proper care to the mentally ill people, while 57% were not afraid to work with the people who are mentally disturbed (Figure 5.4).

5.21 POPULATION AGING IN INDIA

Aging is associated with unavoidable and irreversible demographic transition. Due to advancements in medical science, including declining fertility rates and decrease in mortality rates, there is a spontaneous increase in the percentage of older population that give rise to more cases of dementia (age-related disease) [79].

5.22 CHARACTERISTICS OF DEMENTIA

Table 5.3 summarizes features that distinguish between normal aging, pre-dementia, and dementia.

The life expectancy in India keeps increasing from 1947 to 2019 up to 68.3 years, and it is expected to be 80 years at the end of 2050, due to advancements in medical sciences and implementation of new technologies that are ultimately decreasing mortality and fertility rate and that lead to survival of individuals for longer periods of time. This in turn results in the more cases of dementia associated with a high risk for Alzheimer's [80] (Figures 5.5 and 5.6).

According to ARDSI 2017 report, the Indian population shows great demographic diversity among states that are related to the demographic transition. The rate of elder population also shows a different peak according to their age structure and aging experience within different states. It is clear from the graph that shows a high peak in Kerala; that means the size of elder population is highest, whereas Assam has a lowest peak with a lower rate of elder population. According to the data, in case of population aging, the southern states like Kerala and Tamil Nadu are

Percentage

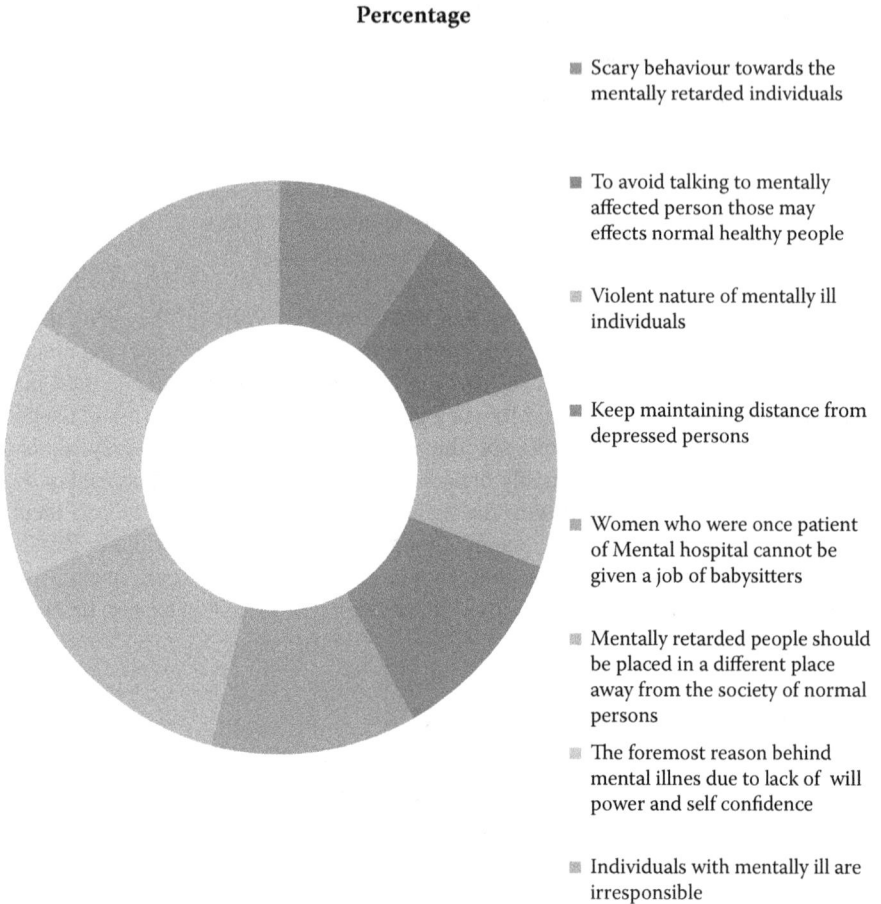

- Scary behaviour towards the mentally retarded individuals

- To avoid talking to mentally affected person those may effects normal healthy people

- Violent nature of mentally ill individuals

- Keep maintaining distance from depressed persons

- Women who were once patient of Mental hospital cannot be given a job of babysitters

- Mentally retarded people should be placed in a different place away from the society of normal persons

- The foremost reason behind mental illnes due to lack of will power and self confidence

- Individuals with mentally ill are irresponsible

FIGURE 5.4   The picture highlighted the doubtful attitude or behavior toward the mentally retarded people.

TABLE 5.3

Distinguishing features between dementia, pre-dementia, and normal aging [65]

S. No.	Features	Dementia	Pre-Dementia	Normal Aging
1.	Hippocampus atrophy	-	+	++
2.	Progressive impairment	-	+	++
3.	Language impairment (aphasia)	-	-	++
4.	Complaints based on subjective perspective	++	+/-	-
5.	Deficit dissimulation	+/-	+/-	+
6.	Anterograde memory treatment	-	+	++
7.	Retrograde memory treatment	-	-	+

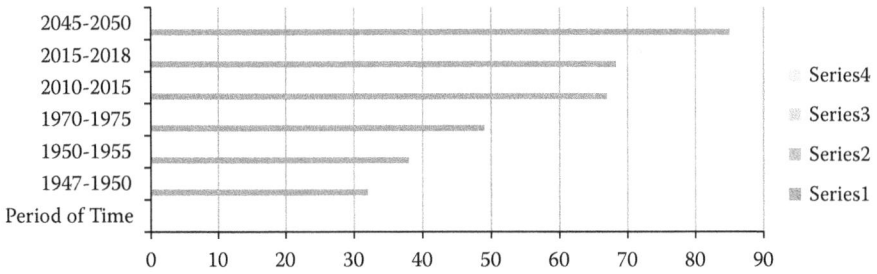

FIGURE 5.5 The graph is showing the life expectancy increasing pattern from 1947 to 2050 [80,81].

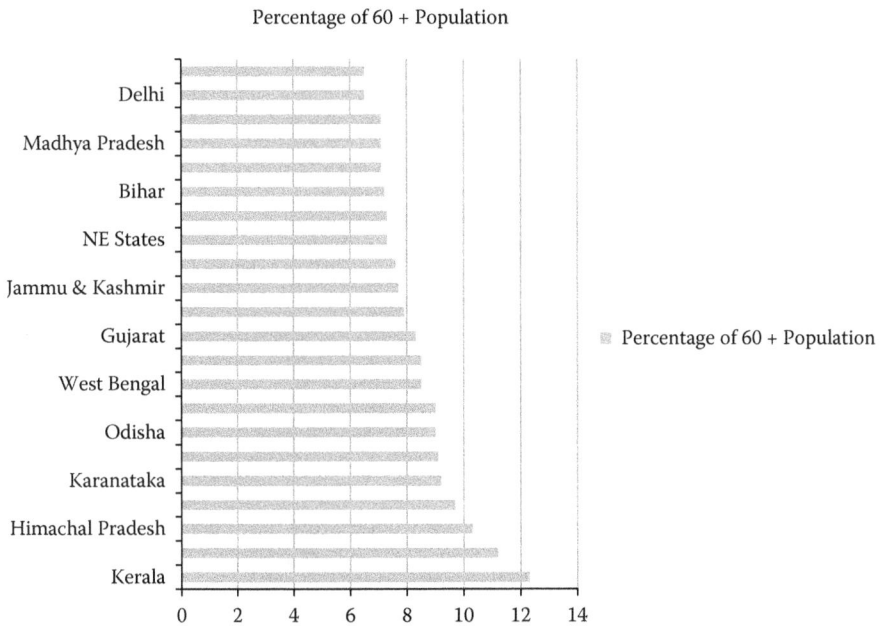

FIGURE 5.6 The graph is showing above 60 population in different states of India [78].

the front runner along with Punjab, Haryana, Himachal Pradesh, Odisha, whereas the less proportion of aged population has been observed in northern states, including Uttar Pradesh, Jammu and Kashmir. The rate of higher old-age population reflects the greater demand with proper facilities, care, and treatment. On the basis of 2011 census, in the case of aging population significantly who is working, it is estimated that the ratio is approximately about 14:100 in which more than 14 are elders. But the rate is over 14 in the case of certain southern states that witness high cases of dementia every year as a result of mores cases of Alzheimer also [76] (Figure 5.7).

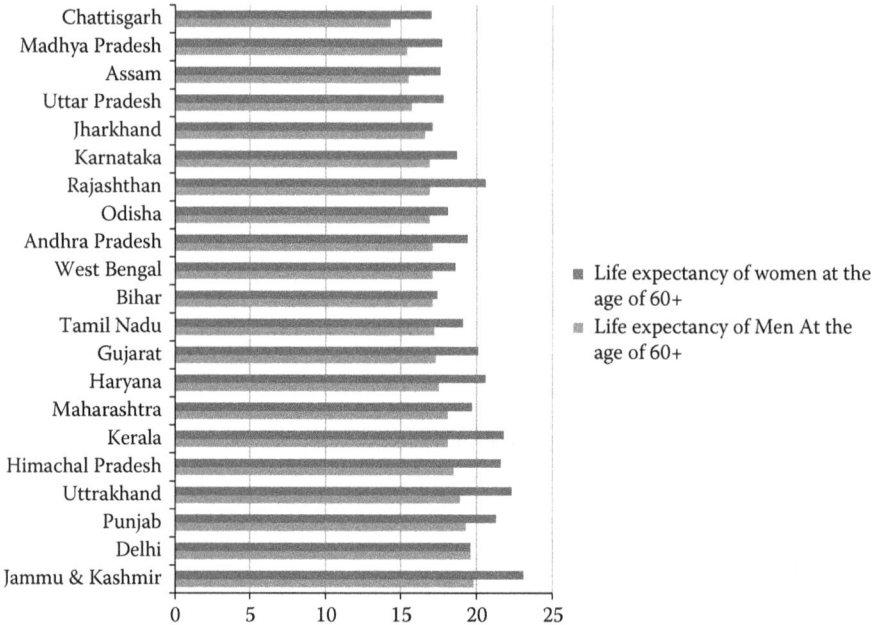

FIGURE 5.7   Differences between the life expectancy of men and women in different states of India [77].

The average life expectancy seen from Figure 5.7 keeps increasing at different rates in different states due to advancements in medical science. High life expectancy has been observed in females when compared to males at old ages (Figure 5.8).

Data of 2011 census has been shown that 66% of total population represents currently married status, 32% population contributes to widowed status, and rest 3% comes under other categories like divorced. In the case of older population of men and women, only 82% and 50% includes the population that comes under the status of currently married, whereas other 48% population of aged women and 15% population of older men come under windowed status (Figure 5.9).

The wide difference within different regions in India mainly depends on a number of factors like multiethnicity, multicultural, adoption of different instruments and techniques, using different methodology, environmental factors. Thus, the more cases of dementia have been found in west India as compared to south India and there is variation in north and east India too.

5.23   CONCLUSION

Alzheimer's is an incurable insidious disease that usually affects the people from all over the world because of the strong reduction in mortality rate and improvement in medical science that results in high life expectancy and ultimately increases the risk of Alzheimer's that is associated with mental illness or dementia. Various

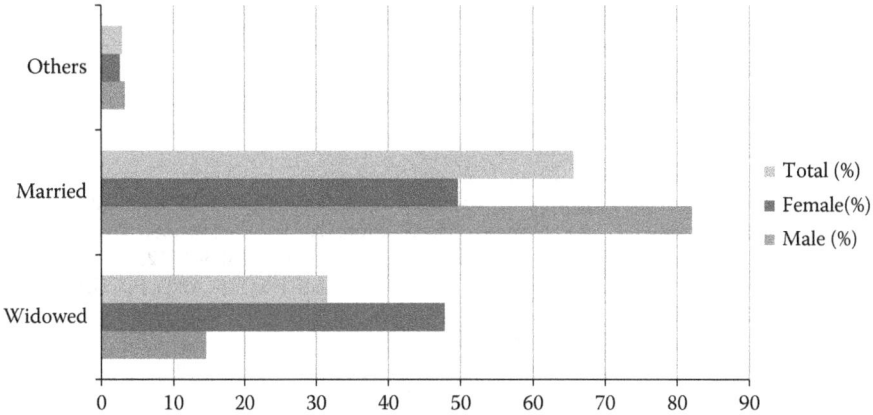

FIGURE 5.8 Older population of men, women, and others who come under different categories including currently married, widowed, and others [78].

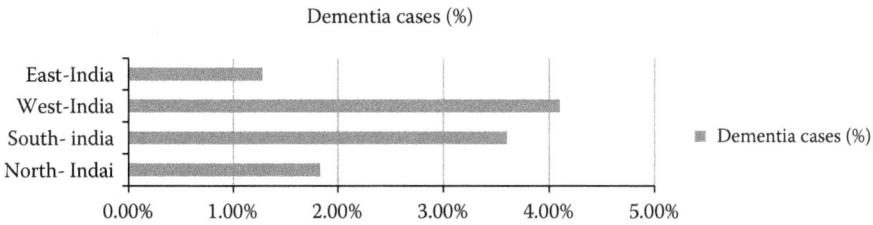

FIGURE 5.9 A huge difference in dementia cases in different regions of India [80].

techniques and drugs are being developed for providing proper treatment to the Alzheimer's patient. But drugs are not much effective. There is need for the effective drugs in order to cure disease. Blood plasma-based biomarkers and other fluid-based biomarkers like cerebrospinal fluid-based biomarkers are being prepared for the diagnosis of disease in which the concentration of different proteins or protein products, like beta-amlyoid protein, is estimated. Several genes that play a vital role in the undesirable production of several proteins, like beta-amyloid and tau proteins, in the hippocampus region of the brain have been identified, but exactly which pathway associated with it is not known. Microglia cells, the phagocytic cells of the brain, are destroyed or undergo apoptosis process, but the exact mechanism associated with the strong decline in the number of microglia is not known. It has been estimated that in the upcoming years, India would have more cases of Alzheimer's because people are not aware of this disease. According to them, loss of memory is the sign of old age, not a disease and in the Indian society a mentally disturbed person is considered as a sign of danger and people start maintaining distance from him instead of helping him. Awareness among the Indian society is necessary because the people have a number of doubts and myths associated with that disease. Rural people have no idea about the medication related to that disease.

There are no effective drugs or biomarkers available in the market to prevent the progression or diagnose the disease in the very early stage.

REFERENCES

[1]. Fox C.N., Johnson A.K., Klunk E.W. and Sperling A.R. Brain imaging in Alzheimer's disease. *Cold Spring Harbor Perspectives in Medicine*, 2(4), 1403–1412 (2012).
[2]. T. B. Winslow, K. M. Onysko, M. C. Stob, A. K. Hazlewood, Treatment of Alzheimer's disease. American Fam Physician, 83 (12), 1403–1412.
[3]. Alzheimer Association: ALZHEIMER'S DISEASE FACTS AND FIGURES., 14 (3), 367–429 (2018).
[4]. Dogan Z. and Kocahan S. Mechanism of Alzheimer's disease pathogenesis and prevention: The brain, neural pathology, N-methyl-D-asparatate receptors, tau protein and other risk factors. *Clinical Psychopharmacology and Neuroscience*, 15(1), 1–8 (2017).
[5]. Jones P.G. and Holtzman D. Cellular/molecular/biomarker studies of Alzheimer's disease and neonatal brain injury. *Science Translational Medicine*, (2011).
[6]. Magalingam B. K., Radhakrishnan A. et al. Current Concepts of Neurodegenerative Mechanisms in Alzheimer's Disease. *Hindawi BioMed Research International*, 5, 1–12 (2018).
[7]. Korolev I. O. Alzheimer's disease: A clinical and basic science review. *Medical Student Research Journal*, 4 (Fall), 24–33 (2014).
[8]. Bauer T., Priller C., Mitteregger G. et al. Synapse formation and function is modulated by the amyloid precursor protein. *The Journal of Neuroscience*, (27), 267212–267221 (2006).
[9]. Abraham W.C., O'Connor K., Turner P.R. and Tate W.P. Roles of amyloid precursor protein and its fragments in regulating neural activity, plasticity and memory. *Progress in Neurobiology*, 70(1), 1–32 (2003).
[10]. Cater M.A., Duce J.A., James S.A., Tsatsanis A., et al. Iron export ferroxidase activity of ß-amyloid precursors protein is inhibited by zinc in Alzheimer's disease. *Cell*, 142(6), 857–867 (2010).
[11]. Doh-Ura K., Furuya H., Sasaki H., Yoshikai S. and Sakaki Y. Genomic organization of the human amyloid beta-protein precursor gene. *Gene*, 87(2), 257–263 (1990).
[12]. Lamb B.T., Lawler A.M., Sisodia S.S., Slunt H.H. et al. Introduction and expression of the 400 kilobase amyloid precursor protein gene in transgenic mice. *Nature Genetics*, 5(1), 22–30 (1993).
[13]. Brown J., Chartier-Harlin M.C. Goate A., Mullan M. et al. Segregation of a missense mutation in the amyloid precursor protein gene with familial Alzheimer's disease. *Nature*, 349(6311), 704–706 (1991).
[14]. Benson M.D., Farlow M., Ghetti B. and Murrell J. A mutation in the amyloid precursor protein associated with hereditary Alzheimer's disease". *Science*, 254 (5028), 97–99 (1991).
[15]. Chartier-Harlin M.C., Crawford F., Houlden H., Warren A. et al. Early-onset Alzheimer's disease caused by mutations at codon 717 of the beta-amyloid precursor protein gene. *Nature*, 353(6347), 844–846 (1991).
[16]. Annaert W. and De Strooper B. Proteolytic processing and cell biological functions of the amyloid precursor protein. *Journal of Science*, 113(11), 1857–1870 (2000).
[17]. Bush A. I., Cho H. H., Rogers J. T., Smith D. H. et al. Iron and the translational of the amyloid precursor protein (APP) and ferritin mRNAs: Riboregulation against neural oxidative damage in Alzheimer's disease. *Biochemistry Society Transactions*, 36(6), 1282–1287 (2008).

[18]. Farhud D. D., Khanahmadi M., et al. Genetic of Alzheimer's disease: A narrative review article. *Iran Journal of Public Health*, 44(7), 892–901 (2015).

[19]. Barber C.R. The genetics of Alzheimer's disease. *Hindawi BioMed Research International*, (2012).

[20]. Ebbert W.T.M., Kauwe S.K.J. and Ridge G.P. Genetics of Alzheimer's disease. *BioMed Research International*, (2013).

[21]. Clarke R.F., Hutton M. and the Alzheimer's Collaborative Group. The structure of the presenilin-1 (S182) gene and identification of six novel mutations in early onset AD families. *Nature Genetics*, 11, 219–222 (1955).

[22]. Fuldner R. A., Lincoln S., Prihar G., Perez-Tur J. et al. Structure and alternative splicing of the presenilin-2 gene. *Neuroreport*, 7, 1680–1684 (1996).

[23]. Levy-Lahad E., Poorkaj P., Wang K. et al. Genomic structure and expression of STM2, the chromosome 1 familial Alzheimer's disease gene. *Genomics*, 34, 198–204 (1996).

[24]. Levesque G., Rogaev E. I., Sherrington R., Wu C., et al. Analysis of the 5' sequence, genomic structure and alternative splicing of the presenilin 1 gene associated with early onset Alzheimer's disease. *Genomics*, 40, 415–424 (1997).

[25]. Liang Y., Rogaev E. I., Rogaeva E. A., Sherrington R., et al. Cloning of a gene bearing missense mutations in early onset familial Alzheimer's disease. *Nature*, 375, 754–760 (1995).

[26]. Levy-Lahad E., Poorkaj P., Romano D. M., Wasco W.. et al. Candidate gene for the chromosome 1 familial Alzheimer's disease locus. *Science*, 269, 973–977 (1995).

[27]. George-Hyslop P.H., Rogaev E.I., Sherrington R., et al. Familial Alzheimer's disease in kindreds with missense mutations in a gene on chromosome 1 related to the Alzheimer's disease type 3 gene. *Nature*, 376, 775–778 (1995).

[28]. Hutton M., Talbot C., Wragg M.. et al. Association between a presenilin 1 polymorphism and late onset Alzheimer's disease. *Lancet*, 347, 509–512 (1996).

[29]. Arai H., Higuchi S., Muramastu T., Mutsushita S., et al. Presenilin 1 polymorphism and Alzheimer's disease. *Lancet*, 347(9009), 1186–1187 (1996).

[30]. Kehoe P., Holmans P., Liddell M., Williams J., et al. Association between a PS-1 intronic polymorphism and late onset Alzheimer's disease. *Neuroreport*, 7, 2155–2158 (1996).

[31]. Adachi Y., Isoe K., Urakami K., et al. Presenilin 1 polymorphism in patients with alzheimer's disease, vascular dementia and alcohol-associated dementia in Japanese population. *Acta Neurologica Scandinavica*, 94, 326–328.

[32]. Growdon J. H., Roses A. D., Scott W. K., et al. Presenilin 1 polymorphism and Alzheimer's disease. *Lancet*, 347, 1186–1187 (1996).

[33]. Cairns N. J., Tysoe C., Whittaker J., et al. Presenilin 1 intron 8 polymorphism is not associated with autopsy-confirmed, late-onset Alzheimer's disease. *Neuroscience Letters*, 222, 68–69 (1997).

[34]. Bayatti N.N., Mann D.M., Pickering-Brown S.M., Wright A.E., et al. An intronic polymorphism in the presenilin 1 gene does not influence the amount or molecular form of the amyloid beta protein deposited in Alzheimer's disease. *Neuroscience Letters*, 222, 57–60 (1997).

[35]. Cai X., Fallin D., Hoyne J., Stanton J., et al. No association between intronic presenilin 1polymorphism and Alzheimer's disease in clinic and population based samples. *Neuropsychiatric Genetics*, 74, 202–203 (1997).

[36]. Hwo S. Y., Kirschner M. W., Lockwood A. H. and Weingarten M. D. A protein factor essential for microtubule assesmbly. *Proceedings of the National Academy of Sciences of the United states of America*, 72(5), 1858–1862 (1975).

[37]. Cleveland D. W., Hwo S. Y., Kirschner M. W. Purification of tau, a microtubule

associated protein that induces assembly of microtubules from purified tubulin. *Journal of Molecular Biology*, 116(2), 207–225 (1977).

[38]. Crowther R. A., Goedert M., Klung A., Wischik C. M. and Walker J. E. Cloning and sequencing of the cDNA encoding a core protein of the paired helical filament of Alzheimer disease: Identification as the microtubule associated protein tau. *Proceedings of the National Academy of Sciences of the United States of America*, 85(11), 4051–4055 (1988).

[39]. Crowther R. A., Goedert M., Jakes R., Rutherford D. and Spillantini M. G. Multiple isoforms of human microtubule-associated protein tau: sequences and localization in neurofibrillary tangles of Alzheimer's disease. *Neuron*, 3(4), 519–526 (1989).

[40]. Mohandas E., Rajmohan V. and Raghunath B. Neurobiology of Alzheimer's disease. *Indian Journal of Psyhiatry*, 51, 55–61 (2009).

[41]. Augustinack J. C., Hyman B. T., Mandelkow E. M. and Schneider. "Specific tau phophorylation sites correlate with severity of neuronal cytopathology in Alzheimer's disease". *Acta Neuropathologica*, 103 (1), 26–35 (2002).

[42]. Weiler N. Early Alzheimer's Brain Pathology Linked to Psychiatric Symptoms. University of Calfornia San Francisco (2018).

[43]. Phillips M. C. " Apoliopoprotein E isoforms and lipoprotein metabolism". *IUBMB Life*, 66(9), 616–623 (2014).

[44]. NCBI, "Entrez Gene: APOE Apolipoprotein E".

[45]. Bu G., Kanekiyo T., Liu C. C. and Xu H. "Apolipoprotein E and Alzheimer disease: risk, mechanism and therapy". *Nature reviews Neurology*, 9(2), 106–118 (2013).

[46]. Stolerman I. P. (Ed). Encyclopedia of Psychopharmacology (online ed.). Berlin: Springer, (2010) ISBN: 978-3540686989.

[47]. Baars H.F., Van der Smagtt J.J. and Doevandans P. (Ed.) (2011) Clinical Cardiogenetics. London: Springer. ISBN: 978-1849964715.

[48]. Dokken C., Ghebranious N., Ivacic L. and Mallum J. Detection of ApoE E2, E3 and E4 alleles using MALDI-TOF mass spectrometry and the homogenous mass-extend technology. *Nucleic Acids Research*, 33(17), e149 (2005).

[49]. Monczor M. Diagnosis and treatment of Alzheimer's disease. *Current Medicinal Chemistry*, 5, 5–13 (2005).

[50]. Streit W. J. Microglial response to injury. *Toxicologic Pathology*, 28(1), 28–30 (2000).

[51]. Jenarius G. R. India is struggling with Alzheimer's and it's set to grow in coming years, Here Are Some Common Myths And Facts About It. Indiatimes.com. (2017, September 22).

[52]. Farhoudi M., Sadigh-Eteghad S., Talebi M. "Association of Apolipoprotein E epsilon 4 allele with sporadic late onset Alzheimer's disease: A meta analysis." *Neurosciences*, 17(4), 321–326 (2012).

[53]. Adams-Campbell L. L., Kamboh M. I., Sepehrnia B. et al. Genetics studies of human Apolipoprotein X: The effect of the Apolipoprotein E polymorphism on quantitative levels of lipoproteins in Nigerian blacks. *American Journal of Human Genetics*, 45(4), 586–591 (1989).

[54]. Notkola I. L., Pekkanen J., Sulkava R.. et al. Serum total cholesterol, Apolipoprotein E epsilon 4 allele, and Alzheimer's disease. *Neuroepidemiology*, 17(1), 14–20 (1998).

[55]. DeRosa S., Petanceska S. S., Sharma A. et al. Changes in Apolipoprotein E expression in response to dietary and pharmacological modulation of cholesterol. *Journal of Molecular Neuroscience*, 20(3), 395–406 (2003).

[56]. Helkala E. L., Kivipelto M., Laasko M. P. et al., Apolipoprotein E epsilon E4 allele, elevated midlife total cholesterol level, and high midlife systolic blood pressure are

independent risk factors for late life Alzheimer disease. *Annals of Internal Medicine*, 137(3), 149–155(2002).

[57]. Corder E. H., Risch N. J. Saunders A. M. et al. Protective effects of Apolipoprotein E type 2 allele for late onset Alzheimer disease. *Nature Genetics*, 7(2), 180–184 (1994).

[58]. Cupples L. A., Farrer L. A., Hainess J. L., Hyman B. et al. Effects of age, sex, and ethinicity on the association between apolipoprotein E genotype and Alzheimer disease: A meta analysis. APOE and Alzheimer Disease Meta Analysis Consortium. *JAMA*, 278(16), 1349–1356 (1997).

[59]. Sherry C. Top 8 Alzheimer's Breakthroughs in 2012. *The AD Plan*. (2012).

[60]. Boado R. J., Hui E. K. W., Lu J. Z., Pardridge W. M. and Zhou Q. H. Pharmacokinetics and brain uptake of a genetically engineered bifunctional fusion antibody targeting the mouse transferring receptor. *Molecular Pharmaceutics*, 7, 237–244 (2010).

[61]. Gill S. S., Hotton G. R., Patel N. K., Mc Carter R., Heywood P. et al. Direct brain infusion of glial cell line derived neurotrophic factor in Parkinson disease. *Nature Medicine*, 9, 589–595 (2003).

[62]. Cohen-Gadol A. A., Hendricks B. K., Miller J. C. Novel delivery methods by passing the blood-brain and blood-tumor barriers. *Neurosurg Focus*, 38(3), E10 (2015).

[63]. Bankiewicz K. S., Forsayeth J. and Yin D. Optimized cannula design and placement for convection enhanced delivery in rat striatum. *Journal of Neuroscience Methods*, 187, 46–51 (2009).

[64]. Salvatore M. F., et al. Point source concentration of GNF may explain failure of phase II clinical trial. *Experimental Neurology*, 202, 497–505 (2006).

[65]. Goecks N., Joers V., Ohshima-Hosoyama S., Simmons H. A., et al. A monoclonal antibody-GDNF fusion protein is not neuroprotective and is associated with pro-liferative pancreatic lesions in parkinsonian Monkeys. *PLoS ONE*, 7(6), e39036 (2012).

[66]. Evans H. T., Leinega G., Nisbet R. M., Vander Jeugd A. et al. Combined effects of scanning ultrasound and a tau-specific single chain antibody in a tau transgenic mouse model. *Brain*, 140, 1220–1230 (2017).

[67]. Jordao J. F., et al. Antibodies targeted to the brain with image-guided focussed ultrasound reduces amyloid beta plaque load in the TgCRND8 mouse model of Alzheimer's disease. *PLoS ONE*, 5(5), e10549 (2010).

[68]. Burgess A., et al. Targeted delivery of neural stem cells to the brain using MRI-guided focussed ultrasound to disrupt the blood-brain barrier. *PLoS ONE*, 6(11), e27877 (2011).

[69]. Thevenot E., et al. Targeted delivery of self-complementary adeno-associated virus serotype 9 to the brain, using magnetic resonance imaging-guided focussed ultra-sound. *Human Gene Theraphy*, 23, 1144–1155 (2012).

[70]. Dewey J. D., Raymond S. B., Treat L. H. et al. Ultrasound enhanced delivery of molecular imaging and therapeutic agents in Alzheimer's disease mouse models. *PLoS ONE*, 3(5), (2008).

[71]. Kinoshita M., Jolesz F. A., McDannold N., and Hynynen K. Non-invasive localized delivery of Herceptin to the mouse brain by MRI-guided focussed ultrasound-induced blood brain barrier disruption. *Proceedings of the National Academy of Sciences of United States of America*, 103, 11719–11723 (2006).

[72]. Aryal M., McDannold N., Vykhodtseva N. and Zhang Y. Z. Multiple sessions of liposomal doxorubicin delivery via focused ultrasound mediated blood-brain barrier disruption: A safety study. *Journal of Controlled Release,* 204, 60–69 (2015).

[73]. Diaz R. J., et al. Focussed ultrasound delivery of Raman nanoparticles across the

blood-brain barrier: potential for targeting experimental brain tumors. *Nanomedicine*, 10, 1075–1087, (2014).

[74]. Tanaka C. P., Teresa M. et al. A qualitative study on the stigma experienced by people with mental health problems and epilepsy in the Philippines. *BMC Psychiatry*, 18, 325 (2018).

[75]. Kantipudi J. S., Sathianathan R. The dementia epidemic: Impact, prevention, and challenges for India. *Indian Journal of Psychiatry*, 60(2), (2018).

[76]. United Nations Population Fund, Caring for Our Elders: Early Responses India Ageing Report – 2017. United Nations Population Fund (UNFPA) 55 Lodi Estate, New Delhi 110003 India.

[77]. Source: Computed from ORGI, Census of India, 2011, Office of the Registrar General and the Census Commissioner of India, *Ministry of Home Affairs*, Government of India. www.censusindia.gov.in. (2011).

[78]. Source: ORGI, SRS Based Life Table 2010–14, Office of the Registrar General and the Census Commissioner of India, *Ministry of Home Affairs*, Government of India. www.censusindia.gov.in. (2016).

[79]. HOW INDIA PERCEIVES MENTAL HEALTH TLLLF 2018 NATIONAL SURVEY REPORT (2018).

[80]. Das K. S., Ghosal K. M. and Pal S. Dementia: Indian scenario. *Neurology India*, 60(6), (2012).

[81]. Swapna Kishore, Dementia in India, 2015: An Infographic (2015).

6 Phytochemicals' Potential to Reverse the Process of Neurodegeneration

Surekha Manhas and Zaved Ahmed Khan

CONTENTS

DOI: 10.1201/9781003171829-6

6.1 INTRODUCTION

Demographic aging is a complex phenomenon that is associated with changes occurring in normal functions with relation to the longer period of time that results in the deficit in the cognitive functions and other brain-related activities [1,2]. Deleterious deterioration in the normal biological functioning leads to several problems, including memory loss, language problem, difficulty in learning and calculating [3]. These all are the identifiable symptoms that are specifically related to Alzheimer's disease (AD). This disease is worsening because it affects the individual's behaviours so badly [2]. Nowadays, approximately 10 million new cases are there every year due to AD and dementia, which are growing issues related to a number of health problems [2]. Regular increase in the older population size leads to a higher risk of Alzheimer's. Many research studies are going on to find a cure for that disease, but there is no effective therapy to properly treat the disease as the mechanism behind AD is not explored yet. The focus of the studies is just trying to control behavioral changes [3]. Thus, a number of research studies are focusing on finding out the potentially risk factors that directly link to the disease. Diet or nutrient concentration plays a crucial role in order to maintain normal functions of the body. For the regularity of systemic functions, nutrients act as a potent factor that helps in the regulation of different biological activities. Researchers are trying to identify the relationship between neurodegenerative diseases like AD and nutrients. In fact, the involvement of nutrients can be seen in a number of biochemical activities as they act as an energy source [4]. Due to this reason, modification in diet leads to various problems that affect central nervous system. This in turn leads to the excessive production of beta amyloid protein in the brain that causes neurodegeneration. From different studies, the relation has been found between cholesterol and apolipoprotein [4].

Researchers have found that the harmful effects occur due to nutrition deficiency on this neurodegenerative disease that causes various health problems like obesity and malnutrition. According to certain studies, the effects of malnutrition have been observed in AD. After macro-specific and micro-specific studies on AD, researchers agree that nutrients or anti-oxidants deficiency may lead to the neurodegenarative disease [5]. Continuous weight loss and depletion in muscles result in the progression of neurodegeneration [6]. In addition, obesity has been identified as one of the common determinant factors for the progression of Alzheimer [5]. A case study had been conducted on 6,853 people and presented the data that shows these individuals had a large waist, and had a higher chance of developing this disorder than those who had a normal waist [7]. Another cohort study has demonstrated that a higher risk of dementia has been observed in those individuals who were obese under the age of 30–39, and it steadily decreased with a decreased in obesity [7].

Moreover, certain nutrients and vitamins have been found to play some role during disease progression. The nutrient deficiency shows a huge impact on AD that has been estimated from a number of different studies. The deficiency of vitamins B, C, and E results in the higher AD risk [5]. However, different reviews related to this topic have demonstrated that the consumption of a single vitamin does not show any noticeable protective effects, but that a combination of different vitamins or multivitamins may enhance the action to generate protective effects toward that disease [8]. These vitamins are the natural antioxidants that exhibit potential to diminish oxidative stress by scavenging free radicals and decrease beta amyloid proteins that are the basic disease-causing factor in AD and aging [5]. Moreover, these effects might be noticed during the consumption of multivitamins [8].

Phytochemicals are chemical compounds extracted from plant sources and have antioxidant properties. Several different studies have been conducted in order to find how antioxidants or polyphenols help in the reduction of beta amyloid content by lowering the oxidative stress particularly in AD patients [5]. A study conducted by Hartman showed that when a mice was supplemented with pomegranates that contains polyphenols, it showed a 50% reduction in developing AD than the normal mice which was kept as a control [9]. A research study on transgenic mouse done by Kim showed that a transgenic mouse that was treated with resveratrol, a polyphenol extracted from grapes, showed a decrease in the process of neurodegeneration and memory loss [10].

The study is focused on the beneficial potent role of various different phytochemicals in AD. For this, the data was collected from different sources that show the association between polyphenols and AD. The aim of this review article is to answer this particular question, 'How phytochemicals or polyphenols act as a potent therapeutic approach for the treatment of AD?'

6.2 ALZHEIMER'S DISEASE

AD affects the central nervous system and is characterized by the destruction of neurons, beta amyloid accumulation, presence of tau fibrils, and excess production of endogenous proteins that settle down as soluble and insoluble aggregates in brain especially in the hippocampus area [11–19]. Certain studies have found that the insoluble form of protein is inert whereas soluble aggregates are toxic forms having a potential to cause disease [20–25]. It is assumed that tau proteins, beta amyloid protein, and other oligomer have beta sheet conformation that play a role in pathogenicity [24–30]. Individuals suffering from AD has an average life of 8 years after diagnosis and this may go up to 20 years depending on the individual's health status [31].

6.3 SYMPTOMS

Typically, AD is distinguished into three stages that vary according to the severity of disease and health status of individuals before being affected with AD [2,3]. Early symptoms of AD are short-term loss of memory and thus result in difficulty to remember latest events or updates, meaning normal forgetfulness. For instance, the central AD stage usually includes symptoms like facing problems in communication, help is needed, proper care is required, forget name of the family members. In late-onset disease, people experience a lot of problems that totally disrupt their daily activities that include difficulty recognizing face of their own family members, forgetting their own homes and feeling lost escalated behavior, difficulty walking [2,31].

6.4   EPIDEMIOLOGY

It is estimated that approximately 15 million people from all over the world are suffering from this chronic disease [32]. Every year 0.5% new cases of AD under the age of 65 and 8% at the age of 85 years rise [32]. The disease growing rate is very high; the pervasiveness of disease keeps increasing from 3% at 65 years of age up to 40% at the age of 85 years or more [32]. Older people, aged 65 years or more, are mostly affected with this disease. Dementia patients have a high risk to develop the disease. AD affects the individuals at the age of 65, but still it is not an age-related disorder [2]. About 9% of cases have been detected in young-age people and are characterized as early-onset AD [2,3]. The risk factors that cause communicable diseases may show a relationship with AD also. Those factors are consumption of tobacco, unhealthy diets, obesity, diabetes, cardiovascular disease, hypertension, alcohol consumption [32]. However, there are no clear similar evidences to prove the effective relationship between these risk factors and AD [32]. Apolipoprotein gene (*APOE* gene) is associated with a high risk of developing AD at later stages; particularly ε4 allele is responsible for the progression of disease [33]. However, the presence of gene is not always related to the development of disease [3,34]. In fact, there are a number of genetic factors related to AD among different families that are not explored yet. Finally, people suffering from Down syndrome have a high risk of developing the disease. Depression, head trauma, social isolation, lack of awareness are the modifiable risk factors. Finally, women are more likely to be affected by this disease than men because life expectancy of women is longer than that of men [34].

6.5   ETIOLOGY

A number of studies that have been conducted have shown that oxidative stress leads to aging under normal metabolic conditions [1]. Oxidative damage and excess production of free radicals result in the mitochondria dysfunctioning because it maintains the oxidative metabolism; any damage in it leads to the failure in energy production; cells lose capacity to perform functions and eventually neurons or cells die [35]. The exact mechanism behind the disease is not known yet, but studies still are going on to identify it [33]. From the studies, it has been described that AD is caused by the mutation in the genes like *APP, PSEN-1,* and *PSEN-II,* but only 0.5 or fewer cases have been detected where the main disease causative factors are these genes [33].

6.5.1   AMYLOID HYPOTHESIS

Accumulation of beta amyloid proteins in the brain occurs due to mutation in specific genes *APP*, *PSEN-1*, *PSEN-2*, *APOE*, *BACE-1*, and *IDE* [33,36]. This accumulation in turns causes synaptic loss and loss of dendrites, and the eventually results in the death of neurons [33]. APP protein exists in two forms: Aß-40 and Aß-42. Under normal conditions, Aß-40 plays a crucial role in the formation of synapses, helps in cellular transmission, and is found in many different proteins, whereas Aß-42 induces toxicity in neuronal cells [37]. The mechanism of how it exactly gets accumulated in the brain is not known yet. Figure 6.1 shows the known explanation about the mechanism behind the disease [38].

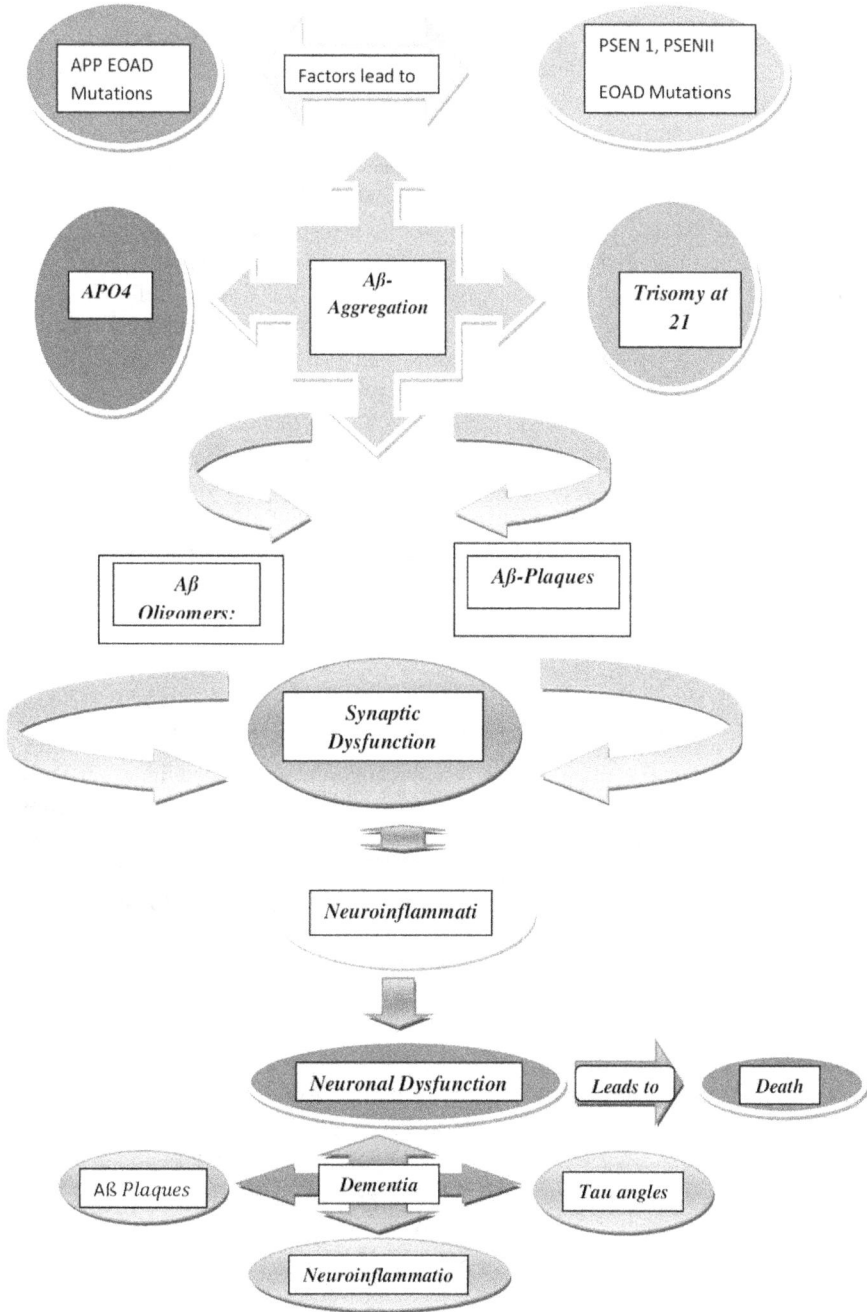

FIGURE 6.1 Brief summary of amyloid hypothesis: APOE: apolioprotein E; APP: amyloid precursor protein; Aß: amyloid beta; PSEN1: presenilin1; PSEN2: presenilin 2.

6.5.2 TAU HYPOTHESIS

Neurons contain tau proteins that play a vital role in the stabilization of microtubules, to maintain cellular morphology and axonal transport [38]. The aggregation and accumulation of tau proteins in the form of neurofibrillary tangles leads to the neurodegeneration [39]. Tau protein loses its normal function when the paired helical filament undergoes hyper-phosphorylation that badly affects the frontotemporal lobe due to neuronal damage [40]. Interestingly, advanced researchers have demonstrated that a high dose of antioxidants decreases the tau hyperphosphorylation [41]. It has been observed that DNA damage increases in double in the neuronal cells in the case of AD patient than normal individuals, and it might be an earlier sign of disease that can be used as a biomarker for further studies [42]. The formation of neuritic plaques in the brain is considered a potent sign of developing disease [43].

6.6 REDUCTION IN ANTIOXIDANT ENZYMES IN BRAIN

Antioxidants enzymes such as superoxide dismutase, glutathionine peroxidise, and catalase play potent roles in order to prevent the accumulation of free radicals, thereby reducing lipid peroxidation [44]. Reduction in these enzyme levels leads to accumulation of reactive oxygen species (ROS), which ultimately damage mitochondrial proteins.

6.7 ROLE OF PHYTOCHEMICALS OR POLYPHENOLS

Phytochemicals are the plant-derived chemical molecules found in a variety of sources like green tea, red wine, fruits, and vegetables [45]. Several polyphenols, like isoflavones, show specificity toward only one individual specific group of food, specifically found in soya, whereas other chemicals like quercetin have been detected mostly in all plants [45]. Various numbers of different phytochemicals are used for the treatment of AD on the basis of varied antioxidant properties.

6.7.1 CURCUMIN

Curcumin is used traditionally in several Indian dishes like curry powder as a spice to enhance the flavor of the dishes and is isolated from *Cucuma longa* (turmeric) [46]. Interestingly, according to different reports, it has been found that AD prevalence between the age of 70 and 79 years in India is less about 4.4-fold than the United States, which indicates that curcumin-rich diet reduces the effect of AD at a certain level [46]. Considerably, the evidences have been found from in-vivo and in-vitro studies that represent antioxidative, anti-inflammatory and anti-amyloidogenic properties having the potential to reduce the risk of AD [47,48]. In addition, when chronic supplementary curcumin was given to transgenic mice (Tg2576) that was 16 months old, reduction in the concentration of beta amyloid was observed [49]. In ayurveda, curcumin is widely used as an anti-inflammatory agent to reduce pain in muscles and has anti-cancerous properties, too. But due to more advancements in science, it has been proved that turmeric

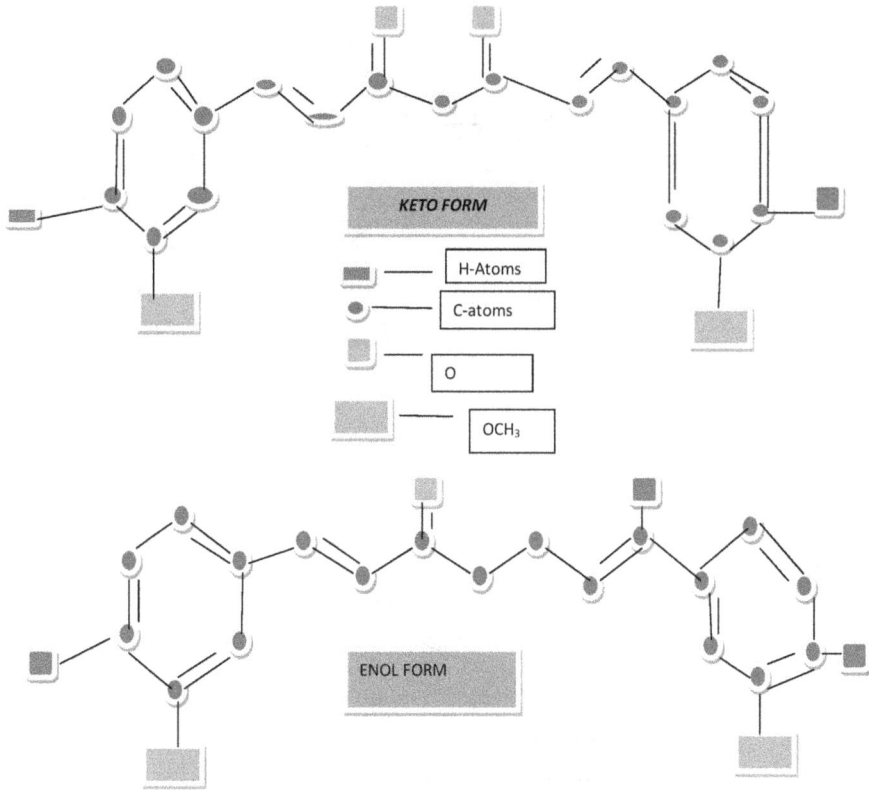

FIGURE 6.2   Structure of curcumin: keto and enol forms.

helps in the cure of certain diseases [50–52]. The different enol and keto forms of curcumin are shown in Figure 6.2 [53].

6.7.1.1   Mechanism of Action of Curcumin

During AD, neuronal cells get degraded due to several different factors, including oxidative damage, high accumulation of beta amyloid or tau protein, metal toxicity, inflammation as shown in Figure 6.3 [43].

6.7.2   AD TREATMENT: CURCUMIN ACT AS THE PLEIOTROPIC AGENT

Considering several factors associated with etiology and various undefined mechanisms of AD, it is entirely sensible that different therapeutic drugs target only one particular factor that shows limited benefits (Figure 6.3). Therefore, now research is focused on the pleiotropic activity of various therapeutic agents in order to target several different affected processes as shown in Figure 6.4 [54,55].

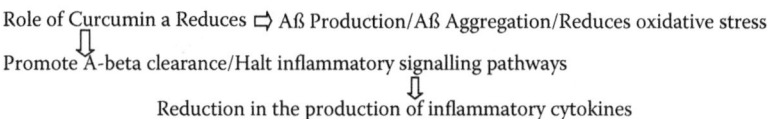

Role of Curcumin a Reduces ⇨ Aß Production/Aß Aggregation/Reduces oxidative stress

Promote A-beta clearance/Halt inflammatory signalling pathways

Reduction in the production of inflammatory cytokines

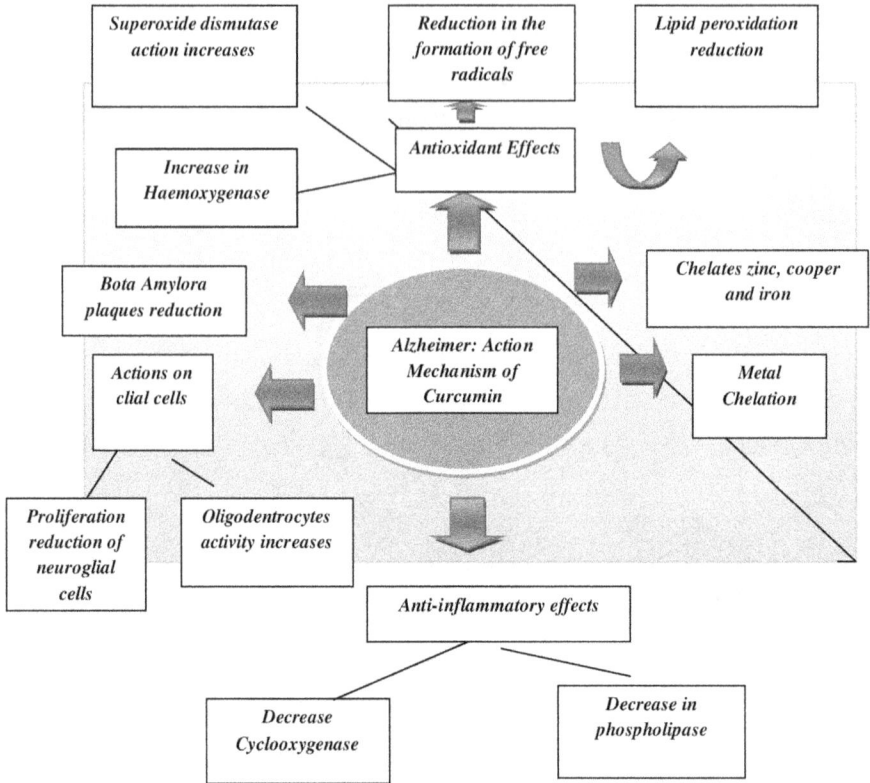

FIGURE 6.3 Various different mechanisms associated with curcumin in AD.

6.7.3 CLINICAL ASPECTS OF CURCUMIN

Past research studies have shown the potent role of curcumin to treat AD where curcumin directly comes into contact with various signaling molecules, including apoptotic proteins, certain pro-inflammatory cytokines, phosphorylase kinase. All these studies give solid evidence that shows the efficacy of curcumin in the clinical field trials [56]. Until now, approximately nine human trials have been done related to curcumin in the case of AD interventions that include diagnosis, therapy, and prevention (Table 6.1).

AD: Alzheimer's disease; Aß: ß$_2$ amyloid; MCI: mild cognitive impairment; MMSE: Mini-Mental State Examination; PET: positron emission tomography; LDL: low density lipoprotein; ^{18}F-FDG: hypometabolism of 2-[18F] fluoro-2-deoxy-D-glucose; FDDNP: 2-(1-[16-](2-[F-(F-18] floroethyl) (methyl) amino]-2-naphthyl)ethylidene)malononitrile; d: day

But still the exact mechanism of action of curcumin is not explored yet: How curcumin helps in the reduction of beta amyloid or what happens exactly when curcumin and beta amyloid or neuronal plaques interact with each other, and how they interact? Therefore, more research is required to understand the effect of curcumin on the treatment of AD.

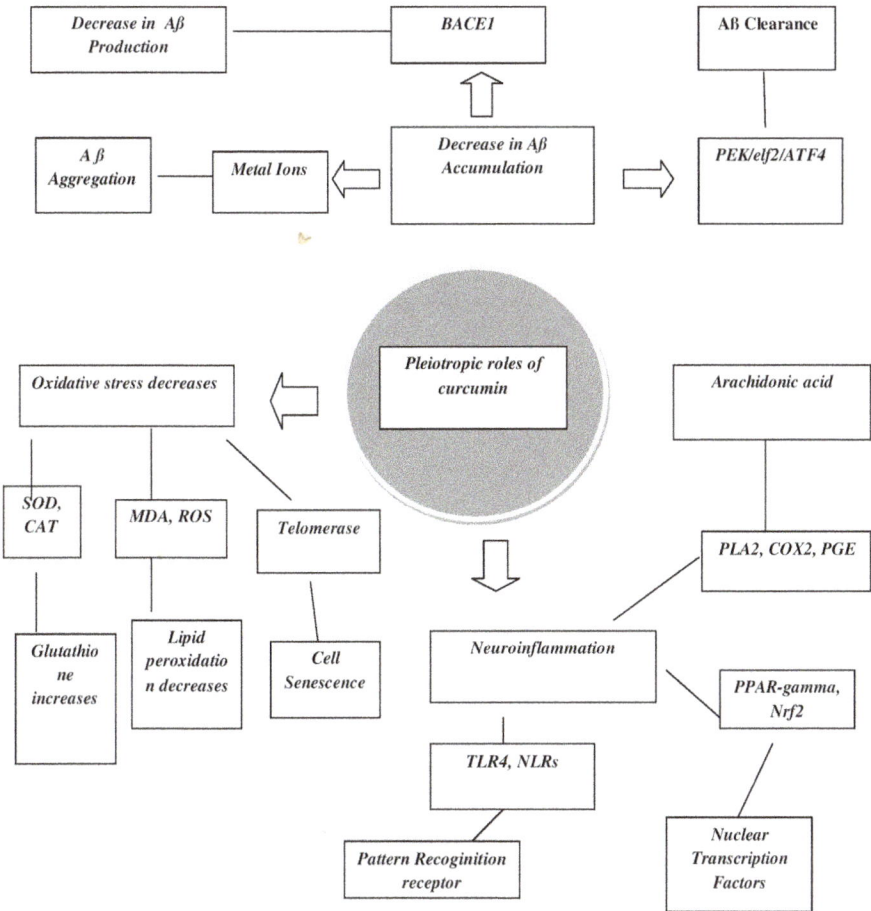

FIGURE 6.4 Curcumin: a pleiotropic agent for the treatment of Alzheimer's disease.

6.7.4 QUERCETIN

3,3',4',5,7-Pentahydroxyflavone (quercetin) is a potent flavonoid (phytochemical) with pharmacological, cardioprotective, antiapoptotic and antioxidant properties that is naturally found in various foods and plants including apples, red wine, broccoli, and onions [61]. Few research studies have demonstrated the role of quercetin in the prevention of neurodegenerative disease [62]. Metabolites of quercetin play a vital role in AD are shown in Figure 6.5 [63]. In addition, the effect of this crucial flavonoid has been evaluated in young rats which had been treated with metals, specifically aluminum, in the isolated mitochondria of the hippo-campus [64]. In this study, ROS reduction was evaluated; however, no changes were observed in the activity of superoxide mutase (MnSOD) [64]. In the fractions of mitochondria, when the apoptotic marker expression was analyzed, the reduction in the Bax levels with an increase in Bcl levels was observed. During the evaluation of cytosolic fractions, Cyt c and Bcl-2 expression that was responsible for inhibition

TABLE 6.1

Clinical trials with curcumin in diagnosis, prevention, and therapy

Study	Cohort	Intervention	Primary Endpoint	Main Results
Clinical trial gov NCT 03085680 [55]	24 older adults with physical and/or cognitive impairment	Curcumin (100 mg/d): 3 months	Physical functions: cognitive function: pain and inflammation	Not yet recruiting
Clinical trials gov NCT01811381 [55]	80 subjects with MCI	Curcumin (800 mg/d) and yoga: 12 months	Blood biomarkers, cerebral biomarkers: cerebral glucose metabolism observation and coginitive changes and associated changes diagnosis	Recruiting
Clinical trials gov NCT01383161 [54]	132 subjects with agar-associated impairment or MCI	Curcumin (180 mg/d): 18 months	Cognitive changes: abnormal accumulation of Aß and tau (FDDNP-PET): inflammatory markers	Active, not recruiting
Clinical trials gov NCT01001637 [55]	26 subjects with AD	Longvida (2 g/d or 3 g/d): 2 months	Cognitive changes: blood concentration of Aß	Unknown status
Clinical trials gov NCT00595582 [55]	10 subjects with MCI	Curcumin (5.4 g/d) and bioperine (900 mg\d): 24 months	MMSE scores: metabolic lesions (PET)	Terminated for various reasons
Baum et al. [56]	36 subjects with AD	Curcumin (1 or 4 g/d) and ginkgo extract (120 mg/d): 6 months	MMSE scores: blood biomarkers (isoprostane, Aß, cholesterol, triglycerides, and metals): plasma curcumin levels	Completed. No difference in MMSE scores or blood biomarkers among groups, but vitamin E increased
Ringman et al. [57]	33 subjects with AD	Curcumin C3 complex (2 or 4 g/d): 6 months	MMSE scores: side effects: plasma and cerebrospinal fluid biomarkers (Aß, tau, and F2-isoprostanes): curcumin and metabolites in plasma	Completed. No difference among groups, and no serious adverse events

TABLE 6.1 *(Continued)*
Clinical trials with curcumin in diagnosis, prevention, and therapy

Study	Cohort	Intervention	Primary Endpoint	Main Results
Frost et al. [58,59]	40 subjects healthy, MCI, AD	Longvida (20 g/d): 7 days	Diagnostics: curcumin fluorescence retinal imaging of Aß plaques	Completely differentiated between AD and non-AD with 80.6% specificity
Cox et al. [60]	60 subjects healthy, aged 60–85 years old	Longvida (400 or 800 mg/d): acute: 1–3 hours:chronic: 4 weeks	Cognition: mood and anxiety; blood biomarkers (lipid profile, inflammatory markers and Aß)	Completed. Cognition and mood were improved. Total and LDL cholesterol decreased

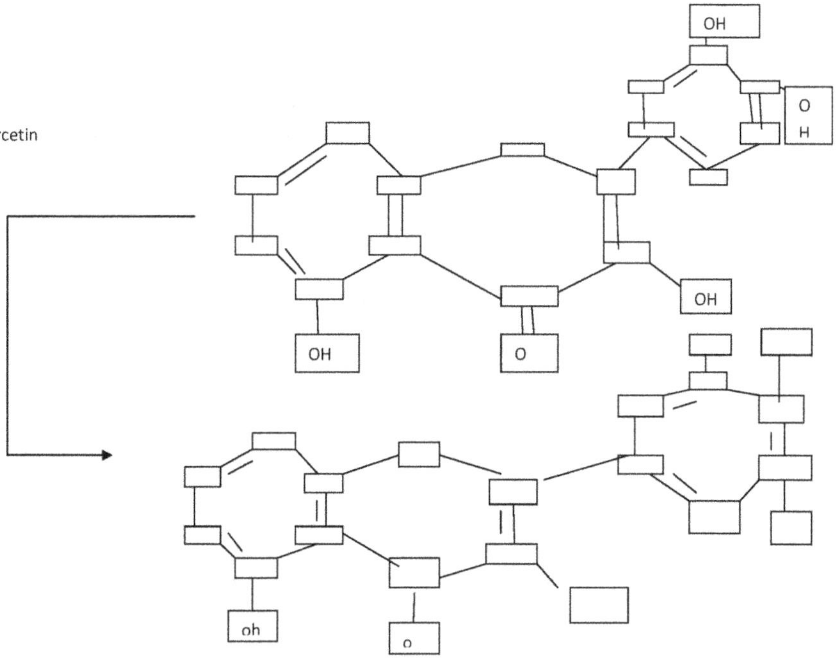

FIGURE 6.5 Structure of quercetin that exhibits various potent properties that reverse the actions of AD.

in caspase-3 activation decreased; this shows that the induction of quercetin leads to apoptosis inhibition [64].

6.7.4.1 Role of Quercetin in Neuroprotection: *In Vivo* Studies on Humans and Animals

Extensive evidence supports the role of quercetin as a neuroprotective agent and antagonistic agent for the oxidative stress [65–67]. Quercetin when taken orally protected the rodents from neurotoxicity that is generated due to oxidative stress [68–70], and it also provided protection from metal toxicity like methyl mercury, tungsten, and lead (Table 6.2) [71–74].

F: female; GPx: glutathione peroxidase; M: male; MeHg: methylmercury; MPTP: 1-methyl-4-phenyl-1,2,3,6-tetrahydropyridine; PCBs: polychlorinated biphenyls; PND: postnatal day; SOD: superoxide dismutase.

Still research studies should focus on the signaling mechanism, including signal transduction pathways, mitochondrial integrity, and proteasome functions and pharmacokinetic effects of quercetin.

6.7.5 EGCG (Epigallocatechin-3-Gallate) and FA (Ferulic Acid)

The green tea and carrots contain crucial polyphenolic compounds that help cure memory impairments. The different structural catechnins extracted from tea are shown in Figure 6.6 [75]. The regular uptake of these dietary components in a daily diet may help in the reduction of the symptoms of AD according to recent study reports. While this study has been focused on the two potent components, epigallocatechin-3-gallate and ferulic acid, that are found in carrots and green tea, and mice having Alzheimer's symptoms were used as a model to determine the effects of these two components. The nutraceuticals have promising anti-amyloidogenic properties. For this study, transgenic mice were used as a study model which expressed human APP and presenilin 1 to check amyloidosis. EGCG and ferulic acid (30 mg/kg each) were given orally to the 12 months old mice with continuous observation for 3 months regularly. After 15 months, the combined effects of EGCG and ferulic acid were evaluated and were found to reduce or show a reversal of cognitive impairments" in these tests. Thus, the combined use of EGCG and ferulic acid has the most promising approach for treating Alzheimer's [76,77].

6.7.6 Supplementation of Choline

Choline is an essential vitamin taken as a dietary supplement and is also found in certain foods. Choline is needed to maintain structural integrity in plants and animals. It is also a source of methyl groups that are required to perform a number of metabolic functions. It, when combined with an acetyl group, forms acetylcholine, a crucial neurotransmitter that helps in signaling processes of the brain by maintaining cognitive functions and maintaining expression of genes. Moreover, choline provides protection toward Alzheimer's by reducing the level of neurotoxin and homocysteine (amino acid) a risk factor of Alzheimer's. A number of studies have evaluated the elevated levels of homocysteine in AD patients that represent the high

TABLE 6.2

Neuroprotection by quercetin against neurotoxicants *in vivo*

S.No.	Animal Model	Neurotoxin	Phytochemical: Quercetin	Quercetin Effects	References
1.	M Wistar rats	100 ppm tungsten in water for about 3 months	Given oral dose: for 3 months: 0.3 mM/d continuously	Results in the reduction of oxidative stress	[70]
2.	M C57BL/6 mice	Exposed with MPTP for 4 d with a continuous dose: 30 mg/kg/d for 4 d (10–14 0 f Q)	50, 100, and 200 mg/kg/d dose of quercetin given continuously for 14 d	Decreased the reduction in the levels of SOD, GPx, and DA	[72]
3.	M Wistar rats	30 mg/kg/d MeHg dose given orally for 45 d	0.5, 5, and 50 mg/kg/d orally dose given for about 45 d	Diminished the reduction levels of GPx and GSH	[69]
4.	M Wistar rats	2 mg/kg/d Endosulfan given orally continuously for 6 d	10 mg/kg/d given orally up to 6 d	Diminished mitochondrial swelling and lipid peroxidation	[73]
5.	M,F Wistar rats	Lead: for pre- and post natal development: 0.2% taken in trough filled with water	Starting from PND 60: dose of 30 mg/kg/d given continuously for 7 d	Diminished the process of lipid peroxidation in the area of hippocampus	[68]
6.	M Wistar rats	2 mg/kg/d PCBs given orally for 30 d.i.p	50 mg/kg/d given orally for 30 d	Decrease the dopaminergic toxicity level and in cerebellum, reduction in oxidative stress	[71]

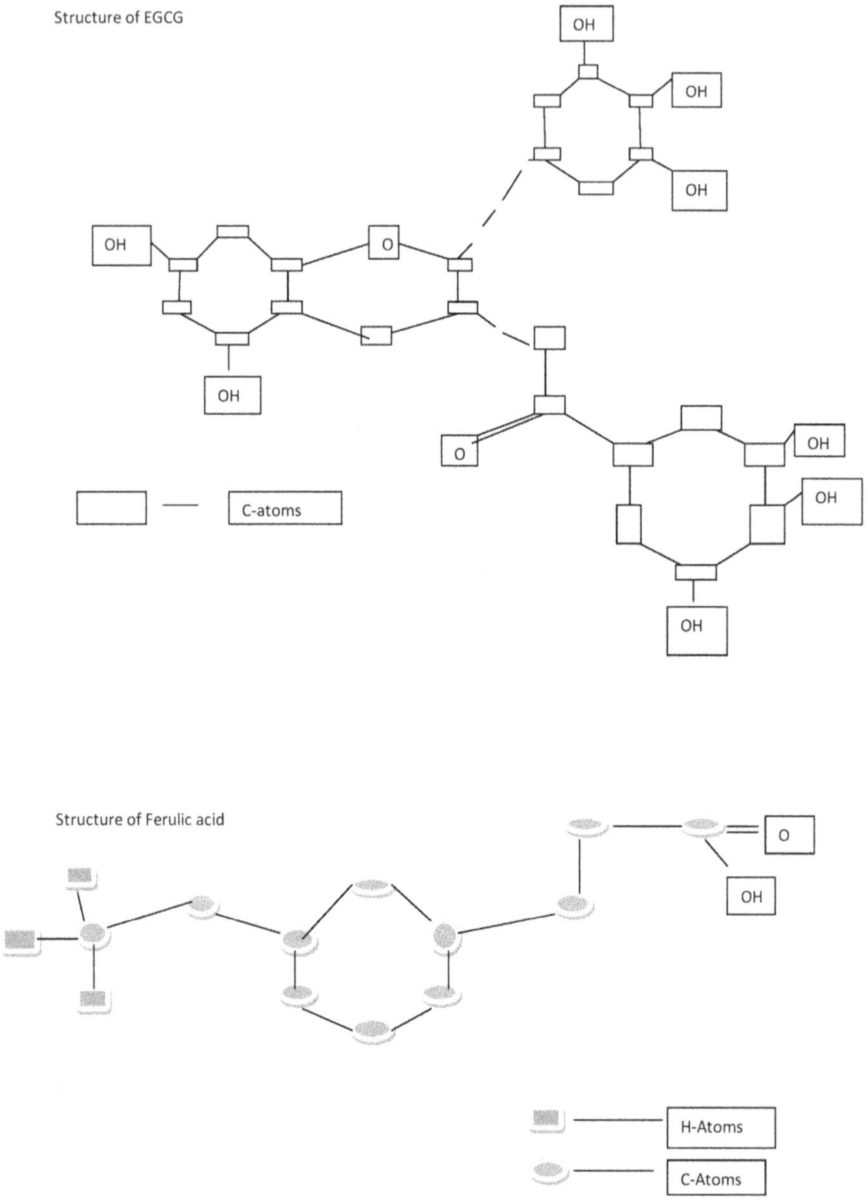
Structure of EGCG
OH
OH
OH
OH
O
OH
O
OH
OH
OH
C-atoms
Structure of Ferulic acid
O
OH
H-Atoms
C-Atoms

FIGURE 6.6 Structure of tea catechnis that shows potent beneficial effects on AD.

risk of AD. Thus, choline acts as a donor which gives the methyl group to homocysteine to convert it into methionine. In AD patients, over-activation of microglia that leads to the chronic inflammation in the brain has been observed; this over-activation of microglia could be controlled by choline. When AD-affected mice was provided the diet with choline, their offsprings exhibited improvements in cognitive activities that test was performed in a water maze. Subsequently, when the hippocampus region of the brain that is responsible for memory and learning was extracted from mice, epigenetic alterations that were induced by the supplementation of choline in diet were observed [78].

All these studies have been carried out on mice or transgenic mice which have shown great effects to treat AD. Future research work should focus on humans to check the choline effects and may act as a promising human welfare approach or therapeutic approach to treat AD.

6.7.7 RESVERATROL

Resveratrol is a phytoalexin phenolic molecule found abundantly in grapes, wine, peanuts, blueberries, mulberries, and tea, and is produced by certain plants when they get injured [79]. It is recognized as a miracle molecule due to its anti-inflammatory and anti-oxidant properties and shows a strong response toward neurodegenerative diseases. Various tests have been done on transgenic mice by inducing cognitive defects in mice, and resveratrol supplementation was shown to have reversal effects toward AD by inhibiting the action of TNF-alpha and levels of IL-1ß with the elevation in the levels of BDNF in the regions of hippocampus. Moreover, it has been found that resveratrol is responsible for the induction in the IL-10 levels that causes inflammation by inhibiting TNF-alpha and levels of NF-kappa beta that leads to the activation of ERK-2/CREB pathways that are associated with signaling processes that promote neuronal survival with the increased level of GDNF and BDNF after administration of this phenolic compound [76,79]. In the new studies, it has been found that treated patient showed a 50% reduction in the levels of metalloproteinase-9 (MMP-9) in the cerebrospinal fluid that is due to the activation of SIRT-1 (sirtuin-1). The increase in the level of MMP-9 responsible for the destruction of blood brain barrier (BBR) that allows the access of certain proteins and other molecules in the brain. Normally, low level of MMP-9 provides maintenance of blood–brain barrier [80]. The normal mechanism of signal transmission in the brain results in the proper functioning of brain (Figure 6.7) [81]. The mechanism of action of resveratrol in the pathogenesis of AD is described in Figure 6.8 [81].

1. Beta and gamma secretase is responsible for the cleavage of *APP* that leads to the production of beta amyloid.
2. Without the involvement of SIRT1, only AMPK activation promotes the potent function of resveratrol that leads to the clearance of the beta amyloid without creating any hindrance in the beta amyloid generation process.
3. Resveratrol also causes the phosphorylation of PKC that plays a crucial role in the neuroprotective functions.
4. The generation of Aß-Cu, Aß-Zn, and Aß-Fe gets reduced due to the protective action of resveratrol.
5. Under oxidative stress, the mitochondria is damaged that leads to the generation of ROS, including iNOS and COX-2, and thus results in apoptosis.
6. The main function of resveratrol is to reduce the expression of particular enzymes that play a role in the production of ROS like Nox4, and in other

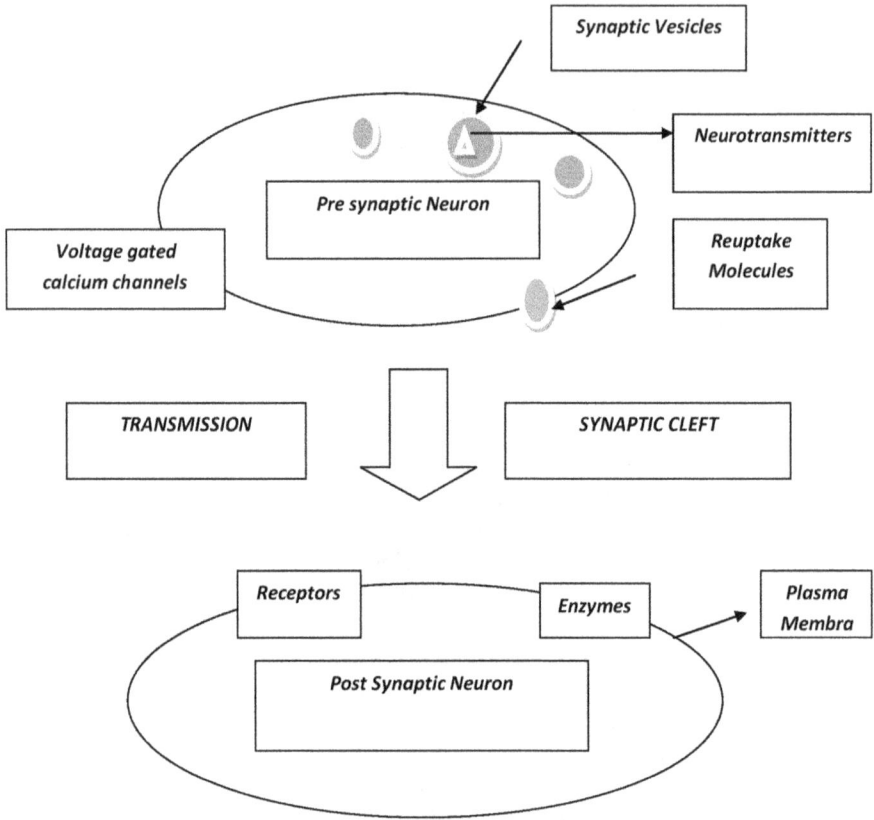

FIGURE 6.7 Mechanism of signal transmission or transfer of neurotransmitters from pre-synaptic neuron to post-synaptic neuron through the synaptic cleft.

ways, it promotes the expression of SOD 1 and GPx 1 (enzymes responsible for ROS inactivation).

7. Wide influences of resveratrol on apoptotic signaling pathways that include NF-kB binding suppression, Bcl-XL expression restoration, Bax expression inhibition, and JNK activation blockage.

8. Through the activation of microglial cells it causes PGE2 inhibition.

9. Accumulation of beta amyloid causes the activation of various cells like microglial cells and astrocytes that produce certain cytokines such as TNF-alpha, IL-ß, IL-6. IκBα, STAT-3 and STAT-1 phosphorylation gets reduced due to inhibitory action of resveratrol.

6.7.8 HOLY SHRUB: YARBA SANTA (STERUBIN)

A holy shrub from California called Yarba Santa has medicinal properties that were used previously to treat fever, respiratory ailments, and headaches. Now, it has been

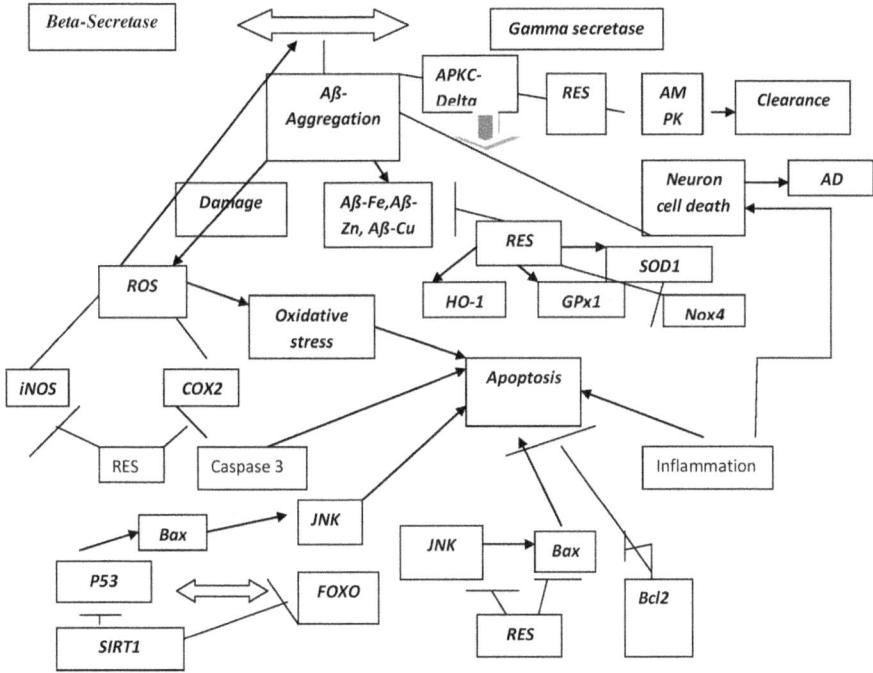

FIGURE 6.8 Mechanism of action of resveratrol on AD.

identified that extracts from this shrub might be flavones having a potential to reverse the neurodegeneration. After the screening of 400 plant extracts, researchers identified an active compound called sterubin. It acts as an iron remover that causes damage to the neurons [81]. The various different properties of sterubin are shown in Figure 6.9 [82].

But more research is needed to check its potential toward controlling AD and its mechanism related to that.

6.7.9 SAFRANAL

Safranal, which exhibits anti-apopotic and antioxidant properties, is extracted from the medicinal plant *Crocus sativus* (saffron) previously used to prepare medicines in Asia, India, and other Mediterranean countries where it had been used as a expectorant, apoptogenic agent, sedative, emmenagogue, anti-astma, anti-cancer, anti-inflammatory, ant-depressant agent. The effective role of safranal has been evaluated on PC12 cell lines in which cells are pre-treated with the extract of saffron (2.5–40 µg/ml), safranal (2,5–40 µM), 2.5–40 µg/ml of essential oil with 5, 10, and 20 µM dopenzil for 120 minutes. After that, treated cells were exposed to either 25 µM of Aß (48 hours) or 150 µM of H_2O_2 (24 hours). At the end of the test, apoptotic reduction was observed. Safranal may act as a promising source of

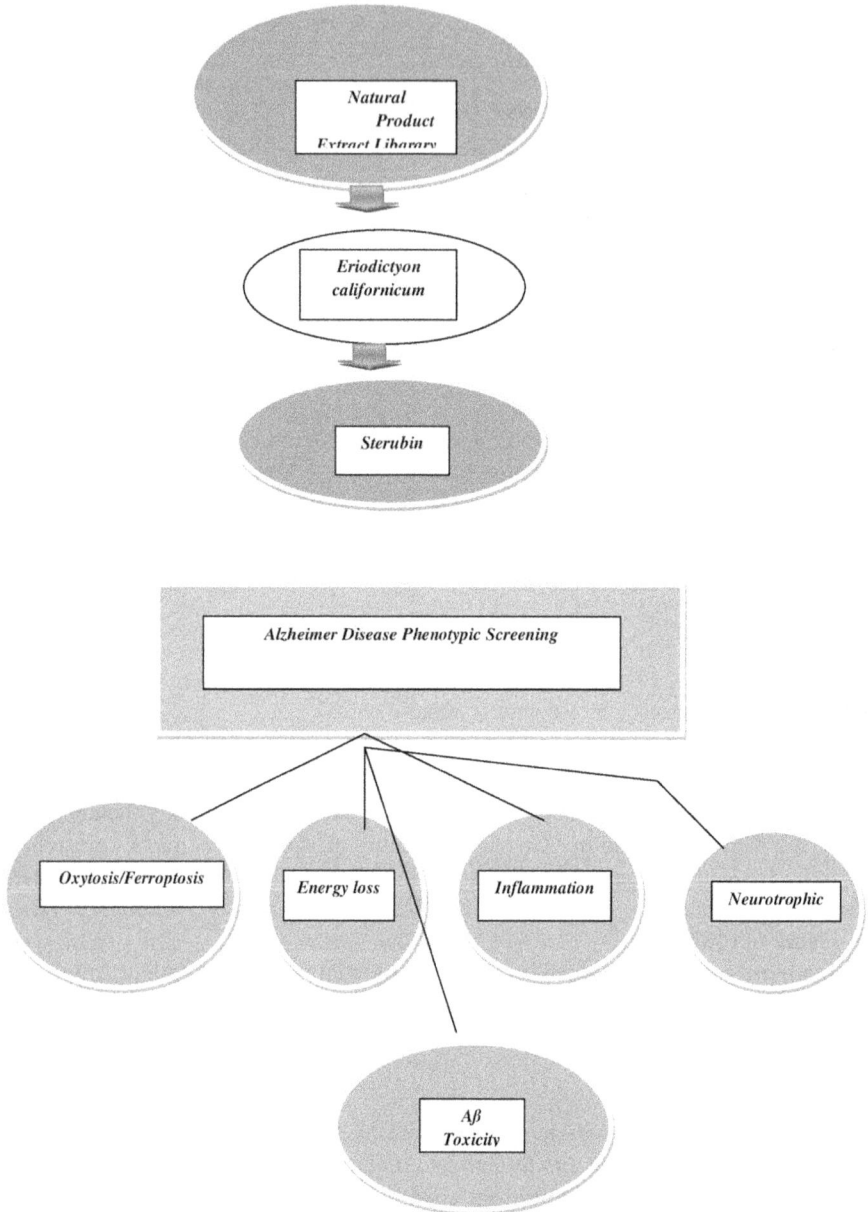

FIGURE 6.9 Beneficial properties of sterubin on AD.

treating AD in the future. Till now, no research has been done to determine the protective role of safranal on Alzheimer's model of research. So, the research should be done on safranal to explore the potential of this compound [83]. In AD pathogenesis, mechanism of action of safranal has been shown in Figure 6.10 [83].

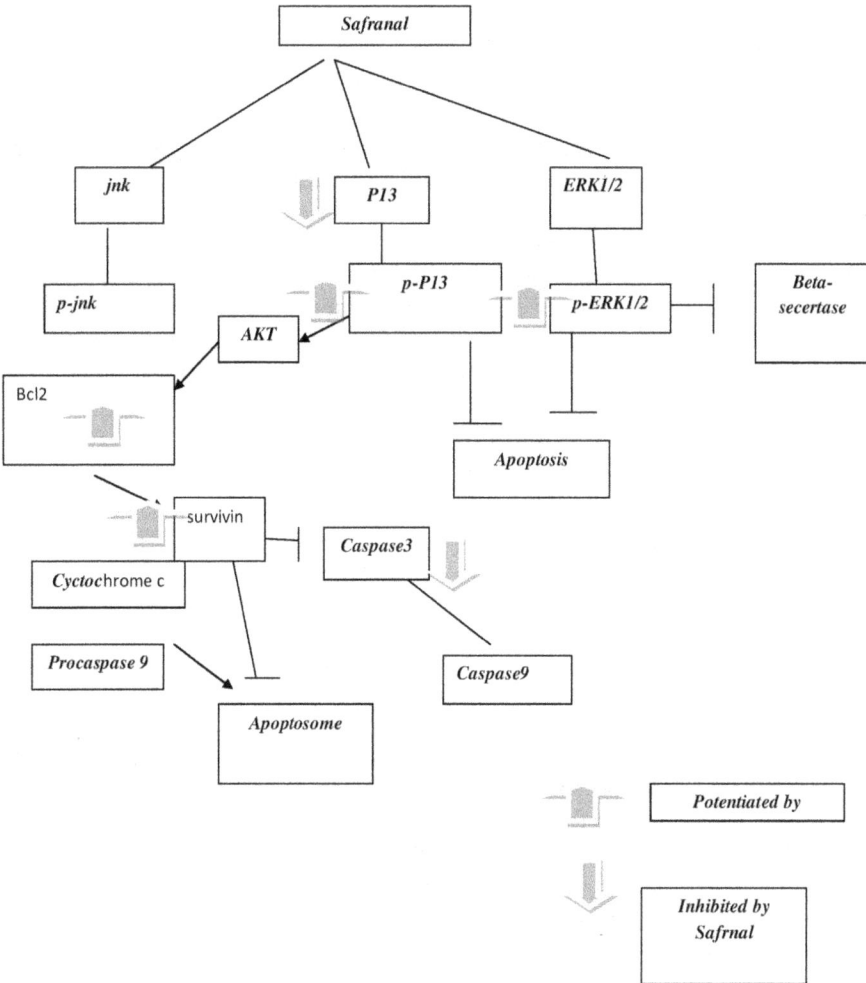

FIGURE 6.10   Mechanism of action of safranal during AD pathogenesis.

6.7.10 ONOSMA TAURICU

According to certain reports, there are approximately 102 *Onosma* species found in Turkey, and maximum species grow naturally in Europe and Asia regions. In addition, these species are not only used to treat various disorders, including fever, strangury, leucoderma, bronchitis, and abdominal pain, but they are also a good source of adulterant which is generally used in chilli powder to enhance the color because of their dying and coloring properties. Few investigations have been done to demonstrate the anti-bacterial, anti-inflammatory, anti-cancerous, anti-nociceptive and wound healing activities of some species of *Onosma*. A study report was performed to analyze the activity of different extracts, ethyl-acetate (OTT-EtOAc), methanol (OTT-MeOH), and water (OTT-W) extracted from *Onosma tauricu*. After evaluation, water extracts were found to be the richest source of flavonoid and other phenolic components: the flavonoid and phenolic concentration in water extracts was 40.88 μmolGAEs/g and also 7.40 μmolREs/g in dry plants. Various compounds rosmarinic acid, caffeic acid, luteolin, *p*-coumaric acid, apigenin, trans-cinnamic acid, cholorogenic acid, rutin, and *p*-hydroxybenzoic acid were found in the extracts of *Onosma tauricu*. OTT-W extracts showed remarkable effects in iron chelation, radical scanvenging, reducing power, and in phosphomolybednum. The methanol extract also showed inhibitory response toward acetylcholinesterase, while butyrlcholinesterase showed no effects. On the contrary, OTT-W extract also exhibited the inhibitory action on ß-glucosidase and tyrosinase too. From the data analysis, it has been found that the disease caused by these enzymes could be cured by using these plant extracts, specifically OTT-W and OTT-MeOH extract [84].

But the beneficial role of these species in the case of AD as a source of therapeutic agents is not explored yet.

6.7.11 *Matricaria chamomilla* L.

This medicinal herb is used as an anxiolytic, antidepressant, anti-viral, anti-microbial, and anti-inflammatory agent. To demonstrate the effects of hydroalco-holic extracts (25–75 mg/kg) that were extracted from *Matricaria chamomilla*, a test was performed on mice that was treated with scopolamine (0.7 mg/kg) 30 minutes and the extract was orally administered for 7 days. The following compounds were observed: luteolin, rutin, chlorogenic acid, apigenin, cynaroside, and apigenin-7-glucoside in the hydroalcholic extract. The results of the test showed the extract helped improve the memory deficit that was induced by the injection of scopolamine through modulating the activity of acetyl cholinesterase with the ac-tivation of BDNF and reduction in the expression of IL1ß in the hippocampus region of brain. Therefore, it might be the propitious therapeutic drug approach in order to prevent neurodegenerative disorders that are associated with memory loss and amnesia [84].

6.7.12 Allylguaiacol

Allylguaiacol is a chemical compound (phytochemical) extracted from a number of plants including cloves, nutmeg, basil, and cinnamon that show anti-bacterial, anti-cancer, anti-inflammatory, and anti-oxidant properties with neuroprotective activ-ities. The study was conducted to examine the effect of allylguaiacol by treating HT22 cells of hippocampus with hydrogen peroxide (H_2O_2). The free radicals such as 2,2-diphenyl-1-picrylhydrazyl (DPPH), 2,2'-azino-bis-(3-ethylbenzothiazoline-6-sulphonic acid) (ABTS) act as scavengers, and their scavenging activities get en-hanced with an increase in the expression of enzymes, like catalase and manganese superoxide dismutase (MnSOD), that act as anti-oxidants. Moreover it inhibits the damage caused by hydrogen peroxide in HT22 cell lines with an increase in the production of the brain-derived neurotrophic factor (BDNF). Allyguaiacol showed potent effects by activating antioxidant enzymes with the regulation of proteins like

P65 and NF-kappa beta and signaling process related to Death Domain Associated Protein (DAXX) [85]. From all these evidences, still there is no one report that describes about the regulatory mechanism of allylguaiacol toward AD.

6.8 CONCLUSION

This chapter reviews all collected information from literature regarding the beneficial effects of phytochemicals on this deadly disease by analyzing the study or tests that have been done to determine the effectiveness of phytochemicals that are isolated from a variety of plants. In addition, several phytochemical studies were examined to understand different roles phytochemicals play in the inhibition of different signaling pathways associated with AD. According to one study, it was evaluated that people who take food with turmeric as a supplement (curcumin) are less likely to develop the disease than those without turmeric. Curcumin exhibited its efficiency in the clinical fields through a number of analytic studies and was found to directly interact with proteins involved in apoptosis, cytokines involved in inflammatory reactions and halting the function of phosphorylase kinase. In spite of that, the exact mechanism behind curcumin interaction with these molecules is not known yet. Quercetin treatment on rodents has shown protective effects against neurotoxicity to diminish the effects of oxidative stress. A number of novel phytochemicals have been extracted from different medicinal plants which show anti-inflammatory, anti-apopotic, and anti-oxidant properties which might be the future therapeutic drug approach to treat AD. But their effectiveness has not been examined on human and animal models. Some phtyochemicals show their effectiveness when used in combination with other phytochemicals. In order to enhance the effects of phytochemicals, properties of compounds should be analyzed thoroughly by using other ways, techniques, or methods. Still there is no single drug in the market yet that has the ability to reverse the disease or control it. All phytochemical-based drugs only slower down the symptoms that appear during disease, but not cure the AD properly. Because the exact mechanism of AD is not known yet, the disease could not be controlled before the development of AD.

REFERENCES

[1]. Queen B. L. and Tollefsbol T. O. Polyphenols and aging. *Current Aging Science*, 3, 34–42 (2010)

[2]. Dementia [online]. World Health Organization Available: http://www.who.int/ mediacentre/factsheets/fs362/en/, (2018).

[3]. Alzheimer's Disease Fact Sheet [online]. National Institute on Aging Available: https://www.nia.nih.gov/alzhe imers/publication/alzheimers-disease-fact-sheet, (2018).

[4]. Dosunmu R., Wu J., Basha M. R. and Zawia N.H. Environmental and dietary risk factors in Alzheimer's disease. *Expert Review of Neurotherapeutics*, 7, 887–900 (2007).

[5]. Hu N., Yu J., Tan L., Wang Y., Sun L. and Tan L. Nutrition and the risk of Alzheimer's disease. *Biomed Research International*, 1–12. (2013). doi:10.1155/ 2013/524820

[6]. Saragat B., Buffa R., Mereu E., Succa V., Cabras S., Mereu R. M., et al. Nutritional and psycho-functional status in elderly patients with Alzheimer's disease. *Journal of Nutrition, Health and Aging*, 16, 231–236 (2012)

[7]. Pugazhenthi S., Qin L. and Reddy P. H. Common neurodegenerative pathways in obesity, diabetes, and Alzheimer's disease. *Biochimica et Biophysica Acta*, 1863, 1037–1045 (2016).

[8]. Shah R. The role of nutrition and diet in Alzheimer's disease: A systematic review. *Journal of the American Medical Directors Association*, 14, 398–402 (2013).

[9]. Hartman R., Shah A., Fagan A., Schwetye K., Parsadanian M., Schulman R., et al. Pomegranate juice decreases amyloid load and improves behaviour in a mouse model of Alzheimer's disease. *Neurobiology of Disease*, 24, 506–515 (2006).

[10]. Kim D., Nguyen M., Dobbin M., Fischer A., Sananbenesi F., Rodgers J., et al. SIRT1 deacetylase protects against neurodegeneration in models for Alzheimer's disease and amyotrophic lateral sclerosis. *EMBO J*, 26, 3169–3179 (2007).

[11]. Hyman B. T., Phelps C. H., Beach T. G., Bigio E. H., Cairns N. J., Carrillo M. C., Dickson D. W., Duyckaerts C., Frosch M. P., Masliah E., Mirra S. S., Nelson P. T., Schneider J. A., Thal D. R., Thies B., Trojanowski J. Q., Vinters H. V. and Montine T. J. National Institute on Aging-Alzheimer's Association guidelines for the neuropathologic assessment of Alzheimer's disease. *Alzheimers Dementia*, 8, 1–13 (2012).

[12]. Braak H. and Braak E. Staging of Alzheimer's disease-related neurofibrillary changes. *Neurobiology of Aging*, 16, 271–8. discussion 278–284 (1995).

[13]. Thal D. R., Rub U., Orantes M. and Braak H. Phases of A beta-deposition in the human brain and its relevance for the development of AD. *Neurology*, 58, 1791–1800 (2002).

[14]. Mirra S. S., Heyman A., McKeel D., Sumi S. M., Crain B. J., Brownlee L. M., Vogel F. S., Hughes J. P., Van Belle G. and Berg L. The consortium to establish a registry for Alzheimer's disease (CERAD). Part II. Standardization of the neuropathologic assessment of Alzheimer's disease. *Neurol*, 41, 479–486 (1991).

[15]. Scheltens P., Blennow K., Breteler M. M., de Strooper B. and Frisoni G. B., Salloway S., Van der Flier W.M. Alzheimer's disease. *Lancet*, 388, 505–517 (2016).

[16]. Nelson P. T., Alafuzoff I., Bigio E. H., Bouras C., Braak H., Cairns N., Davies P., Tredici K. D., Duyckaerts C., Frosch M. P., Hof P. R., Hulette C., Hyman B. T., Iwatsubo T., Jellinger K. A., Jicha G. A., Kovari E., Kukull W. A., Leverenz J. B., Love S., Mackenzie I. R., Mann D. M., Masliah E., McKee A., Montine T. J., Morris J. C., Schneider J. A., Sonnen J. A., Thal D. R., Trojanowski J. Q., Troncoso J. C., Wisniewski T., Woltjer R. L. and Beach T. G. Correlation of Alzheimer's disease neuropathologic changes with cognitive status: A review of the literature. *JNEN*, 71, 362–381 (2012).

[17]. Lane C. A., Hardy J. and Schott J. M., Alzheimer's disease. *European Journal of Neurology* 2018, 25, 59–70 (2018).

[18]. Selkoe D. J. and Hardy J. The amyloid hypothesis of Alzheimer's disease at 25 years. *EMBO Molecular Medicine* 2016, 8(6), 595–608 (2016).

[19]. Silverberg N., Elliott C., Ryan L., Masliah E. and Hodes R. NIA commentary on the NIA-AA Research Framework: Towards a biological definition of Alzheimer's disease. *Alzheimers Dement*, 14, 576–578 (2018).

[20]. Tomic J. L., Pensalfini A., Head E. and Glabe C. G. Soluble fibrillar oligomer levels are elevated in Alzheimer's disease brain and correlate with cognitive dysfunction. *Neurobiology of Disease*, 35, 352–358 (2009).

[21]. McLean C. A., Cherny R. A., Fraser F. W., Fuller S. J., Smith M. J., et al. Soluble pool of Abeta amyloid as a determinant of severity of neurodegeneration in Alzheimer's disease. *Annals of Neurology*, 46, 860–866 (1999).

[22]. Lue L. F., Kuo Y. M., Roher A. E., Brachova L., Shen Y., et al. Soluble amyloid beta peptide concentration as a predictor of synaptic change in Alzheimer's disease. *American Journal of Pathology*, 155, 853–862 (1999).

[23]. Wang J., Dickson D. W., Trojanowski J. Q. and Lee V. M. The levels of soluble versus insoluble brain Abeta distinguish Alzheimer's disease from normal and pathologic aging. *Exp Neurol Acta Neuropathologica*, 158, 328–337 (1999)

[24]. Viola K. L. and Klein W. L. Amyloid beta oligomers in Alzheimer's disease pathogenesis, treatment, and diagnosis. *Journal of Alzheimers Disease* 2018, 64(Suppl 1), S567–S610...129:183–206 (2015)

[25]. Sengupta U., Nilson A. N. and Kayed R. the role of amyloid-beta oligomers in toxicity, propagation, and immunotherapy. *EBioMedicine* 2016, 6, 42–49 (2016)

[26]. Wisniewski T. and Goni F. Immunotherapeutic approaches for Alzheimer's disease. *Neuron* 2016, 85, 1162–1176 (2015)

[27]. Bucciantini M., Giannoni E., Chiti F. et al. Inherent toxicity of aggregates implies a common mechanism for protein misfolding diseases. *Nature* 416, 507–511 (2002)

[28]. Wisniewski T. and Drummond E. Developing therapeutic vaccines against Alzheimer's disease. *Expert Review of Vaccines*, 5, 401–415 (2016)

[29]. Drummond E., Goni F., Liu S., Prelli F., Scholtzova H. and Wisniewski T. Potential novel approaches to understand the pathogenesis and treat Alzheimer's disease. *Journal of Alzheimers Disease, 64*(s1), S299–S312. doi: 10.3233/JAD-179909 (2018).

[30]. Breydo L., Kurouski D., Rasool S., Milton S., Wu J. W. et al., Structural differences between amyloid beta oligomers. *Biochemical and Biophysical Research Communication* 2016, 477, 700–705 (2016)

[31]. Perry G. Alzheimer's Disease: Advances for a New Century. Amsterdam: IOS Press BV (2013)

[32]. Mayeux R. and Yaakov S. Epidemiology of Alzheimer's disease. *Cold Spring Harbor Perspectives in Medicine*, 2, a006239 (2012)

[33]. Pericak-Vance M. A., Bebout J. L., Gaskell P. C. Jr, et al. Linkage studies in familial Alzheimer disease: Evidence for chromosome 19 linkage. *American Journal of Human Genetics*, 48, 1034–1050 (1991)

[34]. Lane C. A., Hardy J. and Schott J. M. Alzheimer's disease. *European Journal of Neurology* 2018, 25, 59–70 (2018)

[35]. Sharma R. D., Wani Y. W., Sunkaria A. et al., Quercetin protects against chronic aluminium induced oxidative stres and ensuing biochemical, cholinergic, and neurobehavioural impairements in Rata. *Neurotoxicity Research* 2013, 23, 336–357 (2013)

[36]. Kim J., Basak M. J. and Holtzman D. M., "Te role of apolipoprotein E in Alzheimer's disease," *Neuron*, 63, 287–303 (2009)

[37]. Priller C., Bauer T., Mitteregger G., Krebs B., Kretzschmar A. H. and J. Herms. "Synapse formation and function is modulated by the amyloid precursor protein," *Te Journal of Neuroscience*, 26(27), 7212–7221 (2006)

[38]. G. P. Morris, I. A. Clark and B. Vissel Inconsistencies and controversies surrounding the amyloid hypothesis of Alzheimer's disease *Acta Neuropathol Commun*, 2, 1–21 (2014)

[39]. M. Goedert and M. G. Spillantini, "A century of Alzheimer's disease," *Science* 2006, 314 (5800), 777–781 (2006).

[40]. E. Kopke, Y.-C. Tung, S. Shaikh, A. D. C. Alonso, K. Iqbal and I. Grundke-Iqbal, "Microtubule-associated protein tau: Abnormal phosphorylation of a non-paired helical flament pool in Alzheimer disease." *Te Journal of Biological Chemistry*, 268 (32), 24374–24384 (1993)

[41]. S. Melov, P. A. Adlard and K. Morten "Mitochondrial oxidative stress causes hyperphosphorylation of tau." *PLoS ONE*, 2 (6), e536 (2007).

[42]. E. Mullaart, M. E. T. I. Boerrigter, R. Ravid, D. F. Swaab, and J. Vijg, "Increased levels of DNA breaks in cerebral cortex of alzheimer's disease patients," *Neurobiology of Aging*, 11(3), 169–173 (1990)

[43]. Shrikant Mishra and kalpana Palanivelu. The effect of Curcumin (turmeric) on Alzheimer's disease: An overview. *Annals of Indian Academy of Neurology*, 11 (1), 13–19 (2008)

[44]. Magalingam B. K., Radhakrishnan A., Ping S. N. and Haleagrahara N. Current concepts of neurodegenerative mechanisms in Alzheimer's disease. *BioMed Research International* (2018).

[45]. Zibadi S., Preedy V. R. and Watson R. R. Polyphenols in Human Health and Disease. London: Academic Press; 2014.

[46]. Singh M., Arseneault M., Sanderson T., Murthy V. and Ramassamy C. Challenges for research on polyphenols from foods in Alzheimer's disease: Bioavailability, metabolism, and cellular and molecular mechanisms. *Journal of Agriculture and Food Chemistry*, 56, 4855–4873 (2008)

[47]. Ganguli M., Chandra V., Kamboh M. I., Johnston J. M., Dodge H. H., Thelma B. K., Juyal R. C., Pandav R., Belle S. H. and DeKosky S. T. Apolipoprotein E polymorphism and Alzheimer disease: The Indo-US Cross-National Dementia Study. *Archives of Neurology*, 57, 824–830 (2000)

[48]. Ringman J. M., Frautschy S. A., Cole G. M., Masterman D. L. and Cummings J. L. A potential role of the curry spice curcumin in Alzheimer's disease. *Current Alzheimer Research*, 2, 131–136 (2005)

[49]. Lim G. P., Chu T., Yang F., Beech W., Frautschy S. A. and Cole G. M. The curry spice curcumin reduces oxidative damage and amyloid pathology in an Alzheimer transgenic mouse. *Journal of Neuroscience*, 21, 8370–8377 (2001)

[50]. Shishodia S., Sethi G. and Aggarwal B. B. Getting back to roots. *Annals of the New York Academy of Sciences*, 1056, 206–217 (2005)

[51]. Ammon H. P. and Wahl M. A. Pharmacology of curcuma longa. *Planta Medicine*, 57,1–7 (1991)

[52]. Youssef K. M. and El-Sherbeny M. A. Synthesis and antitumor activity of some curcumin analogs. *Archiv der Pharmazie* (Weinheim), 338, 181–189 (2005)

[53]. Shrikant Mishra and Kalapana Palanivelu. The effect of curcumin (turmeric) on Alzheimer's disease: An overview. *Annals of Indian Academy of Neurology*, 11 (1), 13–19 (2008)

[54]. Bajda M., Guzior N., Ignasik M. and Malawska B. Multi-target-directed ligands in Alzheimer's disease treatment. *Current Medicinal Chemistry*, 18, 4949–4975 (2011)

[55]. Chen M., Di Y. Z., Zheng X. Li L. D., Zhou P. R. and Zhang K. Use of curcumin in diagnosis, prevention, and treatment of Alzheimer's disease. *Neural Regeneration Research*, 13 (4), 742–752 (2018)

[56]. Gupta S. C., Patchva S. and Aggarwal B. B. Therapeutic roles of curcumin: Lessons learned from clinical trials. *AAPS Journal*, 15, 195–218 (2013)

[57]. Baum L., Lam C. W. K., Cheung S. K., Kwok T., Lui V., Tsoh J., Lam L., Leung V., Hui E. and Ng C. Six-month randomized, placebo-controlled, double-blind, pilot clinical trial of curcumin in patients with Alzheimer disease. *Journal of Clinical Psychopharmacology*, 28, 110–113 (2008)

[58]. Ringman J. M., Frautschy S. A., Teng E., Begum A. N., Bardens J., Beigi M., Gylys K. H., Badmaev V., Heath D. D. and Apostolova L. G. Oral curcumin for Alzheimer's disease: Tolerability and efficacy in a 24-week randomized, double blind, placebo-controlled study. *Alzheimers Research and Therapy*, 4, 43 (2012)

[59]. Frost S., Kanagasingam Y., Macaulay L., Koronyo-Hamaoui M., Koronyo Y., Biggs D., Verdooner S., Black K., Taddei K. and Shah T. Retinal amyloid fluorescence imaging predicts cerebral amyloid burden and Alzheimer's disease. *Alzheimers Dementia*, 10, 234–P235 (2014)

[60]. Cox K. H., Pipingas A. and Scholey A. B. Investigation of the effects of solid lipid curcumin on cognition and mood in a healthy older population. *Journal of Psychopharmacology*, 29, 642–651 (2015)

[61]. Li Y., Yao J., Han C. et al. Quercetin, inflammation and immunity. 2016, 8(3), 167. doi: 10.3390/nu8030167.

[62]. Spagnuolo C., Moccia S. and Russo G. L. Anti-inflammatory effects of flavonoids in neurodegenerativedisorders, 2017, 17, 30683–30689.doi:10.1016/j.ejmech.2017.09.001,

[63]. Costa G. L., Garrick M. J., Roque J. P. and Pellacani C. Mechanism of neuroprotection by Quercetin: Counteracting oxidative stress and more. *Oxidative Medicine and Cellular Longevity*, 10 (2016). 2986796.

[64]. Sharma D. R., Wani W. Y., Sunkaria A. et al. Quercetin attenuates neuronal death against aluminum-induced neurodegeneration in the rat hippocampus. *Journal of Neuroscience*, 324, 163–176 (2016) doi: 10.1016/j.neuroscience.2016.02.055.

[65]. Ossola B., Kääriäinen T. M. and Männistö P. T. The multiple faces of quercetin in neuroprotection. *Expert Opinion on Drug Safety*, 8 (4), 397–409 (2009), doi: 10. 1517/14740330903026944.

[66]. Ishisaka A., Ichikawa S., Sakakibara H., et al. Accumulation of orally administered quercetin in brain tissue and its antioxidative effects in rats. *Free Radical Biology and Medicine*, 51(7), 1329–1336 (2011) doi: 10.1016/j.freeradbiomed.2011.06.017.

[67]. Das S., Mandal A. K., Ghosh A., Panda S., Das N., Sarkar S. Nanoparticulated quercetin in combating age related cerebral oxidative injury. *Current Aging Science*, 1(3),169–174 (2008) doi: 10.2174/1874609810801030169.

[68]. Hu P., Wang M., Chen W. H., et al. Quercetin relieves chronic lead exposure-induced impairment of synaptic plasticity in rat dentate gyrus in vivo. *Naunyn-Schmiedeberg's Archives of Pharmacology*, 378(1), 43–51 (2008) doi: 10.1007/s00210-008-0301-z.

[69]. Barcelos G. R. M., Grotto D., Serpeloni J. M., et al. Protective properties of quercetin against DNA damage and oxidative stress induced by methylmercury in rats. *Archives of Toxicology*, 85(9), 1151–1157 (2011) doi: 10.1007/s00204-011-0652-y.

[70]. Sachdeva S., Pant S. C., Kushwaha P., Bhargava R. and Flora S. J. S. Sodium tungstate induced neurological alterations in rat brain regions and their response to antioxidants. *Food and Chemical Toxicology*, 82, 64–71 (2015) doi: 10.1016/j.fct. 2015.05.003.

[71]. Bavithra S., Selvakumar K., Kumari R. P., Krishnamoorthy G., Venkataraman P., and Arunakaran J. Polychlorinated biphenyl (PCBs)-induced oxidative stress plays a critical role on cerebellar dopaminergic receptor expression: Ameliorative role of quercetin. *Neurotoxicity Research*, 21 (2), 149–159 (2012) doi: 10.1007/s12640-011-9253-z.

[72]. Lv C., Hong T., Yang Z., et al. Effect of quercetin in the 1-methyl-4-phenyl-1, 2, 3, 6-tetrahydropyridine-induced mouse model of Parkinson's disease. *Evidence-Based Complementary and Alternative Medicine* 6, (2012) doi: 10.1155/2012/928643.928643.

[73]. Lakroun Z., Kebieche M., Lahouel A., Zama D., Desor F. and Soulimani R. Oxidative stress and brain mitochondria swelling induced by endosulfan and protective role of quercetin in rat. *Environmental Science and Pollution Research*, 22 (10), 7776–7781 (2015) doi: 10.1007/s11356-014-3885-5

[74]. T. Mori, N. Koyama, J. Tan, T. Segawa, M. Maeda, T. Town. Combined treatment with the phenolics (−)-epigallocatechin-3-gallate and ferulic acid improves cognition and reduces Alzheimer-like pathology in mice. *Journal of Biological Chemistry*, 294 (8), 2714 (2019) DOI: 10.1074/jbc.RA118.004280.

[75]. Ide K., Matsuoka N., Yamada H., Furushima D. and Kawakami K. Effects of Tea Catechins on Alzheimer's Disease: Recent Updates and prospectives. *Moecules*, 23 (9), 2357 (2018)

[76]. Ma T., Tan S. M., Yu T. J. and Tan L. Resveratrol as a therapeutic agents for Alzheimer's disease. *BioMed Research International*, 13 (2014). DOI: 10.1155/2014/350516

[77]. Q. Hiser. Old-age associated phenotypic screening for Alzheimer's Disease drug Candidate identifies sterubin as a potent neuroprotective compound from Yerba santa. *Redox Biology*, 21 (2019).

[78]. Ramon Velazquez, E. Ferreira, W. Winslow, N. Dave, I.S. Piras, M. Naymik, M.J. Huentelman, A. Tran, A. Caccamo,S. Oddo. Maternal choline supplementation ameliorates Alzheimer's disease pathology by reducing brain homocysteine levels across multiple generations. *Molecular Psychiatry*, (2019). DOI: 10.1038/s41380-018-0322-z

[79]. Anastacio J. R., Netto C. A., Castro C. C., Sanches E. F., Ferreira D. C., Noschang C., Krolow R., Dalmaz C. and Pagnussat A. Resveratrol treatment has neuroprotective effects and prevents cognitive impairment after chronic cerebral hypoperfusion. *Neurology of Research*, 36, 627–633 (2014). Doi: 10.1179/1743132813Y.0000000293.

[80]. Georgetown University Medical Center. "Resveratrol appears to restore blood-brain barrier integrity in Alzheimer's disease." ScienceDaily.

[81]. W. Fischer, A. Currais, Z. Liang, A. Pinto, P. Maher, Old age-associated phenotypic screening for Alzheimer's disease drug candidates identifies sterubin as a potent neuroprotective compound from Yerba santa. *Redox Biology*, 21, (2016)

[82]. Rafieipour F., Hadipour E., Emami A. S., Asili J. and Najaran T. Z. Safranal protects against beta-amyloid peptide-induced cell toxicity in PC12 cells via MAPK and PI3 K pathways. *Metabolic Brain Disease*, 34(1), 165–172 (2018).

[83]. Kirkan B., Sarikurkcu C., Ozer S. M., Cengiz M. et al., Phenolic profile, antioxidant and enzyme inhibitory potential of *Onosma tauricum* var. Tauricum. *Industrial Crops & Products*, 125, 549–555 (2018)

[84]. Ionita R., Postu A. P., Mihasan M., Gorgan L. D. et al. Ameliorative effects of *Matricaria chamomilla* L. hydroalcoholic extract on scopolamine-induced memory impairment in rats: A behavioral and molecular study. *Phytomedicine* (2018), doi: 10.1016/j.phymed.2018.04.049.

[85]. Lim S. H., Kim Y. B., Kim J. Y. and Jeong J. S. Phytochemical allylguaiacol exerts a neuroprotective effect on hippocampal cells and ameliorates scopolamine-induced memory impairment in mice. *Behavioural Brain Research,* 339, 261–268 (2017).

7 Existing Methods and Emerging Trends for Novel Coronavirus (COVID-19) Detection Using Residual Network (ResNet): A Review on Deep Learning Analysis

Upasana Bhattacharjya and
Kandarpa Kumar Sarma

CONTENTS

7.1 INTRODUCTION

The novel coronavirus infection, commonly known as COVID-19, caused by SARS-CoV-2, has become a prevalent disease worldwide, leading to a severe global crisis across the world. It is an infectious disease that originated in December

DOI: 10.1201/9781003171829-7

2019 in Wuhan, China, and eventually turned into a pandemic by March 2020 as per World Health Organization (WHO) declaration [1]. With a statistic of more than 118 million positive subjects, and more than 2.62 million deaths, as of March 12, 2021, COVID-19 has marked itself as one of the deadliest pandemics in history across the globe [1–3].

COVID-19 is typically spread via respiratory droplets during sneezing and coughing and during close contact with the infected people, resulting in typical symptoms like fever, cold, cough, shortness of breath, loss of taste, sore throat, diarrhea, abdomen pain, and muscle pain. Although most cases end with mild symptoms, some cases lead to diseases like pneumonia and multi-organ failure. The virus's progression is causing a significant loss worldwide due to massive quarantine procedures and asymptomatic transmission where the symptoms are absent (asymptomatic patients) [4]. Amid the pandemic, many countries are in different phases of the development of the COVID-19 vaccine. As of now, the national regulatory authorities have permitted emergency use for 11 vaccines, but only 6 of those vaccines have been approved for immediate use. The first vaccination program started at the beginning of December 2020 and continuing to 175.3 million as per [1] till February 15, 2021. With the limited diagnosis arrangements across the globe, a proper diagnosis approach for COVID-19 diagnosis is in high demand at the present stage [3–5].

As per the WHO, the primary standard protocol to identify COVID-19 is the reverse transcriptase polymerase chain reaction (RT–PCR) test [4]. Yet, with a high number of cases and limited resources and environment, the screening could not be made fast and effective. Therefore, the practical solution to combat this virus is through vaccination and drug therapy. Moreover, clinical diagnosis methods, which include computer tomography (CT)-scan, X-ray, and ultrasound imaging, are also beneficial. These image modalities are considered powerful techniques for COVID-19 detection as all the hospitals and radiology clinics are equipped with X-ray and CT-scan imaging machines [4,5]. The analysis of these medical images has also gained much interest in the research fraternity. The detection process can be automated, which will be cost-effective, user-friendly, readily deployable, accurate, and time-saving.

In the current era, with various intuitive and innovative technologies, the healthcare sector has been upgraded. The identification and management of COVID-19 are also leveraged with these technologies. The most reliable and practiced techniques in the area are the X-ray and CT-scan analysis [6,7]. We may consider various artificial intelligence (AI) software tools as a solution in the extensive triage condition. AI deals with the research and development of techniques that resemble human intelligence, proving itself as a successful technique in various fields like robotics, computer vision, fraud detection, disease detection, patient monitoring, and drug discovery. With its success in disease detection, AI techniques can be considered a successful path to combat this pandemic. There are many applications where AI techniques can be implemented, which are based on clinical applications, pharmaceutical studies, processing COVID-19 related images, and epidemiology [8]. Deep learning-based approaches have shown noticeable results for the proper diagnosis of the disease in this present crisis. With the advancement in the area of deep learning and computer vision, medical imaging has shown revolutionary changes in recent years [9]. Deep learning-based approaches have proved themselves as successful applications for fast testing and detection of various diseases. Mostly CT-scan imaging is considered over X-ray imaging due to its three-dimensional pulmonary view and versatility [10,11]. Taking CT-scans and X-ray samples, deep learning-based systems investigate COVID-19 samples [12,13]. Many designs are also created using customized learning and also with pre-trained models using transfer learning [14–17]. Computer vision, machine learning (ML), and data science are also few areas for corona detection, outbreak prediction, and forecasting [18–20]. In addition to these techniques, big data, smartphone technology, and the Internet of things (IoT) are primarily used as a control measure for COVID-19 outbreak.

This chapter highlights the recent advancement in the COVID-19 detection system based on the analysis of X-ray and CT-scan samples. Further, the chapter contains a description of various deep learning methods used by researchers, with a focus on the pre-trained model like Residual Network (ResNet), which has been extensively used for diagnosis purposes [21–23]. For training, other models have also been used, which are discussed under the section related to custom deep learning techniques. A nomenclature or taxonomy is presented to properly segregate the methods under discussion. The chapter also focuses on the challenging aspects of the deep learning methods and presents a future research path for further expansion to the COVID-19 diagnosis system.

7.2 MATERIALS

To achieve the automated diagnosis of COVID-19, various datasets are collected from different sources used by the researchers. Among them, few databases are extensively used, whereas many of them are hospital data that are not publicly available. Most of these datasets have variable size images, and the population of the participants is not known. Depending on the frequency used, few databases are reviewed here, which may help the readers. As discussed earlier, the databases are categorized into X-ray and CT-scan images. Among the databases, the most used is the COVID-19 X-ray database [24]. It has a total of 589 samples, with 434 COVID-19 patients and 155 other category patients. It is publicly available, and the images vary in size. Kaggle chest X-ray repository dataset [25,26] consists of 5,856 samples, with 1,583 healthy and 4,273 pneumonia cases of X-ray images of different sizes. Another Kaggle dataset for X-ray images contains 79 samples with 1 COVID-19 case. RSNA pneumonia detection challenge dataset, with 30,227 samples consisting of 8,851 healthy and 21,376 infected cases, is also used for detection purposes [27]. NIH chest X-ray datasets consisting of 5,606 samples with an image size of $1,024 \times 1,024$ are also used [28]. This dataset contains only fixed-size images. Few datasets are collected from Radiopaedia.org, which is an open-edit radiology resource, where cases are put together by radiologists and various health professionals across the globe [29]. A total of 59 samples of various sizes are collected from this source. The database with the highest number of samples (224,316) is obtained from the ChexPert database, consisting of 65,240 samples, which has

14 different sub-categories to choose from [30]. The chest X-ray database contains 108,948 samples with 14 various lung diseases and healthy images. The COVIDDx Dataset comprises 13,870 individuals' data, totaling 13,975 samples, and is sub-categorized into three divisions containing 358 COVID-19, 8,066 healthy, and 5,538 pneumonia cases [31].

Apart from X-ray images, the COVID-CT database, collected from an open-source, consists of 271 patients with 812 samples, where 349 COVID-19 cases and 463 other cases CT-scan are present [32]. Two different COVID-19 named data-bases consist of 68 and 59 samples [29][33].

The variation in these databases makes it quite challenging to place them into some category. Moreover, with the increase in COVID-19 cases and the addition of new cases every day, it is pretty tough to keep track of these databases. Apart from all the limitations, these databases can be used for evaluation and validation purposes.

7.3 METHODS

The application of deep learning provided a helping hand to the researchers for computerized COVID-19 analysis using medical images. Deep learning is popular and presents the exact representation from the learned data. Generally, deep learning–based systems comprise collecting data, feature extraction, data prepara-tion, classification, and, lastly, evaluation of performance. New deep learning al-gorithms have been extensively used on X-ray and CT-scan images for coronavirus detection. Various deep learning pretrained models are designed considering con-volution neural networks (CNNs) for COVID-19 such as ResNet, GoogleNet, AlexNet, SqueezeNet, MobileNet, DenseNet, and U-Net [23][34–39]. Among these models, the preexisting CNN termed as Residual Network (ResNet) has shown outstanding results using various classification tasks. The following discussion will give insights into the ResNet algorithm and its advantages.

7.3.1 Residual Network

ResNet is a type of CNN introduced by Kaiming He and others in 2015 [23]. ResNet provides fast training of data and gives better performance of the parameters taken into consideration during the research work. Another advantage of con-sidering ResNet architecture is its ability to feed images of sizes other than that they are trained with [40].

Some additional layers are stacked in the deep neural network (DNN) to solve complex problems, resulting in better performance and accuracy. CNN, like AlexNet, has five convolution layers; the VGG network [41] has 19 layers; and GoogleNet (also codenamed Inception_v1) [42] has 22 layers. The reason behind adding more layers in these models is that these layers continuously learn more complex features. In image recognition, the layers may be divided as follows: layer one detects an image, layer two identifies textures, layer three detects objects, and so on. On the contrary, the traditional CNN models exhibit a maximum threshold for depth. Figure 7.1 describes the error percentage on training and testing data for a 20- and 56-layer network.

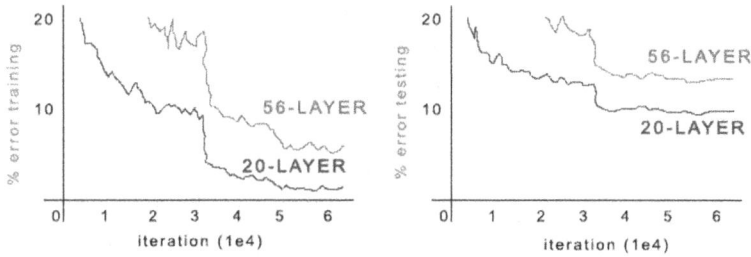

FIGURE 7.1 Test error (right) with training error (left) on CIFAR-10 with 56- and 20-layer "plain" networks [23].

From Figure 7.1, it is found that the 56-layer network gives more error percentage than that of a 20-layer network in the case of both training and testing data. The decrease in gradients due to backpropagation turns out to be the de-accelerating of the deep network algorithms with the increase in layers. Hence with an increase in the number of layers increases the error percentage in both training and testing data. Therefore, adding more layers on top of a network degrades the performance of the network. Since the error percentage of 56-layer networks lacks training and testing data, overfitting is not considered an issue. Instead, the network's initialization, optimization function, and vanishing gradient problem may be an issue [43].

The basic concept of ResNet is to initiate "identity shortcut connection," which helps to skip one or more layers in the system, as shown in Figure 7.2.

The stacking of identity mapping over the present network does not deteriorate the network performance, maintaining the architecture performance [23]. This means that deeper models are more training error-free than their shallower counterparts. Thus, the fitting of stacked layers to residual mapping is more spartan than the direct fit of desired underlying mapping. Hence, we may say residual blocks make it easier for layers to learn identity functions. The use of ResNet has significantly improved the performance of neural networks with one or more layers.

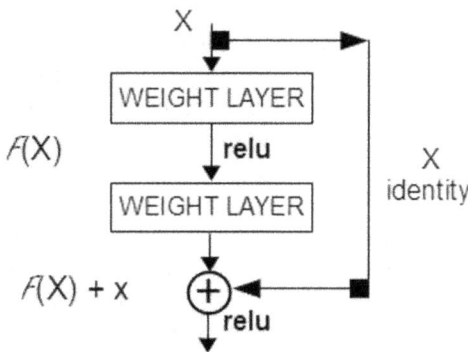

FIGURE 7.2 Residual learning: a building block [23].

The difference is more in the networks with 34 layers. ResNet-34 has a much lesser error percentage than plain-34. Also, from the plot, it is observed that the error percentage of ResNet-18 and plain-18 is almost the same.

7.3.1.1 ResNet Architecture

Inspired by VGG-19, the architecture of ResNet uses a 34-layer plain network in addition to its so-called identity shortcut connection. The shortcut connections then transform the architecture into a residual network, as referred by [23].

7.3.1.2 Using ResNet with Keras

Keras is a neural network library designed in Python and is skilled in controlling over TensorFlow, Microsoft Cognitive Toolkit, R, Theano, or PlaidML [40] during implementation. The primary purpose behind Keras is to increase the execution time of deep neural networks. Keras applications include the following implementations of ResNet and provide ResNet V1 and ResNet V2 with 50, 101, or 152 layers.

- ResNet50
- ResNet101
- ResNet152
- ResNet50V2
- ResNet101V2
- ResNet152V2

ResNetV2 is an updated version of the original ResNet V1 and uses batch normalization before each weight layer.

There are various updated ResNet networks proposed, which may be referred from Xie et al. [44], Huang et al. [38], Huang et al. [45], and Srivastava et al. [46]. With the recent advancement and efficiency of the ResNet algorithm, it is extensively used for COVID-19 detection with various Keras such as ResNet 18, ResNet 50, and ResNet 152, which is elaborated in the next section.

7.4 REVIEW AND DISCUSSION

The generalized representation for the COVID-19 diagnosis system is shown in Figure 7.3 about the deep learning technique. The data collected from the COVID-suspected patients from the hospitals may be of various types, but for analysis purposes, X-ray and CT-scan images are mainly taken into consideration. The next step is data pre-processing, where the collected data of the patients are converted into an appropriate format by using operations like noise removal and resizing. Next, the data are partitioned using a cross-validation technique with segments of training, validation, and testing. The training data are then evaluated by a validation process followed by the test data. The primary step of diagnosis process is based on feature extraction, which is followed by the classification into class with the labels of COVID-positive and COVID-negative. Finally, the overall diagnosis setup is evaluated using parameters like accuracy, precision, and specificity sensitivity.

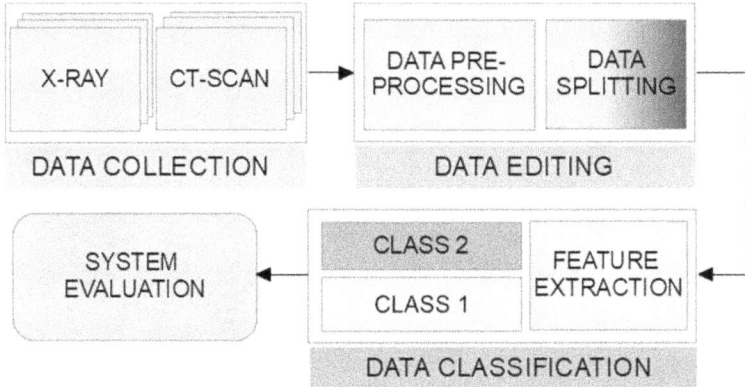

FIGURE 7.3   General block diagram for COVID-19 diagnosis system using deep learning.

Deep learning–based detection can be categorized based on two different perspectives:

- Pre-trained model with deep learning
- Deep learning on custom based

Pre-trained models are those where the data are already trained in the area that is similar to the application context. Deep transfer learning involves transferring weight and bias for training and retraining purposes to a new model similar to the trained parent model. General training models require more time and high computational power. Utilizing a pre-trained model advances the facility to accelerate convergence with network generalization [47,48]. Another technique, which is the custom deep learning technique, requires no previous weight and bias; hence, it is time-consuming and requires high computational power. Due to its specific application of interest, custom deep learning models deal with feasible architecture development, which is consistent and gives more accurate performance [5].

With its advantage over custom deep learning techniques, we focus on the pre-existing CNN, ResNet, and its utilization by various researchers to classify and diagnose COVID-19. The following section elaborates on the application of ResNet using both imaging modalities.

7.4.1   PRE-TRAINED MODEL WITH DEEP LEARNING RESNET

This section details on the application of ResNet on chest region X-ray and CT-scan images of probable COVID-19 diagnostic patients.

7.4.1.1   X-Ray and ResNet

Various methods based on X-ray image analysis using ResNet are presented in Table 7.1 [5], which summarizes the research findings. Almost all the algorithms have used the database COVID-19 X-ray image as the standard. Apart from COVID-19 X-ray image databases, other sources are used with multiple source

TABLE 7.1

Summary of Pre-Trained Deep Learning ResNet algorithm evaluation methods for COVID-19 detection on X-ray image [5]

Authors	Apostolopoulos and Bessiana [49]	Loey et al. [50]	Horry et al. [51]	Ozcan [52]	Sethy and Behra [53]	Minaee et al. [54]	Punn and Agarwal [55]	Narin et al. [56]	Bukharia et al. [57]	Abbas et al. [58]	Moutounet-Cartan [59]
Techniques	VGG19, MobileNetv2, Inception, Xception, Inception-ResNetv2	GAN, AlexNet, GoogleNet, ResNet18	VGG16, VGG19, ResNet50, Xception, Inception V3	ResNet50, ResNet18, GoogleNet	AlexNet, VGG-16, VGG-19, GoogleNet, ResNet18, 50, 101, InceptionV3, InceptionResNetV2, DenseNet201, XceptionNet, SVM	ResNet50, ResNet18, SqueezeNet, DenseNet-121	ResNet, Inception-v3, Inception, ResNet-v2, DenseNet169, NASNetL	ResNet50, Inception V3, Inception-ResNetv2	ResNet50	DeTraC-ResNet18	VGG16, VGG19, Inception, ResNetV2, Inception V3, Xception
Data Source	COVID-19 X-ray image database, Kaggle database, Kermany et al	COVID-19 X-ray image database, Database, Kermany et al	COVID-19 X-ray image database, NIH Chest X-ray	COVID-19 X-ray image database, Kaggle chest x-ray repository	COVID-19 X-ray image database, NIH Chest X-ray, Kaggle chest x-ray repository	COVID-19 X-ray image database, ChexPert	COVID-19 X-ray image database, RSNA	COVID-19 X-ray image database, Kaggle chest x-ray repository	COVID-19 X-ray image database, NIH Chest X-ray	COVID-19 X-ray image database, Japanese Society of Radiological Technology	COVID-19 X-ray image database, Kermany et al
Number of samples (Images)	Total-1442 COVID-19-224 Pneumonia-714 Normal-504	Total-307 COVID-19-69 Normal-79 Pneumonia bac-79 Pneumonia vir-79	Total-400 COVID-19-100 Pneumonia-100 Normal-200	Total-721 COVID-19-131 Normal-300 Bacteria-242 Virus-148	316	Total-5071 COVID-19-71 Non-COVID-19-5000	Total-1076 COVID-19-108 Pneumonia-515 Normal-453	Total-100 COVID-19-50 Normal-50	Total-278 COVID-19-89 Pneumonia-96 Normal-93	Total-196 COVID-19-105 SARS-11 Normal-80	Total-327 COVID-19-125 Pneumonia-50 Normal-152
Data partitioning	10-fold cross-validation	Training-80% Validation-10% Testing-10%	Training-80% Testing-20%	Training-50% Validation-20% Testing-30%	Training-60% Validation-20% Testing-20%	Training-40% Testing-60%	Training-80% Validation-10% Testing-10%	5-fold cross-validation	Training-80% Testing-20%	Training-70% Testing-30%	5-fold cross-validation
Performance Evaluation (%)	Accuracy-96.87 Specificity-96.46 Sensitivity-98.66	Sensitivity-100 Precision-100 Accuracy-100 F1-Score-100	Precision-83 F1-Score-80 Sensitivity-80	Accuracy-97.69 Specificity-97.90 Precision-95.95 Sensitivity-97.26 F1-Score-96.60	Accuracy-95.38 Sensitivity-97.47 F1-Score-95.52 MCC-91.41 FPR-95.52 Specificity-93.47 Precision-95.95 Kappa-90.76	Sensitivity-100 AUC-99.6 Specificity-95.6	Specificity-91 Precision-98 AUC-99 F1-Score-89 Accuracy-98 Sensitivity-91	Accuracy-98 Sensitivity-96 Specificity-100 Precision-100 F1-Score-98	Accuracy-98.18 Sensitivity-98.24 Precision-98.14 F1-Score-98.19	Accuracy-95.12 Sensitivity-97.91 Specificity-91.87 Precision-93.36	Accuracy-84.1 Sensitivity-87.7 AUC-97.4

data. Although the databases are composed of many images, the COVID-19 cases are deficient in number. The application of ResNet allows classifying the images with high accuracy and sensitivity. Cross-validation of 10-fold and 5-fold enhances the classification.

7.4.1.2 CT-scan and ResNet

Table 7.2 sums up almost every deep learning–based pre-trained model using ResNet technique on COVID-19 suspected CT-scan images.

The table highlights some specific factors like the total number of images used, data collection source, data partitioning techniques, and performance evaluation of various CNN networks.

7.4.2 CUSTOMIZED DEEP LEARNING METHODS

As discussed earlier, the customized deep learning methods are not pre-trained and do not require previous weights and bias. Various deep learning techniques used include support vector machine (SVM), CNN, radio frequency (RF), and capsule neural network (CAPS) [66–71].

The detailing of the methods used in COVID-19 diagnosis is summarized in Tables 7.3 and 7.4. The detail of the data source of X-ray and CT-scan images with image class partitioning and evaluation measures is referred to in these tables.

From Table 7.4, it is found that few custom network–based systems have shown better performance. The system's efficiency could not be compared as the databases are varied in nature, and most are not publicly available. Although the X-ray images exhibit better results, the CT-scan images provide more real-time information. Thus, analyzing CT images turn out to be more effective.

7.5 FUTURE SCOPE AND LIMITATIONS OF THIS STUDY

Deep learning algorithms, in general, are automated, robust systems but seek large amounts of data for evaluation. The application of the ResNet algorithm for COVID-19 detection is efficient in determining automated classification. Still, with the limitation of valid data, the efficiency gets reduced. These limitations of the COVID-19 datasets are mentioned in twofolds. First, the data available were not in any proper format, including inconclusive, noisy, incomplete, and unmarked formats. They lead to variation in preparations of the data before applying ResNet by varied authors. Also, during training, we encounter issues like data redundancy, sparsity, and non-availability of values. The second limitation is the availability of a minimal dataset of actual COVID patient data. With this limitation, the ResNet algorithm causes underfit or overfit problems when pre-trained models are not considered. The following limitation of the reviews lies in the evaluation parameter selection. Due to a standard database's unavailability, the authors have used varied images, and various parameters like sensitivity, specificity, F1-score, AUC, and ROC are evaluated. Therefore, we may not estimate which database or algorithm has high efficiency. Although we are moving ahead with using the X-ray and CT-scan analysis, the PCR-based RT–PCR method is still the standard and fast

TABLE 7.2

Summary of pre-trained deep learning ResNet algorithm evaluation methods for COVID-19 detection using CT-scan image [5]

Authors	Wu et al. [60]	Li et al. [61]	Yousefza deh et al. [62]	Jin et al. [63]	Xu et al. [64]	Jin et al. [65]
Techniques	ResNet50	ResNet50	DenseNet, ResNet, Xception, Efficient Net	ResNet152	ResNet18	DPN-92, Inception-V3, ResNet50, Attention ResNet50 with 3D U-NET++
Data Source	China Medical University and Beijing Youan Hospital	Multiple Hospitals	Real-time data from Hospitals	Three Different Hospitals of China, LIDC-IDRI, ILD-HUG	Zhejiang University, Hospital of Wenzhou, Hospital of Wenling	Five Different Hospitals of China
Number of samples (Images)	Total-495 COVID-19-368 Pneumonia-127	Total-4536 COVID-19-1296 CAP-1735 Non-pneumonia-1325	Total-2124 COVID-19-706 Non-COVID-19-1418	Total-1881 COVID-19-496 Non-COVID-19-1385	Total-618 COVID-19-219 Influenza-A-viral-pneumonia-224 Irrelevant-to-infection-175	Total-1391 COVID-19-850 Non-COVID-19-541
Data partitioning	Training-80% Validation-10% Testing-10%	Training-90% Testing-10%	Training-80% Validation-20%	Random partition	Training+Validation-85.4% Testing-14.6%	Random partition
Performance Evaluation (%)	Accuracy-76 Sensitivity-81.1 Specificity-61.5 AUC-81.9	Sensitivity-90 Specificity-96 AUC-96	Accuracy-96.4 Sensitivity-92.4 Specificity-98.3 AUC-98.9 F1-Score-95.3 Kappa-91.7	Accuracy-94.98 Sensitivity-94.06 Specificity-95.47 Precision-91.53 AUC-97.91 F1-Score-92.78 NPV-96.86 Youden Index89.53	Accuracy-86.7 Sensitivity-81.5 Precision-80.8 F1-Score-81.1	Sensitivity-97.04 Specificity-92.2 AUC-99.1

procedure for identifying COVID-19. Hence, we may also consider the image-based evaluation as an assistive measure. With these limitations and hindrances, we may suggest the proper formation and labeling of databases so that researchers may evaluate the ResNet or any other methods to its total capacity. Otherwise we may work on algorithms which may function on small size database. Another limitation of this review is the nonavailability of picture comparison of the results to

TABLE 7.3

Summary of customized deep learning algorithm evaluation methods for COVID-19 detection on X-Ray image [5]

Authors	Wang et al. [66]	Khan et al. [67]	Rahimzade h and Attar [68]	Alqudah et al. [69]	Farooq and Hafeez [70]	Afshar et al. [71]
Techniques	COVID-Net (CNN)	CoroNet (CNN)	Concatenated CNN	CNN, SVM, RF	COVID-ResNet (CNN)	COVID-CAPS (Capsule Network)
Data Source	COVID-19 X-ray image database, RSNA Pneumonia Detection challenge dataset	COVID-19 X-ray image database, Kaggle chest x-ray repository	COVID-19 X-ray image database, RSNA Pneumonia Detection challenge dataset	COVID-19 X-ray image database,	COVIDx Dataset	COVIDx Dataset
Number of samples (Images)	13,800	Total-1251 COVID-19-284 Normal-310 Pneumonia_bac-330 Pneumonia_vir-327	Total-15085 COVID-19-180 Pneumonia-6054 Normal-8851	Total-71 COVID-19-48 Non-COVID-23	13,800	13,800
Data partitioning	Training-90% Testing-10%	Training-80% Validation-20%	5-fold cross-validation	Training-70% Testing-30%	Training-90% Testing-10%	Training-90% Testing-10%
Performance Evaluation (%)	Accuracy-92.4 Sensitivity-80 Precision-88.9	Accuracy-89.5 Sensitivity-100 Precision-97 F1-Score-98	Accuracy-99.50 Sensitivity-80.53 Specificity-99.56 Precision-35.27	Accuracy-95.2 Sensitivity-93.3 Specificity-100 Precision-100	Accuracy-96.23 Sensitivity-100 Precision-100 F1-Score-100	Accuracy-95.7 Sensitivity-90 Precision-95.8 AUC-97

understand the detection process visually. Also, this review gives a glimpse of algorithms other than ResNet.

7.6 CONCLUSION

The COVID-19 continues to spread and mark its presence all over the world with evolutional new strains as time is progressing. In the present state, although most of the countries are equipped with vaccines, there is still no cure for the virus's progression and effects. The effect of the virus is more dangerous because asymptomatic patients who do not show any symptoms spread the virus unknowingly. Therefore, the steeping in of the AI systems to at least detect and isolate the patients is of utmost importance. Various AI and IoT devices have provided promising

TABLE 7.4

Summary of customized deep learning algorithm evaluation methods for COVID-19 detection using CT-scan image [5]

Authors	He et al. [72]	Zheng et al. [73]	Singh et al. [74]	Farid et al. [75]
Techniques	CRNet	DeCoVNet	MODE-CNN	CNN
Data Source	Italian Society of Medical and Interventional Radiology COVID-19 Database COvid-CT	Union Hospital Tongji Medical College Huazhong University of Science and Technology	Covid-19 patient chest CT images	Kaggle benchmark dataset
Number of samples (Images)	Total-746 COVID-19-349 Non-COVID-397	630	Total-150 COVID-19-75 Non-COVID-75	Total-102 COVID-19-51 SARS-51
Data partitioning	Training-60% Validation-15% Testing-25%	Training-80% Testing-20%	Various portions of training and testing dataset	10-fold-cross-validation
Performance Evaluation (%)	Accuracy-95.2 Sensitivity-93.3 Specificity-100 Precision-100	Accuracy-95.2 Sensitivity-93.3 Specificity-100 Precision-100	Accuracy-95.2 Sensitivity-93.3 Specificity-100 Precision-100	Accuracy-95.2 Sensitivity-93.3 Specificity-100 Precision-100

solutions for COVID-19, yet the detection of the patients by means of processes other than RT–PCR is still within research. The detection process using X-ray and CT-scan images is still referred to as an additional measure to the RT–PCR test. This chapter reviews the AI application in the area of deep learning algorithms with the stress into the rapidly explored method ResNet for COVID-19 analysis. The robustness of ResNet provides promising results, but still there is room for improvements. The chapter review provides discussion based on the taxonomy considered for the classification of the methods. The methods are primarily classified into the pretrained model, where the already -trained models with the similar type of the disease are retrained with the addition of COVID-19 data. The second method is the customized deep learning method to train the systems from scratch. The review also provides insights into the databases, which are publicly available for evaluation, and it is expected to be of great help for the researchers working in the area. The limitations in the present study are also outlined with respect to non-uniform valid databases and the hazards caused due to the lack of real-time COVID-19 data, which are a high necessity for the deep learning methods. The nonavailability of gold standards for evaluation is also reported. Further, the probable solutions and outcomes were also discussed. Although the deep learning algorithms on medical images for COVID-19 can be considered an additional measure of identification, in recent times they may also provide highly efficient and faster solution to the conventional RT–PCR screening. If not then, at least with early detection with AI, they may be helpful in reducing the spread of the virus.

REFERENCES

[1]. WHO COVID-19 Situation Reports. [Online]. Available: March 2021 https://www.who.int/emergencies/diseases/novel-coronavirus-2019/situation-reports, (2021).

[2]. Cascella M, Rajnik M, Cuomo A, Dulebohn SC and Di Napoli R. *Features, evaluation and treatment of coronavirus (covid-19). Statpearls [internet].* StatPearls Publishing, 2020.

[3]. Forni, D., Cagliani, R., Clerici, M. and Sironi, M. Molecular evolution of human coronavirus genomes. *Trends in Microbiology,* 25 (1), 35–48, (2017).

[4]. Harapan, H., Itoh, N., Yufika, A., Winardi, W., Keam, S., Te, H., Megawati, D., Hayati, Z., Wanger, A.L. and Mudatsir, M. Coronavirus disease 2019 (COVID-19): A literature review. *Journal of Infection and Public Health,* 13 (5), 667–673 doi: 10.1016/j.jiph.2020.03.01, 2020.

[5]. Islam, M. M., Karray, F., Alhajj, R. and Zeng, J. A review on deep learning techniques for the diagnosis of novel coronavirus (covid-19). *IEEE Access,* 9, 30551–30572, (2021).

[6]. J. P. Kanne, "Chest CT findings in 2019 novel coronavirus (2019-nCoV) infections from Wuhan, China: Key points for the radiologist." *Radiology,* 295 (1), 16–17, (Apr. 2020).

[7]. J. P. Kanne, "Chest CT findings in 2019 novel coronavirus (2019-nCoV) infections from Wuhan, China: Key points for the radiologist." *Radiology,* 295 (1), 16–17, (Apr. 2020).

[8]. Tayarani-N, M. H. Applications of artificial intelligence in battling against Covid-19: A literature review. *Chaos, Solitons & Fractals,* 110338, 1–60 (2020).

[9]. Mishra, A. K., Das, S. K., Roy, P. and Bandyopadhyay, S. Identifying COVID19 from chest CT images: A deep convolutional neural networks-based approach. *Journal of Healthcare Engineering,* 2020, 1–7 (2020).

[10]. H. Kim, H. Hong, S. H. Yoon, Diagnostic performance of CT and reverse transcriptase polymerase chain reaction for coronavirus disease 2019: A meta-analysis. *Radiology,* 296 (3), E145–E155 (Sep. 2020).

[11]. Z. Ye, Y. Zhang, Y. Wang, Z. Huang and B. Song, Chest CT manifestations of new coronavirus disease 2019 (COVID-19): A pictorial review. *European Radiology,* 30, (8), 4381–4389 (Aug. 2020).

[12]. X. Mei, H. C. Lee, K. Diao, M. Huang, B. Lin, C. Liu and Z. Xie, Artificial intelligence–enabled rapid diagnosis of patients with COVID19. *Nature Medicine,* 26 (8),1224–1228 (Aug. 2020).

[13]. L. Huang, R. Han, T. Ai, P. Yu, H. Kang, Q. Tao and L. Xia, Serial quantitative chest CT assessment of COVID-19: A deep learning approach. *Radiology: Cardiothoracic Imaging,* 2 (2), Art. no. e200075 (Apr. 2020).

[14]. H. Panwar, P. K. Gupta, M. K. Siddiqui, R. Morales-Menendez and V. Singh, Application of deep learning for fast detection of COVID-19 in X-rays using nCOVnet. *Chaos, Solitons & Fractals,* 138, Art. no. 109944, (Sep. 2020).

[15]. K. El Asnaoui and Y. Chawki, Using X-ray images and deep learning for automated detection of coronavirus disease. *Journal of Biomolecular Structure and Dynamics,* 7, 1–12 doi: 10.1080/07391102.2020.1767212, (May 2020).

[16]. Y. Oh, S. Park and J. C. Ye, Deep learning COVID-19 features on CXR using limited training data sets. *IEEE Transactions on Medical Imaging,* 39 (8), 2688–2700 (Aug. 2020).

[17]. R. M. Pereira, D. Bertolini, L. O. Teixeira, C. N. Silla and Y. M. G. Costa, COVID-19 identification in chest X-ray images on flat and hierarchical classification scenarios. *Computer Methods and Programs in Biomedicine,* 194, Art. no. 105532 (Oct 2020).

[18]. A. S. Albahri, R. A. Hamid, J. K. Alwan, Z. T. Al-Qays, A. A. Zaidan, B. B. Zaidan, A. O. S. Albahri, A. H. Alamoodi, J. M. Khlaf, E. M. Almahdi, E. Thabet, S. M. Hadi, K. I. Mohammed, M. A. Alsalem, J. R. Al-Obaidi and H. T. Madhloom, Role of biological data mining and machine learning techniques in detecting and diagnosing the novel coronavirus (COVID-19): A systematic review. *Journal of Medical Systems*, 44 (7), Art. no. 122 (Jul 2020).

[19]. L. J. Muhammad, M. M. Islam, S. S. Usman and S. I. Ayon, Predictive data mining models for novel coronavirus (COVID-19) infected patients' recovery. *Social Network Computer Science*, 1(4), Art. no. 206 (2020).

[20]. S. Latif, M. Usman, S. Manzoor, W. Iqbal and J. Qadir, Leveraging data science to combat COVID-19: A comprehensive review. *IEEE Transactions on Artificial Intelligence*, 1 (1), 85–103 (Aug. 2020).

[21]. Wu, X., Hui, H., Niu, M., Li, L., Wang, L., He, B., … and Zha, Y. Deep learning-based multi-view fusion model for screening 2019 novel coronavirus pneumonia: A multicentre study. *European Journal of Radiology*, 128, 109041 (2020).

[22]. Farooq, M. and Hafeez, A. Covid-resnet: A deep learning framework for screening of covid19 from radiographs. *arXiv preprint arXiv*: 2003, 14395 (2020).

[23]. K. He, X. Zhang, S. Ren and J. Sun, Deep residual learning for image recognition, arXiv:1512.03385. [Online]. Available: http://arxiv.org/abs/1512.03385, (2015).

[24]. J. P. Cohen, P. Morrison and L. Dao, "COVID-19 image data collection," arXiv:2003.11597. [Online]. Available: https://arxiv.org/abs/2003.11597, (2020).

[25]. Kaggle Chest X-ray Repository. Accessed:. [Online]. Available: https://www.kaggle.com/ paultimothymooney/chest-xraypneumonia, (Mar. 20, 2020).

[26]. Kaggle Dataset. Accessed: [Online]. Available: https://www.kaggle.com/andrewmvd/convid19-x-rays, (Mar. 15, 2020).

[27]. Radiological Society of North America. RSNA Pneumo-Nia Detection Challenge. Accessed:[Online].Available: https://www.kaggle.com/c/rsna-pneumoniadetection-challenge/data, (Mar. 10, 2020).

[28]. NIH Chest X-Ray. Accessed: [Online]. Available: https://openi.nlm.nih.gov/, (Mar. 16, 2020).

[29]. COVID-19. Accessed: [Online]. Available: https://radiopaedia.org, (Apr. 9, 2020).

[30]. J. Irvin, P. Rajpurkar, M. Ko, Y. Yu, C. Chute, R. Ball, J. Seekins, S. S. Halabi, R. Jones, D. B. Larson, C. P. Langlotz, B. N. Patel and M. P. Lungren, "CheXpert: A large chest radiograph dataset with uncertainty labels and expert comparison," In Proceedings of the AAAI Conference on Artificial Intelligence. 33, 590–597 (Jul. 2019).

[31]. L. Wang, Z. Q. Lin and A. Wong, COVID-net: A tailored deep convolutional neural network design for detection of COVID-19 cases from chest X-ray images. *Scientific Reports*, 10 (1), Art. no. 19549, (Dec. 2020).

[32]. X. Yang, X. He, J. Zhao, Y. Zhang, S. Zhang and P. Xie, COVID-CTdataset: A CT scan dataset about COVID-19, arXiv:2003.13865. [Online]. Available: http://arxiv.org/abs/2003.13865, (2020).

[33]. Italian Society of Medical and Interventional Radiology: COVID-19 Database. Accessed: [Online]. Available: https://www.sirm.org, (Mar. 28, 2020).

[34]. G. Zeng, Y. He, Z. Yu, X. Yang, R. Yang and L. Zhang, Preparation of novel high copper ions removal membranes by embedding organosilane-functionalized multi-walled carbon nanotube. *Journal of Chemical Technology & Biotechnology*, 91(8), 2322–2330 (Aug. 2016).

[35]. S. Das. CNN Architectures: LeNet, AlexNet, VGG, GoogLeNet, ResNet and More. [Online].Available: https://medium.com/analyticsvidhya/cnns-architectures-lenetalexnet-vgg-googlenet-resnet-andmore-666091488df5, (2017).

[36]. F. N. Iandola, S. Han, M. W. Moskewicz, K. Ashraf, W. J. Dally and K. Keutzer, SqueezeNet: AlexNet-level accuracy with 50x fewer parameters and <0.5MB model size, arXiv:1602.07360. [Online]. Available: http://arxiv.org/abs/1602.07360, (2016).

[37]. Z. Qin, Z. Zhang, X. Chen, C. Wang and Y. Peng, Fd-mobilenet: Improved mobilenet with a fast downsampling strategy, In Proceedings of the 25th IEEE International Conference on Image Processing (ICIP), 1363–1367, (Oct. 2018).

[38]. G. Huang, Z. Liu, L. Van Der Maaten and K. Q. Weinberger, Densely connected convolutional networks, In Proceedings of the IEEE Conference on Computer Vision and Pattern Recognition (CVPR), 2261–2269, (Jul. 2017).

[39]. O. Ronneberger, P. Fischer and T. Brox, U-Net: Convolutional networks for biomedical image segmentation, In Proceedings of the International Conference on Medical Image Computing and Computer-Assisted Intervention, 234–241, (2015).

[40]. Resnet [Online]. Available: https://www.mygreatlearning.com/blog/resnet/, (March 2021).

[41]. K. Simonyan and A. Zisserman. Very deep convolutional networks for large-scale image recognition. *arXiv preprint arXiv*, 1409, 1556 (2014).

[42]. C. Szegedy, W. Liu, Y. Jia, P. Sermanet, S. Reed, D. Anguelov, D. Erhan, V. Vanhoucke, A. Rabinovich. Going deeper with convolutions. In Proceedings of the IEEE Conference on Computer Vision and Pattern Recognition, pp. 1–9 (2015).

[43]. Resnet [Online]. Available: https://towardsdatascience.com/an-overview-of-resnet-andits- variants-5281e2f56035, (March 2021).

[44]. S. Xie, R. Girshick, P. Dollar, Z. Tu and K. He. Aggregated residual transformations for deep neural networks. *arXiv preprint arXiv*, 1611, 05431v1 (2016).

[45]. G. Huang, Y. Sun, Z. Liu, D. Sedra and K. Q. Weinberger. Deep Networks with Stochastic Depth. *arXiv*, 1603, 09382v3 (2016).

[46]. N. Srivastava, G. Hinton, A. Krizhevsky, I. Sutskever and R. Salakhutdinov. Dropout: A Simple Way to Prevent Neural Networks from Overfitting. *The Journal of Machine Learning Research,* 15 (1), 1929–1958 (2014)

[47]. A. Elhassouny and F. Smarandache, ''Trends in deep convolutional neural networks architectures: A review,'' In Proceedings of the International Conference on Computer Science and Renewable Energies (ICCSRE), 1–8, doi: 10.1109/ICCSRE.2019.8807741, (Jul. 2019).

[48]. M. Z. Alom, T. M. Taha, C. Yakopcic, S. Westberg, P. Sidike, M. S. Nasrin, M. Hasan, B. C. Van Essen, A. A. S. Awwal and V. K. Asari, A State of-the-Art survey on deep learning theory and architectures. *Electronics*, 8 (3), 292 (Mar. 2019).

[49]. D. Apostolopoulos and T. A. Mpesiana, COVID-19: Automatic detection from X-ray images utilizing transfer learning with convolutional neural networks. *Physical and Engineering Sciences in Medicine*, 43 (2), 635–640 (Jun. 2020).

[50]. M. Loey, F. Smarandache and N. E. M. Khalifa, Within the lack of chest COVID-19 X-ray dataset: A novel detection model based on GAN and deep transfer learning. *Symmetry*, 12 (4), 651 (Apr. 2020).

[51]. M. J. Horry, M. Paul, A. Ulhaq, B. Pradhan and M. Saha, X-ray image based COVID-19 detection using pre-trained deep learning models, Engrxiv, to be published. [Online]. Available: https://engrxiv.org/wx89s/

[52]. T. Ozcan. A Deep Learning Framework for Coronavirus Disease (COVID-19) Detection in X-Ray Images. [Online]. Available: https://www.researchsquare.com/article/rs-26500/v1, (2020).

[53]. S. K. B. Sethy and P. Kumar. Detection of Coronavirus Disease (COVID-19) Based on Deep Features. [Online]. Available: https://www.preprints.org/manuscript/202003.0300/ v1, (2020).

[54]. S. Minaee, R. Kafieh, M. Sonka, S. Yazdani and G. Jamalipour Soufi, Deep-COVID: Predicting COVID-19 from chest X-ray images using deep transfer learning. *Medical Image Analysis*, 65, Art. no. 101794, (Oct. 2020).

[55]. N. S. Punn and S. Agarwal, Automated diagnosis of COVID-19 with limited posteroanterior chest X-ray images using fine-tuned deep neural networks. *International Journal of Speech Technology*, 15, 1–14, doi: 10.1007/s10489-020-01900-3, (Oct. 2020).

[56]. A. Narin, C. Kaya and Z. Pamuk, Automatic detection of coronavirus disease (COVID-19) using X-ray images and deep convolutional neural networks, arXiv:2003.10849. [Online]. Available: http://arxiv.org/abs/2003.10849, (2020).

[57]. S. Bukhari, S. Bukhari, A. Syed and S. Shah, The diagnostic evaluation of Convolutional Neural Network (CNN) for the assessment of chest X-ray of patients infected with COVID-19,'' MedRxiv, [Online]. Available: https://www.medrxiv.org/content/10.1101/2020.03.26.20044610v1, (Jan. 2020).

[58]. A. Abbas, M. M. Abdelsamea and M. M. Gaber, Classification of COVID-19 in chest X-ray images using DeTraC deep convolutional neural network. *Applied Intelligence*, 8, 1–11, [Online]. Available: 10.1007/s10489-020-01829-7, (Sep. 2020).

[59]. P. G. Moutounet-Cartan, Deep convolutional neural networks to diagnose covid-19 and other pneumonia diseases from posteroanterior chest x-rays, *arXiv preprint arXiv*, 2005.00845, 1–17, (2020).

[60]. X. Wu, H. Hui, M. Niu, L. Li, L. Wang, B. He and X. Yang, Deep learning-based multi-view fusion model for screening 2019 novel coronavirus pneumonia: A multi-centre study. *European Journal of Radiology*, 128, Art. no. 109041, (Jul. 2020).

[61]. L. Li, L. Qin, Z. Xu, Y. Yin, X. Wang, B. Kong, J. Bai and Y. Lu, Artificial intelligence distinguishes COVID-19 from community acquired pneumonia on chest CT. *Radiology*, 19, Art. no. 200905 (Mar. 2020).

[62]. M. Yousefzadeh, P. Esfahanian and S. Movahed, Ai-corona: Radiologist-assistant deep learning framework for COVID-19 diagnosis in chest ct scans, MedRxiv, [Online]. Available: https://www.medrxiv.org/content/10.1101/2020.05.04.20082081v1, (Jan. 2020).

[63]. C. Jin et al., Development and evaluation of an artificial intelligence system for COVID-19 diagnosis. *Nature Communications*, 11 (1), 5088 (Dec. 2020).

[64]. X. Xu, X. Jiang, C. Ma, P. Du, X. Li, S. Lv, L. Yu, Y. Chen, J. Su, G. Lang, Y. Li, H. Zhao, K. Xu, L. Ruan and W. Wu, Deep learning system to screen coronavirus disease 2019 pneumonia, arXiv:2002.09334. [Online]. Available: http://arxiv.org/abs/2002. 09334, (2020).

[65]. S. Jin, B. Wang, H. Xu, C. Luo, L. Wei, W. Zhao and X. Hou, AI-assisted CT imaging analysis for COVID-19 screening: Building and deploying a medical AI system in four weeks, MedRxiv, [Online]. Available: https://www.medrxiv.org/content/10.1101/ 2020.03.19.20039354v1, (2020).

[66]. L. Wang, Z. Q. Lin and A. Wong, COVID-net: A tailored deep convolutional neural network design for detection of COVID-19 cases from chest X-ray images. *Scientific Reports*, 10 (1), Art. no. 19549 (Dec. 2020).

[67]. A. I. Khan, J. L. Shah and M. M. Bhat, CoroNet: A deep neural network for detection and diagnosis of COVID-19 from chest X-ray images, *Computer Methods and Programs in Biomedicine*, 196, Art. no. 105581 (Nov. 2020).

[68]. M. Rahimzadeh and A. Attar, A modified deep convolutional neural network for detecting COVID-19 and pneumonia from chest X-ray images based on the concatenation of xception and ResNet50 V2. *Informatics in Medicine Unlocked*, 19, Art. no. 100360 (2020).

[69]. A. M. Alqudah, S. Qazan, H. Alquran, I. A. Qasmieh and A. Alqudah. COVID-2019 detection using X-ray images and artificial intelligence hybrid systems. [Online].

Available: https://www.researchgate.net/publication/340232556_Covid-2019_Detection_Using_XRay_Images_And_Artificial_Intelligence_Hybrid_Systems, (2020).

[70]. M. Farooq and A. Hafeez, COVID-ResNet: A deep learning framework for screening of COVID19 from radiographs, arXiv:2003.14395. [Online]. Available: http://arxiv.org/abs/2003.14395, (2020).

[71]. P. Afshar, S. Heidarian, F. Naderkhani, A. Oikonomou, K. N. Plataniotis and A. Mohammadi, COVID-CAPS: A capsule network-based framework for identification of COVID-19 cases from X-ray images. *Pattern Recognition Letters*, 138, 638–643 (Oct. 2020).

[72]. S. Wang, B. Kang, J. Ma, X. Zeng, M. Xiao, J. Guo ... and B. Xu, A deep learning algorithm using CT images to screen for Corona Virus Disease (COVID-19). *European Radiology*, 1–9 (Jan. 2020).

[73]. C. Zheng, X. Deng, Q. Fu, Q. Zhou, J. Feng, H. Ma ... and X. Wang, Deep learning-based detection for COVID-19 from chest CT using weak label. *MedRxiv*, 1–13 (2020).

[74]. D. Singh, V. Kumar, M. Kaur, Classification of COVID-19 patients from chest CT images using multi-objective differential evolution–based convolutional neural networks, *European Journal of Clinical Microbiology & Infectious Diseases*. 39 (7), 1379–1389 (2020).

[75]. A. A. Farid, G. I. Selim and H. A. A. Khater, A novel approach of CT images feature analysis and prediction to screen for coronavirus disease (COVID-19). [Online]. Available: https://www.preprints.org/manuscript/202003.0284/v1, (2020).

8 Clinical Impact of COVID on Diabetic Patients

Surekha Manhas, Zaved Ahmed Khan, and Meenu Gupta

CONTENTS

8.1 BACKGROUND

The current disastrous outbreak of dreadful, rapidly spread COVID-19 (coronavirus disease), caused by SARS-CoV-2 (severe acute respiratory syndrome coronavirus-2), spreads continuously. On August 5, the cumulative number of COVID19 cases worldwide exceeded 200 million, and it was only six months before reaching 100 million cases. This week alone, more than 4.2 million new cases and more than 65,000 new deaths were reported, a slight increase compared to the previous week.

DOI: 10.1201/9781003171829-8

149

The Americas Region (14%) and the Western Pacific Region (19%) reported the largest increase in the proportion of new cases, reporting 1.3 million and more than 375,000 new cases, respectively. In addition, the number of new deaths reported in the Western Pacific Region increased significantly this week (46%) .Of the 228 member states and territories, 38 (17%) reported a 50% increase in new cases from the previous week, and 34 (15%) reported a 50% increase in new deaths. Reference: WHO COVID-19 REPORTS Weekly epidemiological update on COVID-19 - 10 August 2021 (who.int). As of April 2, 2020, it has overtaken 205 countries with 900,306 confirmed cases and 45,693 deaths [1,2]. On December 31, 2019, the office of the World Health Organization (WHO) of China was informed about the pneumonia cases associated with unknown etiology that were identified in Wuhan city, Hubei Province of China. National Authentic of China reported 44 total cases of pneumonia with unknown etiology to the WHO [2]. At that time, the disease causative agent was not identified. WHO came in contact with other detailed information about the cases of unknown causes provided by the National Health Commission of China that the outbreak of this unknown disease was associated with the seafood market in Wuhan city. Director General of WHO, Tedras Ahamon Ghebreyesus, on March 5, stated that at this moment, the outbreak situation might be unable to control in some settings. Yet it is not uncontrollable, and it would be the beginning to pass for a statement of the meaning of a pandemic [1].

8.2   INTRODUCTION

Coronaviruses are positive-sense RNA viruses that are enveloped and non-segmented and belong to Coronaviridae family, Nidovirales order. The highly contagious beta-coronavirus has the potential to cause COVID-19, named by WHO on February 11, 2020. The entire population is highly prone to this alarming disease; contact and respiratory droplets are the primary routes of transmission [3,4]. COVID-19 targets the epithelial cells of the alveoli of lungs by using receptor-mediated endocytosis like all other viruses via ACE2 (angiotensin-converting enzyme II) as an opening receptor. In the case of symptomatic patients, symptoms start appearing after not more than a week, including cough, fever, fatigue, nasal congestion, and other signs associated with the infection of the upper respiratory tract. The infection could progress to a severe state with dyspnea and pneumonia with severe chest pain, symptoms that could be seen by computer tomography which have been seen in case of 75% of infected individuals approximately. After second and third weeks in the case of symptomatic infection, pneumonia occurs mostly [5].

8.3   REPLICATION AND PATHOGENESIS OF CORONAVIRUS

In humans, cell receptor ACE is found in the lower respiratory tract. Also known as SARS-CoV cell receptor, it plays a role in the regulation of transmission among human beings or within cross-species [6,7]. After examining the isolated bronchoalveolar lavage fluid (BALF) taken from COVID-19 patients, it was confirmed that SARS-CoV-2 uses the same cellular receptor for entry as SARS-CoV [8].

Coronavirus carries virion S-glycoprotein on its surface that can attach to the cellular ACE receptor present on the human cell surface [9]. S-glycoprotein consists of two main subunits S1 and S2 in which S1 determines cellular tropism and a range of host susceptibility for virus. The role of S2 is not clearly mentioned in paper. RBD domain plays a vital role, while tandem domains, HR1 (heptad repeats 1) and HR2, fuse with the cell membrane of the virus, a process mediated by the S2 subunit [10,11]. After the fusion of cellular membranes, the viral RNA get s released into the cellular matrix or cytoplasm, and pp1a and pp1ab, two polypeptides, are translated by the uncoated viral RNA, which encode unstructured proteins to form RTC (replication transcription complex) in double-membrane vesicles [12,13].

Subgenomic RNAs get synthesized by the continuous replication of RTC that encodes structural proteins and accessory proteins. Mediating Golgi, endoplasmic reticulum (ER), nucleocapsids protein, envelope glycoproteins, and genomic RNA (newly formed) assemble and then form buds of viral particles. At last, the virion consists of vesicle fuse with the cellular membrane to deliver the virus. Spike (S)-glycoprotein and ACE receptor binding is a very crucial step for the entry of the virus; binding between the virus and the ACE receptor is an intensively studied approaches. β-CoV receptor detection was done systematically, which showed that ACE-2 was expressed in human cells but not APN (aminopeptidase N) and peptidase-4 (DPP4) improved SARS-CoV-2 entrance, while other studies showed that the binding efficiency of ACE-2 and the virus is 10–20 folds higher than that of SARS-CoV [14].

In case of SARS-CoV, trimer S protein cleavage is triggered by cathepsin and TMPRSS2 (transmembrane protease serine 2), when membrane invagination is facilitated by other possible molecules for the endocytosis of SARS-CoV-2; still, it's not clear yet [15,16]. Available data stated that the virulence of SARS-CoV-2 might be less than that of MERS-SoV and SARS-CoV; COVID-19 mortality is 3.9% lower than the MERS death rate (35%) and SARS-CoV (9.6%) [17]. Thus, SARS-CoV-2 pathogenic mechanisms and transmission mechanisms are covered by extensive studies.

8.4 COVID-19 TRANSMISSION

Various studies suggested that bat might be the potent source of SARS-CoV-2 infection occurred in the seafood market in China. The genome sequencing of the deadly virus showed 96.2% genome similarities with bat genome sequence. Studies proposed that there might be the same ancestor for SARS-CoV-2 in humans and bat CoV, although in seafood market bats are usually not sold. SARS-CoV-2 transmission among humans mainly occurs between members of a family when one member comes in contact with an infected one or a carrier one or any other COVID patient [4].

8.5 CLINICAL COURSE (COVID-19)

The median incubated period is estimated to be around 5–6 days (within the range of 0–14 days). The median estimated age of confirmed cases was about 59 years. By the analysis of the initial data, it was found that around more than 80% patients had the mild disease or asymptomatic disease and recovered, except that only 15% had severe infection, including pneumonia; the rest of 15% was critically unwell with respiratory and multiorgan failure. Although the estimated fatality rate was about 2% overall, it was 14.8% in people over age 80, 0.2% in cases of those under age 50, and higher in people with chronic comorbid conditions [18].

8.6   CRITERIA FOR DIAGNOSIS

SARS-CoV-2 preliminary identification was done by electron microscopy in the viral research institute (China) to examine its morphology. So far, another golden clinical approach for COVID-19 diagnosis is the detection of the nucleic acid in respiratory tract samples, nasal swabs, and throat samples by using RT-PCR. Further confirmation is done by next-generation sequencing [4].

8.7   AVAILABLE CLINICAL THERAPIES FOR COVID-19 PATIENTS

Till now, no therapeutic drug is approved by US Food and Drug Administration (FDA) to treat or prevent COVID-19. Current approaches in clinical management to somehow control the disease include the control and preventive measures with supportive care, along with supplemental oxygen or mechanical ventilator support when needed. A number of different antiviral drugs are being used to treat COVID-19 infection, for example, remdesivir (intravenous antiviral drug) that has activity against SARS-CoV-2 in vitro. Chloroquine and hydroxychloroquine are under clinical trials for pre- or post-exposure of SARS-CoV-2 infection prophylaxis. Other drugs are also under clinical trials. Numerous immunotherapies, antiviral agents, and vaccines are being explored and developed as potent therapies [19,20].

8.8   CURRENT UPDATED STATUS OF CORONAVIRUS

8.8.1   Situation Report 1: January 31, 2020

In China, there were totally 9,720 cases, in which 213 deaths have been reported. On January 31, 2020, Wuhan city is the epicentre of this initial commencement, which has extended promptly to all regions of China. Along with China, 19 other countries—Nepal, Canada, Australia, India, UAE, Vietnam, Sri Lanka, USA, Philippines, South Korea, Malaysia, Finland, Cambodia, Thailand, Singapore, France, Italy, Germany, and Japan—had reported 106 confirmed COVID cases.

In India, on January 30, 2020, a case was confirmed in the laboratory that was reported in Kerala. It was a student who returned from china (Wuhan city), and his health condition was stable. The 2019-nCoV situation has been closely monitored by the Prime Minister's Office and MoHFW (the Ministry of Health, Family and Welfare) and to reinforce preparedness efforts.

Preparedness efforts for the public health, including infection preventive measures, surveillance, hospital preparedness and diagnostic preparedness, diagnostics are regularly surveyed by national and state health authorities to lower the risk. SHOC (Strategic Health Operations Centre room) has activated by NCDC (National Centre for Disease Control) in order to give instructions to control functions along with the helpline facility (+91-11-23978046) to resolve public queries. The Pune National Institute of Virology has been equipped with the expertise of international standards and capacity in which 49 nCoV samples were tested of which 48 samples were reported negative. From January 31, 2020, 12 additional laboratories have commenced functioning: those are KIPMR, Chennai; SMS, Jaipur; ICMR—NICED, Kolkata; NCDC, New Delhi; Victoria Hospital Campus, Bengaluru; NIV, Kerala; GGMC, Nagpur; NIV, Bengaluru; NIV, Nagpur; KGMU, Lucknow; Kasturba Hospital for Infectious Diseases, Mumbai; and GMC, Secunderabad [21].

8.8.2 SITUATION REPORT 2: FEBRUARY 6, 2020

On February 6, 2020, 28,267 COVID cases had been confirmed among 28 different countries in which 565 deaths were reported (563 in china, 1 in Hong Kong, and 1 in the Philippines). In India, three cases were confirmed in Kerala: one was from Kasaragod, another one from Thrissur, and the third one from Alapuzha. Samples of 223 suspected cases had been sent to ICMR-NIV for confirmation in which 193 samples were marked as negative, and only 3 were positive. Results of the rest of samples were pending [22].

8.8.3 SITUATION REPORT 3: FEBRUARY 13, 2020

According to WHO global updated data, there were 45,177 total cases confirmed in 25 different countries in which a number of reported deaths was 1,369 (1,368 in China and 1 in the Philippines). From January 30 to February 3, three cases of COVID-19 were reported in India. These infected patients were in stable condition and regularly monitored by expertise in isolation. As on February 13, 389 samples had been sent to NIV in Kerala in which 354 examples had been tested negative and other remaining tested samples were pending [23].

8.8.4 SITUATION REPORT 4: FEBRUARY 21, 2020

As on February 20, 2020, 74,748 COVID cases (548 new) had been confirmed in which China was at the top level,with the total cases of 74,675 (399 new); 2,121 deaths were reported in China, in which 115 were from the latest cases. Outside China, a total of 1,073 cases had been confirmed (149 new), among 26 different countries that led to 8 deaths. Between January 30 and February 3, 2020, only three cases had been confirmed that had recovered fully and discharged from the hospital. No further new COVID cases were reported till February 21 [24].

8.8.5 SITUATION REPORT 5: FEBRUARY 28, 2020

Till February 28, this deadly virus had infected 82,294 people globally, with 1,185 new suspected cases. On the other hand, China had reached up to 78,630 cases, in which 439 were new, and it reported 2,747 deaths. In India, till then, no new cases were reported [25].

8.8.6 SITUATION REPORT 6: MARCH 9, 2020

As of March 9, 2020, 109,577 people had been exposed to the viral infection, with 3,809 deaths. Forty-four cases had been confirmed in different states of India, including Uttar Pradesh (9), Tamil Nadu (1), Ladakh (2), Telangana (1), Rajasthan (2), Delhi (4), Punjab (1), Jammu (1), Kerala (9), and Haryana (14) [26].

8.8.7 SITUATION REPORT 7: MARCH 14, 2020

As of March 14, 2020, a total of 132,758 cases had been reported along with 4,955 deaths worldwide. On March 14, 84 cases were confirmed, in which 17 were foreign nationals; 10 were cured, and reported deaths were 2, in which one was a 76-year-old male who was from Karnataka and the other one was a 68-year-old female who was from Delhi [27].

8.8.8 SITUATION REPORT 8: MARCH 22, 2020

On March 22, 2020, globally, 266,073 individuals had lapsed into the chronic infection, with 11,184 deaths. Confirmed cases had reached up to 360 from 84, with 7 deaths including Punjab (1), Maharashtra (2), Gujarat (1), Delhi (1), Karnataka (1), and Bihar (1) [28].

8.8.9 SITUATION REPORT 9: MARCH 28, 2020

Globally the world had reached up to 462,684 confirmed COVID-19 cases and 20,834 deaths till March 28. In India, 909 cases were confirmed, and 19 deaths were reported [29]. Indian Prime Minister Mr. Narendra Modi issued an order under section 6(2)(i), Disaster Management Act, 2005, which prescribed lockdown for 21 days for the containment of the virus epidemic.

8.8.10 SITUATION REPORT 10: APRIL 5, 2020

As of April 5, 2020, 1,051,635 COVID cases had been confirmed, along with 56,985 deaths all over the world. In India, cases had raised up to 3,577 confirmed cases and 83 deaths; 274 had been discharged [30]. An order was issued by MoHFW for insurance cover to health workers up to 90 days under the scheme "Pradhan Mantri Garib Kalyan Package: Insurance Scheme for Health Workers Fighting COVID-19."

8.8.11 SITUATION REPORT 11: APRIL 9, 2020

In 31 different states of India, 5,734 cases had confirmed and 166 deaths were reported on April 9 [31]. WHO representative, Dr. Henk Bekedam, to overcome this unprecedented health challenge situation, announced that WHO stood together with the government of India in its firm resolve (Tables 8.1 and 8.2).

TABLE 8.1
Number of confirmed cases and deaths globally

Date	Number of confirmed cases	Deaths
January 31	9,826	213
February 6	28,276 (3,722 new)	565
February 13	46,997 (1,826)	1,369
February 21	76,769 (1,021)	2,247
February 28	83,652 (1,358)	2,858
March 9	109,577 (3,993)	3,809
March 14	142,534 (9,764)	5,392
March 22	292142(26,069)	12,783
April 5	1,133,758 (82,061)	62,784
April 8	1,353,361 (73,639)	79,235

[1]   The mortality rate was 3.4% on March 9, but it increased up to 5.8% on April 8, 2020 [21–31].

TABLE 8.2
Number of confirmed COVID-19 cases and deaths in India

Date	Number of Confirmed Cases	Deaths
January 31	1	0
February 6	3	0
February 13	3	0
February 21	3	0
March 9	3	0
March 14	84	2
March 22	360	7
March 28	909	19
April 5	3,577	83
April 9	5,734	166

[1]   On March 14, the mortality rate was 2.3% in India and has reached up to 2.89% on April 9 [21–31].

8.9   ANY POSSIBLE RELATIONSHIP OF COVID-19 INFECTION WITH DIABETIC PATIENTS

By January 2, 41 patients were identified to have 2019-nCOV infection in the laboratory in Wuhan, 49% (20) of infected individuals were aged between 25 and 49 years, 34% (14) of the patients were aged between 50 and 64 years. The median age of infected patients was found to be 49 years. Within the first 41 patients, no adolescents or children were infected; men were mostly infected (73%) in which less than half of the patients (32%) already had underlying diseases including hypertension (15%), diabetes (20%), and cardiovascular diseases (15%) [32]. At the onset of the illness, most common symptoms were fever (98%), fatigue, or myalgia and cough, whereas symptoms that were less common included sputum production (28%), headache, diarrhea, and haemoptysis. Dyspnea was developed by more than half of the infected persons. The median duration from the onset of the illness to dyspnea was 8 days [32].

Since March 28, 2020, 122,653 total cases of COVID-19 were confirmed in the lab and 2,113 deaths were reported to the CDC (Centre for Disease Control) in the US. Case report forms of 60.7% (74,439) cases were submitted to the CDC, based on the available data of 7,162 (5.8%) patients analyzed to identify other underlying health conditions with other recognized risk-causing factors, which might be responsible for more disease severity or respiratory infections. Approximately, 2,692 (37.6%) of patients had already suffered from at least one underlying health condition or any other risk factors, in which 784 (10.9%) were reported with diabetes mellitus, 656 (9.2%) with other chronic health condition, and 647 (9.0%) with cardiovascular diseases [33].

Among 72,314 total case records, confirmed COVID-19 cases were 44,672, contributed up to 62%; 16,186 (22%) were considered suspected cases; 10,567 (15%) cases were diagnosed and 889 (1%) cases were reported as asymptomatic cases. Overall case fatality rate (CFR) was 2.3% that encompassed 1,023 deaths among confirmed cases (44,672). At age 9 years or younger, no deaths were reported. The case fatality rate was 8% for the ages of 70–74 years and 14.8% in those who were 80 years old and older. Those who had underlying comorbid health conditions, the case fatality rate was elevated, 7.3% in cases of diabetes, 5.6% in cases of cancer, 10.5% in cases of cardiovascular diseases, 6% for hypertension, and 6.3% for chronic respiratory infections [34].

The severity of diseases has varied from moderate self-limiting symptoms of flu-type illness that leads to fulminant pneumonia and death due to respiratory failure. Mortality rate varies with regional variations. It is estimated that COVID-19 data keeps changing due to increasing number of cases. Diabetic patients are at high risk of infections, especially of pneumonia and influenza. By glycemic control, risk cannot be eliminated but can be controlled or reduced to some extent. According to previously available data, diabetes had also been seen as one of the important risk aspects of mortality in infected patients of MERS-CoV (Middle East respiratory syndrome coronavirus), HINI (pandemic influenza A 2009), and SARS (severe acute respiratory syndrome). At present, data related to COVID-19-infected diabetic patients is limited [35]. Data from studies of smaller cohorts comprising of 140 patients from Wuhan city, China, suggested that in case of disease-severity cases, diabetes was not considered as a risk factor [36].

From the new data released by Centers for Disease Control and Prevention, it was found that individuals, who are already associated with other chronic medical health challenges including diabetes or other heart diseases, face higher chances of being hospitalized when infected with COVID-19 and being admitted into intensive care. Although the severity of the disease has been seen among older ones, risk also gets increased in people with underlying health conditions if they come in contact with the virus in future. Seven thousand confirmed cases of COVID-19 were analyzed by the CDC across the country, and records had been written by health officials about the presence of any other pre-existing underlying health challenges. The pre-existing health challenges covered in the official records include neurological disorders, intellectual disability, diabetes, immunocompromised conditions, and lung diseases. After analyzing the available data, 10.9% of patients already had diabetes mellitus (DM), 9% had cardiovascular disease, and 9.2% had chronic lung disease. But the official report could not reach to the conclusion about whether people with underlying health conditions are correlated to a serious COVID-19 illness condition [37].

Available data is not enough that could show whether diabetic patients are more prone to get COVID-19 infection than the general population. In China more cases of diabetic people are associated with serious complications and death at a very high rate compared to other non-diabetic patients. Risk of getting infected from COVID-19 is reduced when diabetes is well managed or controlled, whereas other diabetic patients who does not control their diabetes experience fluctuation in their blood sugar level that ultimately increases the risk of several other diabetes-related complications. COVID-19 infection in a diabetic patient could increase inflammation and internal swelling too, which might be due to the above-target blood glucose level that leads to more severe health complications [38].

From February 24 to March 9, 2020, 24 critically ill COVID-19 patients' cases were identified at the survey of nine hospitals. The common thing was a chronic health condition in critically infected population in which 14 patients (58%) already had DM, 3 (14%) patients had asthma, 5 (21%) had kidney disease, 5 (22%) were smokers, 1 (4%) with chronic obstructive pulmonary disease, and the rest had more than one single health condition [39].

8.10   CONCLUSION

COVID-19 outbreak swept across disease originated country China and has spread to 210 countries/areas/territories, with total confirmed cases of about 1,700,378 and 102,755 reported deaths till April 11. On August 5, the cumulative number of COVID19 cases worldwide exceeded 200 million, and it was only six months before reaching 100 million cases. This week alone, more than 4.2 million new cases and more than 65,000 new deaths were reported, a slight increase compared to the previous week. The Americas Region (14%) and the Western Pacific Region (19%) reported the largest increase in the proportion of new cases, reporting 1.3 million and more than 375,000 new cases, respectively. In addition, the number of new deaths reported in the Western Pacific Region increased significantly this week (46%). Of the 228 member states and territories, 38 (17%) reported a 50% increase in new cases from the previous week, and 34 (15%) reported a 50% increase in new deaths.

REFERENCES

[1]. COVID-19, a pandemic or not? *Lancet Infectious Diseases* (2020). 10.1016/S1473-3099(20)30180-8.

[2]. WHO, Novel Coronavirus Situation report 1 (January 21 2020), https://www.who.int/docs/default-source/coronaviruse/situation-reports/20200121-sitrep-1-2019-ncov.pdf?sfvrsn=20a99c10_4 . (2019-nCoV).

[3]. Hong H., Wang Y., Chung T. H. and Chen J. C., Clinical characteristics of noval coronavirus disease 2019 (COVID-19) in newborns, infants and children. *Pediatrics & Neonatology* (2020). doi: 10.1016/j.pedneo.2020.03.001.

[4]. Guo R. Y., Cao D. Q., Hong S. Z., Tan Y. Y., Chen D. S., Jin J. H., et al., The origin, transmission and clinical therapies on coronavirus disease 2019 (COVID-19) outbreak—an update on the status. *Military Medical Research*, 7, 11 (2020). doi: 10.1186/s40779-020-00240-0.

[5]. Velavan P. T. and Meyer G. C. The COVID-19 epidemic (2020) doi: 10.1111/TMI.13383.

[6]. Jia H. P., Look D. C., Shi L., Hickey M., Pewe L., Netland J., et al., ACE2 receptor expression and severe acute respiratory syndrome coronavirus infection depend on differentiation of human airway epithelia. *Journal of Virology*, 79(23), 14614–14621 (2005).

[7]. Wan Y., Shang J., Graham R., Baric R. S. and Li F., Receptor recognition by novel Coronavirus from Wuhan: An analysis based on decade-long structural studies of SARS. *Journal of Virology*, 94(7), e00127-20 (2020) doi: 10.1128/JVI.00127-20.

[8]. PengZ, Lou X. Y., Guang X. W., Ben H., Lei Z., et al., A pneumonia outbreak associated with a new coronavirus of probable bat origin. *Nature*, 579(7798), 270–273 (2020) doi: 10.1038/s41586-020-2012-7.

[9]. Tortorici M. A. and Veesler D.Structural insights into coronavirus entry. *Advances in Virus Research*, 105, 93–116 (2019) doi: 10.1016/bs.aivir.2019.08.002.

[10]. Xia S., Zhu Y., Liu M., Lan Q., Xu W., Wu Y., et al., Fusion mechanism of 2019-nCoV and fusion inhibitors targeting HR1 domain in spike protein. *Cellular & Molecular Immunology* (2020) 10.1038/s41423-020-0374-2.

[11]. Fei Y., Lanying D., David O. M., Chungen P. and Shibo J., Measures for diagnosing and treating infections by a novel coronavirus responsible for a pneumonia outbreak originating in Wuhan, China. *Microbes and Infection*, 22(2), 74–79 (2020) doi: 10.1016/j.micinf.2020.01.003.

[12]. de Wilde A. H., Snijder E. J., Kikkert M. and van Hemert M. J., Host factors in coronavirus replication. *Current Topics in Microbiology and Immunology*, 419, 1–42 (2018).

[13]. Sawicki S. G. and Sawicki D. L., Coronavirus transcription: a perspective. *Current Topics in Microbiology and Immunology*, 287, 31–55 (2005).

[14]. Song W., Gui M., Wang X. and Xiang Y., Cryo-EM structure of the SARS coronavirus spike glycoprotein in complex with its host cell receptor ACE2. *PLoS Pathogens*, 14 (8), e1007236 (2018). doi: 10.1371/journal.ppat.1007236.

[15]. Millet J. K. and Whittaker G. R., Host cell proteases: Critical determinants of coronavirus tropism and pathogenesis. *Virus Research*, 202, 120–134 (2015). doi: 10.1016/j.virusres.2014.11.021.

[16]. Simmons G., Gosalia D. N., Rennekamp A. J., Reeves J. D., Diamond S. L. and Bates P., Inhibitors of cathepsin L prevent severe acute respiratory syndrome

coronavirus entry. *Proceedings of the National Academy of Sciences of the United States of America*, 102(33), 11876–11881 (2005). doi: 10.1073/pnas.0505577102.

[17]. de Wit E., van Doremalen N., Falzarano D., Munster V. J., SARS and MERS: Recent insights into emerging coronaviruses. *Nature Reviews Microbiology*, 14 (8), 523–534 2016 doi: 10.1038/nrmicro.2016.81.

[18]. Razai S. M., Doerholt K., Ladhani S. and Oakeshott P., Coronavirus disease 2019 (covid-19): A guide for UK GPs. *BMJ* (2020). doi: 10.1136/bmj.m800.

[19]. CDC, Information for clinicians on therapeutic options for patients with COVID-19, https://www.cdc.gov/coronavirus/2019-ncov/hcp/therapeutic-options.html. (2020).

[20]. Scott, J. B., Treatment of coronavirus disease 2019 (COVID-19): Investigational Drugs and Other Therapies. *Medscape*, https://emedicine.medscape.com/article/2500116-overview (2020).

[21]. WHO India, Novel Corona virus (2019-nCoV). Situation Report 1, https://www.who.int/docs/default-source/wrindia/india-situation-report-1.pdf?sfvrsn=5ca2a672_0.

[22]. WHO India, Novel Corona virus (2019-nCoV). Situation Report-11, https://www.who.int/docs/default-source/wrindia/india-situation-report-2.pdf?sfvrsn=962f294b_0.

[23]. WHO India, Novel Corona virus (2019-nCoV). Situation Report-111, https://www.who.int/docs/default-source/wrindia/india-situation-report-2.pdf?sfvrsn=962f294b_0.

[24]. WHO India, Novel Corona virus (2019-nCoV). Situation Report-1V, https://www.who.int/docs/default-source/wrindia/india-situation-report-2.pdf?sfvrsn=962f294b_0.

[25]. WHO India, Novel Corona virus (2019-nCoV). Situation Report-V, https://www.who.int/docs/default-source/wrindia/india-situation-report-2.pdf?sfvrsn=962f294b_0.

[26]. WHO India, Novel Corona virus (2019-nCoV). Situation Report-VI, https://www.who.int/docs/default-source/wrindia/india-situation-report-2.pdf?sfvrsn=962f294b_0.

[27]. WHO India, Novel Corona virus (2019-nCoV). Situation Report-VII, https://www.who.int/docs/default-source/wrindia/india-situation-report-2.pdf?sfvrsn=962f294b_0.

[28]. WHO India, Novel Corona virus (2019-nCoV). Situation Report-VIII, https://www.who.int/docs/default-source/wrindia/india-situation-report-2.pdf?sfvrsn=962f294b_0.

[29]. WHO India, Novel Corona virus (2019-nCoV). Situation Report-IX, https://www.who.int/docs/default-source/wrindia/india-situation-report-2.pdf?sfvrsn=962f294b_0.

[30]. WHO India, Novel Corona virus (2019-nCoV). Situation Report-X, https://www.who.int/docs/default-source/wrindia/india-situation-report-2.pdf?sfvrsn=962f294b_0.

[31]. WHO, India Ramps up efforts to contain the spread of novel Coronavirus, https://www.who.int/india/emergencies/novel-coronavirus-2019.

[32]. Huang C., Wang Y., Li X., Ren L., Zhao J., et al., Clinical features of patients infected with 2019 novel coronavirus in Wuhan, China. *Lancet*, 395, 497–506 (2020). 10.1016/S0140-6736(20)30183-5.

[33]. Preliminary Estimates of the Prevalence of Selected Underlying Health Conditions Among Patients with Coronavirus Disease 2019 — United States, February 12–March 28, 2020. Morbidity and Mortality Weekly Report, 69 (13).

[34]. Wu Y. Z. and Mc Googan, M. J., Characteristics of and important lessons from the coronavirus disease 2019 (COVID-19) outbreak in China. *JAMA*, 323(13), 1239–1242 (2020) doi:10.1001/jama.2020.2648.

[35]. Gupta R., Ghosh A., Singh K. W. and Mishra K., Considerations for patients with diabetes in times of COVID-19 epidemic. *Diabetes & Metabolic Syndrome: Clinical Research & Reviews* (2020). 10.1016/j.dsx.2020.03.002.

[36]. Zhang J. J., Dang X., Cao Y. Y., Yuan D. Y., Yang B. Y. and Yan Q. Y., Clinical

characteristics of 140 patients infected with SARS-CoV-2 in Wuhan, China. *Allergy*, 75(7), 1730–1741 (2020).

[37]. J. Achenbach and W. Wan, New CDC data shows danger of Coronavirus for those with diabetes, heart or lung diseases, other chronic conditions. *The Washington Post* (2020).

[38]. American Diabetes Association. Diabetes and Coronavirus, https://www.diabetes.org/coronavirus-covid-19.

[39]. Bhatraju K. P., Ghassemieh J. B., Nichols M., Kim R., Jerome R. K., et al., COVID-19 in critically Ill patients in the Seattle Region-case series. *The New England Journal of Medicine*, 382(21), 2012–2022 (2020).

9 Smart Hospitals Using Artificial Intelligence and Internet of Things for COVID-19 Pandemic

*Suman Mann, Deepa Gupta, Yukti Arora,
Shivanka Priyanka Chugh, and Akash Gupta*

CONTENTS

DOI: 10.1201/9781003171829-9

9.1 INTRODUCTION

Cloud computing can be defined as the interconnection of devices, which can be accessed and maintained remotely through the Internet. IoT as the platform can capture the real-time data, analyze the gathered data, and provide the environment to examine it. Both IoT and cloud technology are collectively dependent on each other.

IoT, on the other hand, saves time and enhances the quality of life to a great extent. Primary healthcare systems around the world are stretched to a critical moment, especially in the developing countries where they have high patient-per-doctor ratios. In healthcare, interconnected devices have been introduced for patients in various forms such as ECG monitors, sleep monitors, body temperature monitors, electrocardiograms, or blood glucose level monitors, which require follow-up interaction with a healthcare professional.

This makes a strong reason why one should opt for smart hospitals. Patients require constant monitoring of their glucose levels. Due to the high patient-per-doctor ratio, patients are often than not left unattended. This can be fatal as if the glucose bottle is mistakenly fed completely and not removed in time, the pressure difference between the empty bottle and the patient's blood will cause an air embolism (outward flow of blood into the saline bottle). Figure 9.1 represents the essential elements of a smart healthcare system.

In this chapter with the help of the cloud computing technology, Internet of Things (IoT), artificial intelligence (AI), and Android Operating System, the patient can seek help by clicking on the button and can alert the nurse and doctors; moreover, if the patient is in the unstable state, then the sensors will take care of the patient in case of emergency and normal monitoring of the patient's health. The chapter presents a literature review, followed by a discussion over why one should opt for smart hospitals; then the technologies used and methodology will be discussed, followed by the proposed system, which enables us to understand the result and conclusions.

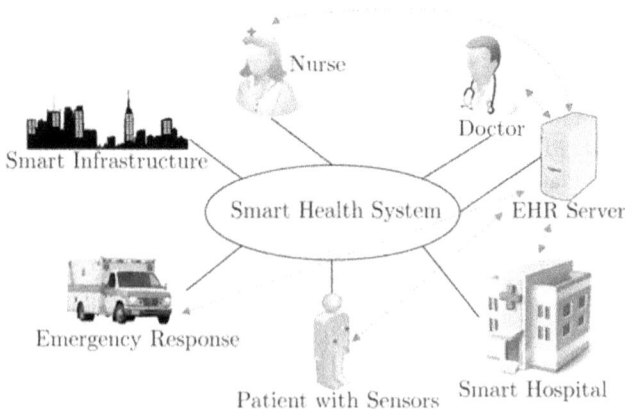

FIGURE 9.1 Smart healthcare system.

9.2 LITERATURE REVIEW

In literature [1], Paritosh Khubchandani states that the AI domain provides a large diversity of solution for reasoning problems. The system is purely based on probabilistic reasoning; it is used to handle large and complex problems and simplifies physician's work, saving their time and energy. In literature [2], Andreas Svanstom states that information gathering and analysis are done in this system. Using an android application and a.NET web service, they developed a working prototype of a personal health device integration. The prototype was created by an integration of personal health devices using ISO/IEEE 11073 protocol family with a web service using a gateway device for an adapter to connect the two terminals.

In literature [3], R. Balasubramaniam states that, in the healthcare area, recently, ElGamal elliptic curve cryptography (EECC)–based RFID authentication schemes have been used. The modified method reduces the number of doubling and adding, making ECC as one of the most efficient cryptosystems being used; it is secured against any kinds of attacks, does fast computations, and consumes less power and low bandwidth. In literature [4], Patan Rizwan states that in previous times this system behaves like a middle patient and their user maintenance application (UMA) authentication system smart device as a resource, which is maintained by Electronic Health Records (EHR). All record information provided should be connected with the cloud, in between observing a trusted network of the object.

In literature [5], R. Babu states that sensors and actuators encapsulated in physical objects are coupled through the wired and wireless network along with IoT and cloud. This model majorly depends on patient participation and consequent data analysis by microprocessor and microcontroller. In literature [6], Gipsa Alex states that the main focus of the medicine box is to regulate the accessibility of medicines and to implement remote prescription in a simpler and user-friendly way. Both need to install an android application health IOT, and log in details are provided at the time of registration. Both can view details easily. Hardware unit includes LEDs, buzzer, and Arduino board with Ethernet shield. This model helps the hospital management to continuously monitor the patients and reminds the patients to have the medicines on time.

In literature [7], B. Sobhan Babu states that this model includes RFID, a study of protocols in IoT. IoT combined with AI can be of help in improving the healthcare system. It results in the prediction of easy health problems at the beginning stage based on the IoT healthcare system. In literature [8], Mingzhe Jiang states that the proposed system allows remote monitoring of biopotentials using a technology named multi-channel biopotential measurement device. This device is operated by battery and transmits data to the cloud via the eHealth gateway. The IoT is based on remote multichannel biopotential monitoring system with supervised machine learning.

In literature [9], Stephanie B. Baker states that an extensive survey is presented, which is focused on commercial solutions, existing applications, and unsolved problems. This chapter gradually makes an important contribution in the field that identifies all key requirements of an end-to-end IoT medical care system and proposes a generic standard model that could be applied to all IoT-based medical care systems. This is an important research as there is still no known end-to-end systems is available for remote monitoring of health care. It further provides a comprehensive survey of the technologies that come within the proposed model. Sensors for monitoring various health parameters, short- and long-range communications standards, and cloud technologies are its main focus.

In literature [10], Sandeep Reddy states that AI applications have solved problems with possible results comparable to that of manual clinicians. As the healthcare system is becoming more expensive, stakeholders started looking for solutions that can replace the costly elements of inpatient care and AI solutions that will be solved after this model in such situations. However, the current technology cannot replace the human touch inpatient care, and a model that comprises both technological innovations and human care has to be investigated.

In literature [11], Kevin Patel states that IoT is continuously providing exclusive tools and abilities that all together build an integrated medical care system with the combination of the clinch to patients so that they have cared for betterment. Medical care costs are reduced significantly and treatment results are in a better way. Thus, it is a combination of multiple scopes that comprises wellness supporters, promoters, and hospitals that can tap after optimizing resources through automated work. For example, a majority of hospitals use IoT for asset management and controlling moisture and temperature within operating rooms.

In literature [12], Graysen Christopher states that by embedding IoT-enabled devices in medical devices, medical care professionals can easily watch patients more efficiently and the use the data obtained from the observations to figure out how one needs close attention. But there are certain obstacles in place that scare to slow and steady adaptation. One such matter of concern is trust: people sometimes feel uncomfortable knowing that their highly confidential data is being stored and accessed. Patient record systems need to be heavily safe because these devices access all the necessary information.

In literature [13], Brad Anderson states that setting an appointment, running diagnostic tests, sorting out insurance coverage, filling prescriptions, and paying for everything make getting care difficult. For many patients, the cutting-edge clinicians and medical centers that make the system great might as well operate in different countries. The challenge confronting providers remains clear: match the advanced treatment available with the communities who need it most. Then, streamline medical care so everyone benefits. In recent years, mobile platforms have helped address the question of accessibility in innovative ways. They make crucial services available remotely. Providers find they create workflow efficiencies. Patients get more engaged in their health, and the quality of care delivered through an app doesn't suffer. Mobile apps are transforming both the quality and accessibility of healthcare. From heart disease to birth control, these innovative platforms put everything that our system provides at patients' fingertips. This is a revolutionary development that's helping our care to catch up with our resources—one app at a time.

In literature [14], Jessica Burton states that there is a need to build and adapt a more efficient and sustainable healthcare infrastructure. It is the adaptation of smart cities and technology that can turn the global healthcare challenge into an opportunity. In literature [15], Iuliana Chiuchisan states that the monitoring in the ICU is made through ICU monitors, and all patients are connected to a bedside monitor. This monitoring system includes a diagnosis of the disease and monitoring of vital symptoms and parameters, like the treatment of all the body organs. The patients will have various types of sensors or sensing devices attached to the body that are connected through wires to the ICU monitor. The sensing devices send electronic signals via wires to the ICU monitor. The main purpose of the system is to increase the quality of the medical treatment for people who need permanent monitoring and to decrease obstacles for monitoring important medical parameters.

In literature [16], Sapna Tyagi states that with the development of technologies like IoT and cloud computing, with increasing adoption of bring-your-own-device (BYOD) working practices, sharing among services will have a transformed impact on human medical care. The proposed systems represent a technology for many medical care providers and frontline warriors to face many challenges such as rising medical care treatment costs, information sharing, and shortage of better treatment and enhanced care for the patients by the medical care professional. In literature [17], Rahul N. states that the Smart IoT Chair implemented by this research can be used in various medical fields. This system is proposed to be responsible for the transmission of data with low power consumption by applying both the node MCU and Bluetooth 4.0 connection mode communication. As a result, the Smart IoT -enabled chair can analyze users in a sitting posture with more accuracy and appropriate readings.

In literature [18], Shubham Banka proposed an automatic system to monitor the patient's body temperature, heart rate, body movements, and blood pressure. Further, they extend the existing system to predict whether the patient is suffering for a small duration. The proposed system can be installed in the hospitals, and a huge amount of data can be obtained and stored in the online database. The desired data can also be shown on the mobile-based application.

In literature [19], Hrishikesh P. Pandharkame states that in the system, sensors are used like LDR, ultrasonic sensor, and temperature sensor. The data obtained by all the sensors will be transmitted by the USB port to Arduino circuit board, and data is published to MQTT server. Whenever the data is needed to be checked, just subscribe to the MQTT server, making the hospitals energy efficient with enhanced treatment results. The system controls the electrical appliances from a webpage or mobile app, and it is user friendly. There is no need to manually ON and OFF the electrical appliances. AI system components accommodate the doctors and the patients.

In literature [20], Prashant Salunke states that after having various equipment in the operating rooms, there are some instances where doctors are not available. Also, the data cannot be shared. The existing solutions are very large and expensive. So they use biomedical sensors that are easy to wear by patients, IoT devices using microcontrollers, and cloud, which results in an IoT-based system which not only provides an appropriate diagnosis of the patient's condition but gives them medical suggestions that detect and prevent health problems with the help of carefully captured data and describe the health strains recorded from physiological and contextual sensors.

In literature [21], Prashob Bharathan states that to help the medical personnel and logistics personnel, patients and their family members can use personalized services based on their roles. To connect various departments of hospitals with the patient, technologies such as IoT, RFID, and sensors can be used. The data gathered from these technologies are combined and implemented to a layered architecture, which results in implementing the layered architecture and interconnecting the departments, patients, and doctor with each other to make things easy and precise.

In literature [22], Lie Yu states that a low power ECG monitoring system using PSOC is used to sense the ECG signal from the human body. ECG monitoring system is connected to less-power, high-speed WICED that will transmit the data directly on to the AWS IoT cloud, which results in an ECG system based on edge cypress WICED IoT technology. In Literature [23], U. U. Deshpande states that a less-power ECG monitoring system with PSOC is used to sense the ECG signal from the human heart. It is connected to low-power WICED that transmits the data to the IoT cloud.

In literature [24], Hamidur Rahman states that a contactless remote HRV monitoring system is developed using the face emotions or the variation of the face skin color caused by the cardiac pulse, which in turn gives variations on the device. In Literature [25], Pooja Kanse states that with the help of IoT, difficulties related to the excessive use of electricity by lights, fans, and various medical equipment can be measured and the proper monitoring of patients in hospitals can be achieved by using various sensors such as MQTT and IoT, resulting in low cost and low power consumption.

In literature [26], Shubham Sagar proposes an android OS–controlled wheelchair with the use of a manual joystick, which uses an android application that is connected via Wi-Fi module, which will decrease the dependency of the user on another person. In literature [27], Syed Muhammad Waqas Shah suggests using IoT and a variety of sensors to monitor the health of the person. Doctors at the remote site can communicate with the patient via the Internet, resulting in smart health care unit for patients to treat them remotely when doctors are not available. In literature [28], Punit Gupta states that IoT data elasticity provides support to emergency medical services like ICU. IoT data elasticity reduces mortality rate and decreases the medical care costs by collecting, recording and analyzing data in real-time. This helps the system to provide subtly and capable medical services to the patient.

9.3 INTRODUCTION TO SMART HOSPITALS: A DIGITAL TRANSFORMATION IN HEALTHCARE

A smart hospital is a hospital that relies on smartly optimized and self-driven procedure built on an optimized environment of interconnected devices, particularly based on IoT, to improve existing patient care technologies and introduce new opportunities. Figure 9.2 represents some key ideas behind the smart hospitals.

Sensors and actuators are capable of managing the smart hospital. Wired or wireless sensors are incorporated into ECG monitors, smart thermostats, and blood pressure monitors. Here are some reasons that one should opt for smart hospitals.

Customization—Smart hospitals enable the management to control the hospital equipment to ease the doctors so that they can be more productive in saving the patient's life.

> I. **Comfort**—Smart hospitals help in making the responsibilities of doctors and medical staff easy so that they can be more productive and can devote their skills to save patient's lives.

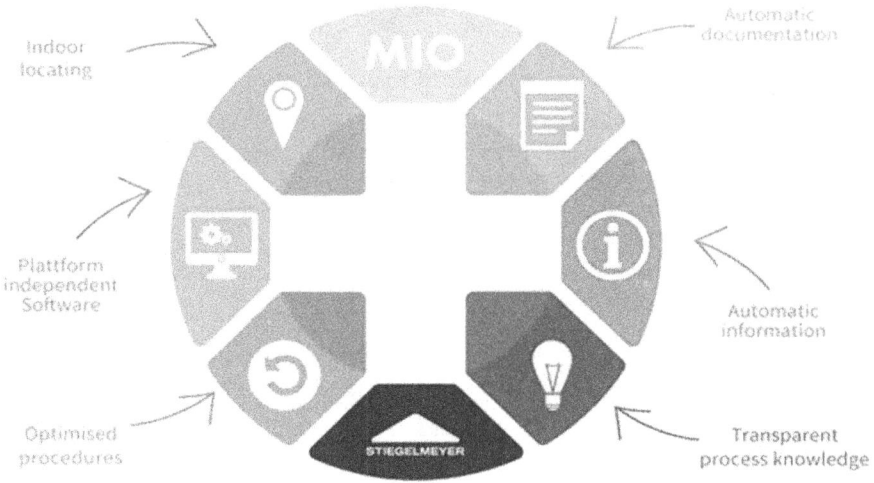

FIGURE 9.2 Key Ideas behind the smart hospital [29].

II. **Life saver**—Smart hospitals can save the patient's life by monitoring their health status and can alert nurses and doctors if any abnormal condition is found.

III. **Cost-efficient**—Power consumption can be monitored and controlled using smart IoT, resulting in money-saving and environment-friendliness.

IV. **Easy to use**—The easy-to-understand GUI will be a blessing for those patients and guardians who have less awareness about technology and smartphones.

Table 9.1 represents the assets that are considered most critical for the successful operation of smart hospitals. This data is collected via interviews and surveys.

There are various threats faced by the smart hospitals. These include malicious actions like Hijacking, medical device tampering, Skimming, and denial-of-service attacks. They also include human errors, system failures, supply chain failures, and even natural phenomena like earthquake, flood, and fires. Table 9.2 represents the likelihood and criticality of these threats.

9.4 TECHNOLOGIES INVOLVED IN THE CONSTRUCTION OF SMART HOSPITALS

In this section, we will discuss the technology required in each phase of the hospital in detail. In this system, we have used Google Cloud platform—Firebase, IoT, AI, and Android Operating System. Figure 9.3 represents some of the emerging technologies involved in the construction of smart hospitals.

9.4.1 GOOGLE CLOUD PLATFORMS—FIREBASE

Firebase is an example of backend-as-a-service (BaaS) by YC11 start-up, which results in a next-era app dev tool on Google Cloud platform. Firebase enables the

TABLE 9.1

Criticality of the various assets required for smart Hospitals

S. No	Assets required for smart hospitals	Criticality (%)
1	Interconnected Clinical Information Systems	67
2	Network Medical Devices	67
3	Networking Equipment	43
4	Remote Care Systems	40
5	Data	30
6	Mobile Client Devices	30
7	Identification Systems	30
8	Buildings	10

TABLE 9.2

Likelihood and criticality of the threats faced by smart hospitals

S. No	Threats	Likelihood (%)	Criticality (%)
1	Human errors	84.2	77
2	Malicious actions	75.8	70
3	System failures	67.2	53
4	Supply chain failures	47.2	17
5	Natural phenomena	22.8	0

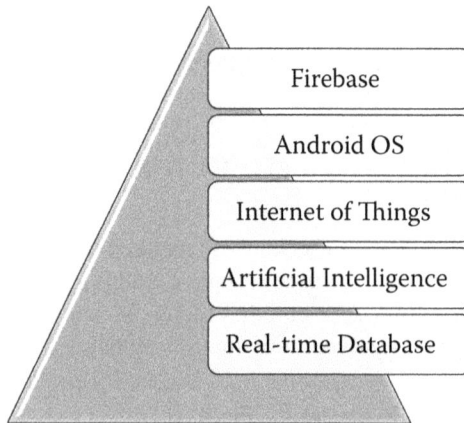

FIGURE 9.3   Emerging technologies involved in the construction of smart hospitals.

developers to remain focused on implementing a good user experience. Firebase is the developer's server, API, and data-store all written so generically that it can be modified to what is required.

9.4.2 Real-Time Database Concept

The real-time database is hosted by cloud NoSQL system. It can be seen as a big JSON object, which helps the developers manage the data in real time. With the help of a single API, the firebase database provides the app with both the present value of data and any future update of data.

9.4.3 Internet of Things

IoT is based on the concept of connecting devices to the Internet, which makes them interconnected devices. Devices have already built-in sensors, which are connected by an Internet platform that combines the data from various devices and follow the procedure to analyze the data to form useful information to fulfil specific needs. The information gathered can be used to analyze patterns, make recommendations, and detect possible situations and warn us. Figure 9.4 represents the role of IoT in the construction of smart hospitals.

9.4.4 Artificial Intelligence

AI refers to the replica of human intelligence in machines, which are programmed such that they tend to think and analyze like the human brain and can solve simple

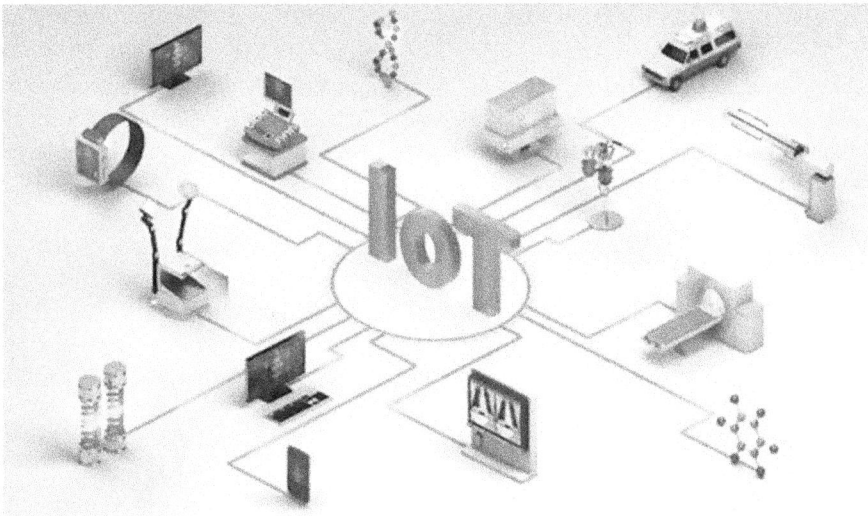

FIGURE 9.4   Role of IoT in the construction of smart hospitals [30].

to difficult and complex problems. It can also be defined as any device that carries qualities like the human mind and replicates their actions. AI uses step-by-step instructions, which are also known as an algorithm,

9.4.5 ANDROID OPERATING SYSTEM

It is a Google-developed operating system exclusively for android phones, tablets, and so on.

9.5 IMPLEMENTATION OF THE SMART HOSPITAL SYSTEM

In a smart hospital, the system operates in two important phases. The first includes the installing of devices. The second phase includes developing a mobile application with AI, android operating system, and Google cloud platform—Firebase.

9.5.1 INITIAL PHASE: INSTALLATION OF SMART DEVICES IN HOSPITALS

The first phase includes the installation of devices in the hospital; these devices will be: Raspberry Pi, pcDuino, Beagle bone Black, and Cubie Board.

9.5.2 RASPBERRY PI

Raspberry Pi will be installed in the circuit board IoT of the hospital, which operates all the sensors that are installed in the hospital building. It can be operated with the help of a mobile application, where the router will send wireless signals, which will be stored in the database/cloud.

9.5.3 PCDUINO

It is a Arduino-based individual board minicomputer with the configuration of 1 GHz ARM cortex-A8 processor. It is a low-cost and low-maintenance device, which is compatible with various programming languages like C, C++, and Java having standard android SDK and Python.

9.5.4 BEAGLE BONE BLACK

It is a more powerful device than any other device, having the configuration of 1 GHz ARM Cortex-A8 processor, which supports both Linux and IoS, and is compatible with HDMI, video audio interface, VSB, and ethernet ports.

9.5.5 CUBIE BOARD

It is configured as a dual-core ARM CortexA7 processor and has a range of input–output interface including USB, HDMI, IR, serial, Ethernet, SATA, and 96 pins extended interface.

9.5.6 SENSORS

These sensors are used to make a system fully automated, secured, and connected:

- **Heart rate sensors**—The fluctuation of blood can be detected through sensing technology placed around the patient's fingertip. The signals can be transferred further for the Raspberry Pi or any other.
- **Temperature sensors**—They will be used to measure the body temperature with an electrical pulse equivalent to a temperature measured in Celsius.
- **Bubble detectors**—These devices detect bubbles in a fluid containing container or bottle. They play an important role in many fields including medical technology, process control, pharma, and the petrol industry.
- **Humidity sensors**—These sensors measure the moisture and temperature of the air inside the operating room.
- **Sleep monitors**—They will sense the sleep time of the patient and will also sense whether the patient is sleeping at the moment.

9.5.7 SUBSEQUENT PHASE: DEVELOPMENT OF MOBILE APPLICATION

This will be a mobile application, which will send alert signals from:

Patient -> nurse, nurse -> doctor in emergency situations. It will send the alert signals which will be received in the form of vibrations on the receiver's device. Also, the devices will be connected with IoT platforms that will gather the data and store it in the cloud; the data will be retrieved from the cloud for analysis, and also the notifications of EMERGENCY will be sent from the firebase and cloud functions itself to other interconnected devices. This will make the quality of care to the patients more efficient. Thus, this application will make the patient safer and connected to nurses and doctors. Figure 9.5 represents the human–computer interaction of smart healthcare mobile applications.

9.6 DOCTOR'S PLATFORM

As we know a doctor's platform in our project is concerned with the doctor. A single doctor can have more than one critical patient, and a doctor also has a large number of patients who visit the doctor for their routine check-ups, so it is not possible for the doctor to devote all of his or her time for the critical patients. So doctors have the solution of having nurses record their situations who visit the patients more frequently. The record given by the nurses to the doctor is not real time as it is manual. Therefore, we created a system which rules out for the mentioned problem, allowing quick and efficient means of communication between the doctors and other health line workers.

9.7 NURSE'S PLATFORM

Similarly, there is a platform specially designed for the nurse as well in the system developed. As nurses also have a lot of patients to deal with and their

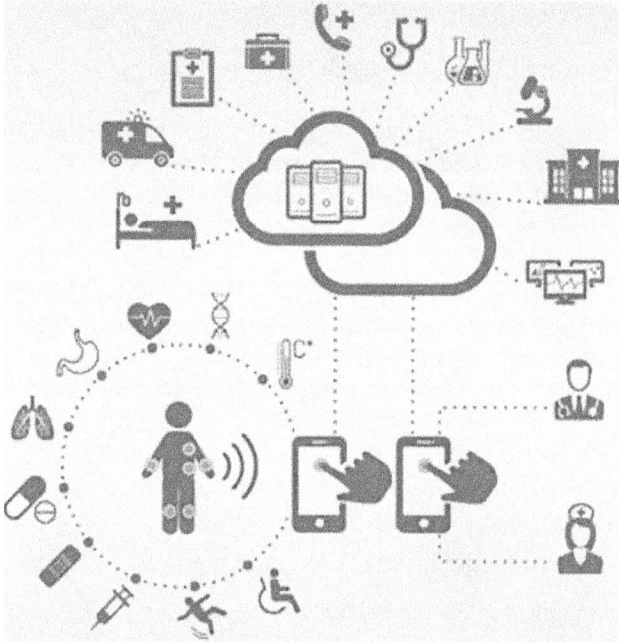

FIGURE 9.5 Human–computer interaction of smart healthcare mobile applications [31].

duties are also changed frequently, it is impossible for them to pay full attention to each patient. So there is a need for nurse's platform to make nurses manage their work easily. They also have to keep track of each patient. With less and more critical situations, they cannot neglect the patient with the less critical situation. Also they need to pay full attention to each patient, so it is essential to have a nurse's platform. Nurse's platform works in such a way that in a critical situation the data is being shared to the doctor, but when there is no need of the doctor or the need of the patient is common, the data is not shared with the doctor. On the nurse side of the platform, the system gets vibrated and all of the patient's information with the name of concerned doctor will be notified on the screen, and any on-duty nurse can attend them. The specific need of the patient is also mentioned on the screen. In case of emergency, the nurses just simply pass on the data and call the doctor.

9.8   PATIENT'S PLATFORM

In any health-related system, it is necessary to have a patient's platform. In the patient's platform, the patients with the less critical situation and those who have no attendant can easily take care of themselves as they easily call the nurses whenever they needed. But for the patients with a more critical situation and who are not in their consciousness, their attendees/relatives can use this platform to call nurses whenever needed. This patient's platform is very useful as their real-time health condition will be recorded and shared with the nurses and doctors. This will prove to be very helpful as it allows critical patients to communicate efficiently.

9.9 THE LAYOUT OF THE SMART HOSPITAL SYSTEM: DESIGNING THE FUTURE HEALTHCARE

In this framework, the patient's platform can send alarming signals to the nurse and doctors, which will be seen as a vibration in the devices. In addition, with the help of the sensors, the patient's health can be monitored in real time.

In the critical case, the nurse itself can send alarming signals to the doctor in real-time, so that the patient can be treated immediately. The information sent by the sensors will be stored in the cloud and will also help in the effective examination of the patient, including the patient's health history and earlier diagnosis. The layout can be represented in Figures 9.6–9.9.

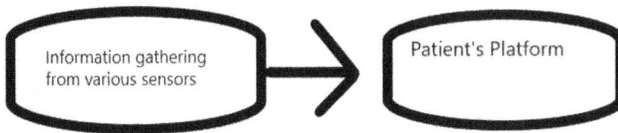

FIGURE 9.6   Information gathering from various sensors to the patient's platform.

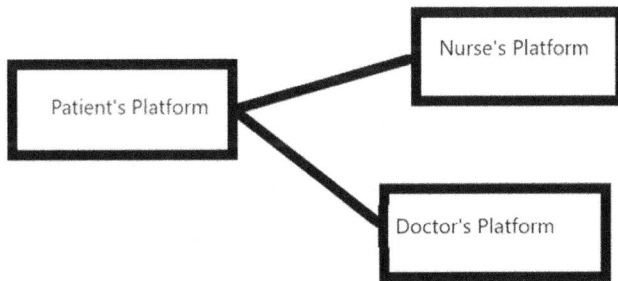

FIGURE 9.7   Patient's platform is connected with nurse's platform and doctor's platform.

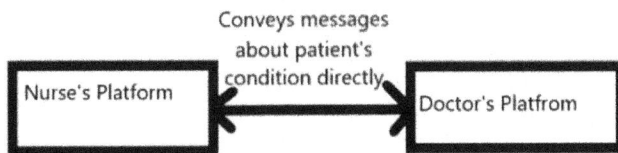

FIGURE 9.8   Nurse's and doctor's platform interconnection.

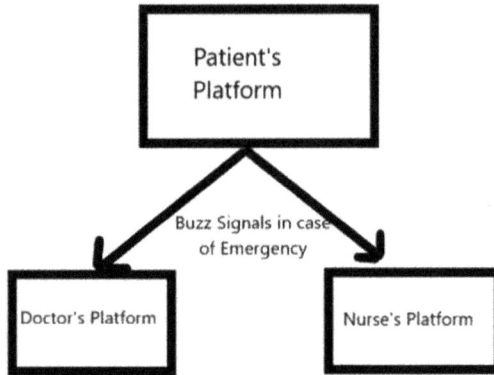

FIGURE 9.9   Buzz signals in case of emergencies.

9.10   CONCLUSION

This project is capable of monitoring and generating an alarming signal in the form of high-alert vibrations and emergency notifications to the nurse and doctor about the patient's health condition at a minimal cost. The android application is used to provide a platform that notifies the nurse and doctor about the alarming situation of the patient in a simple GUI.

REFERENCES

[1]. Khubchandani, P., Jha, K., Bijani, R., Lala, S. and Saindane, P., Medical prediction using artificial intelligence. *International Journal of Engineering Science*, 4898–4900 (2017).

[2]. Svanström, A., IoT communication protocols in healthcare (Master's thesis) (2016).

[3]. Balasubramaniam, M. R., Sathya, R., Ashicka, S. and SenthilKumar, S., An analysis of RFID authentication schemes for Internet of Things (IOT) in healthcare environment using Elgamal Elliptic Curve cryptosystem. *International Journal of Recent Trends in Engineering & Research (IJRTER)*, 2 (3) (2016).

[4]. Rizwan, P., Rajasekhara Babu, M. and Suresh, K., Design and development of low investment smart hospital using internet of things through innovative approaches. *Biomedical Research-Tokyo*, 28, 4979–4985 (2017).

[5]. Babu, R. and Dr. K. Jayashree, Prominence of IoT and cloud in health care. International Journal of Advanced Research in Computer Engineering & Technology (IJARCET), 5(2), 420–424 (2016).

[6]. Alex, G., Varghese, B., Jose, J.G. and Abraham, A., A modern health care system using IoT and Android. *International Journal on Computer Science and Engineering (IJCSE)*, 8(4) 98–101 (2016).

[7]. B. Sobhan Babu, K. Srikanth, T. Ramanjaneyulu and I. Lakshmi Narayana, IoT for Healthcare. *International Journal of Engineering Science and Research (IJSR)*, 2 (5), 322–326 (2016).

[8]. Jiang, M., Gia, T. N., Anzanpour, A., Rahmani, A. M., Westerlund, T., Salanterä, S., Liljeberg, P. and Tenhunen, H., IoT-based remote facial expression monitoring system with sEMG signal. In 2016 IEEE sensors applications symposium (SAS) (pp. 1–6). IEEE (2016, April).

[9]. Baker, S. B., Xiang, W. and Atkinson, I., 2017. Internet of things for smart healthcare: Technologies, challenges, and opportunities. *IEEE Access*, 5, pp. 26521–26544.

[10]. S. Reddy, Use of artificial intelligence in healthcare delivery, eHealth – making health care smarter, Thomas F. Heston, IntechOpen (November 5th 2018). 10.5772/intechopen.74714.

[11]. K. Patel, Benefits of IOT for hospitals and healthcare (2016).

[12]. Christopher, G., Internet of things in healthcare: What's next for IoT technology in the health sector (2016).

[13]. B. Anderson, How mobile apps are improving access to healthcare services (2020).

[14]. J. Burton, Smart cities solving today's healthcare challenges (2020).

[15]. Chiuchisan, I., Costin, H. and Geman, O., Adopting the internet of things technologies in health care systems (2014). 10.1109/ICEPE.2014.6969965.

[16]. Tyagi, S., Agarwal, A. and Maheshwari, P., A conceptual framework for IoT-based healthcare system using cloud computing. In 2016 6th International Conference-Cloud System and Big Data Engineering (Confluence) (pp. 503–507). IEEE (2016, January).

[17]. R. R. Biswas, Calibrating wastewater hydraulic model during post earthquake rapid rebuild works, Volume 5, Issue VI, International Journal for Research in Applied Science and Engineering Technology (IJRASET), pp. 461–470, ISSN: 2321-9653.

[18]. Banka, S., Madan, I. and Saranya, S. S., Smart healthcare monitoring using IoT. *International Journal of Applied Engineering Research*, 13 (15), 11984–11989 (2018).

[19]. Pandharkame and Hrishikesh P., Smart Hospitals using Internet of Things (IoT) (2017).

[20]. P. Salunke and R. Nerkar, IoT driven healthcare system for remote monitoring of patients. *International Journal for Modern Trends in Science and Technology*, 3 (6), 100–103 (2017).

[21]. Bharathan, M. P., Nadar, M. V. and Wayal, M. S. Remote health monitoring using IoT. *International Journal of Advance Research, Ideas and Innovations in Technology* (2017).

[22]. Yu, L., Lu, Y. and Zhu, X., Smart hospital based on internet of things. *Journal of Networks*, 7 (10), 1654 (2012).

[23]. Deshpande, U. and Kulkarni, M. (2017). IoT based real time ECG monitoring system using cypress WICED. 10.15662/IJAREEIE.2017.0602035.

[24]. Rahman, H., Begum, S. and Ahmed, M. U., Ins and outs of big data: A review. In International Conference on IoT Technologies for HealthCare (pp. 44–51). Springer: Cham (2016, October).

[25]. Kanase, P. and Gaikwad, S., Smart hospitals using internet of things (IoT). *International Research Journal of Engineering and Technology (IRJET)*, 3 (03), 1735–1737 (2016).

[26]. Nayak, S. S., Gupta, P., Upasana, A. B. W. and Wani, A. B., Wheel Chair with Health Monitoring System Using IoT. *International Research Journal of Engineering and Technology (IRJET)*, 4 (05) (2017).

[27]. S. M. W. Shah, and M. Pasha, IoT-based smart health unit. *Journal of Software*, 12 (1), 45–52 (2017).

[28]. Gupta, P., Agrawal, D., Chhabra, J. and Dhir, P. K., IoT based smart healthcare kit. In 2016 International Conference on Computational Techniques in Information and Communication Technologies (ICCTICT) (pp. 237–242). IEEE (2016, March).

[29]. Holzinger, A., Röcker, C. and Ziefle, M., From smart health to smart hospitals. In: Smart health (pp. 1–20). Springer: Cham (2015).

[30]. Budida, D. A. M. and Mangrulkar, R. S., Design and implementation of smart HealthCare system using IoT. In 2017 International Conference on Innovations in

Information, Embedded and Communication Systems (ICIIECS) (pp. 1–7). IEEE (2017, March).

[31]. Liu, P., Fels, S., West, N. and Görges, M., Human computer interaction design for mobile devices based on a smart healthcare architecture. *Advances in Computers and Software Engineering*, 2, 99–31 (2019).

10 Researcher Issues and Future Directions in Healthcare Using IoT and Machine Learning

Sharad Chauhan, Ritika Arora, and Neha Arora

CONTENTS

DOI: 10.1201/9781003171829-10

10.1   INTRODUCTION

The utmost requirement of life is medical care as it is the support and improvement of wellbeing. Any deformity that occurred inside the body that is not visible can be determined with the help of equipment like CT, MRI, PET, and SPECT. Additionally, irregular conditions like coronary failure and epilepsy can be determined even before they happen. The consistent expansion of population and the spread of constant sickness among the masses have made strain on the current medical services as the demand for hospital resources is extremely high and the solution should be taken to reduce the pressure and maintain both the standard and the quality of healthcare. Recent research has come to conclusion to reduce pressure on healthcare system. Various wearable frameworks are there to give the dependable remote transmission of data. The doctor can monitor the cardiac impulse of the patient by using health care monitoring devices.

Although there are numerous advantages of Internet of Things (IoT) in the medical field, both the medical clinical chiefs and IT are worried about the information security and IoT gadget management. Machine learning is an arrangement to acquire from the points of reference experience and without being explicitly adjusted. It is used in web searches, spam filtering, stock exchange, and so on. Artificial intelligence (AI) acquires equivalent significance and acknowledgment as that of enormous information and distributed computing in a systematic process [1]. Extensive scale enlightening assortments are assembled and analyzed in different phases from planning sciences to relational associations, business, bio-atomic exploration, and security. AI methods have been generally embraced in various fields, for example, medication, cosmology, and science. Thus, machine learning will be the name of new innovation and development.

10.2   LITERATURE SURVEY

In [2], the author has designed a framework, which is intended for large information application with the point of considering the weakness of patients. The main function of the framework is to draw connections between enthusiastic reaction and physiological changes to perceive how the state of being changes depending upon the patient's emotional state. As a result, a large amount of patient's data gets accumulated on the cloud, which requires efficient data mining techniques for the extraction of the required information. Here the essential point of the distributed storage is not only to keep up the record of the patient's wellbeing but also to apply a proficient AI calculation to keep such immense collection of information.

An exhaustive study of IoT medical care frameworks is given in [3]. It gives a top-to-bottom examination about security prerequisites and the difficulties looked by IoT security. The patient reliably needs their data to be ensured, and in the end, everyone needs their data to be protected from unapproved clients, as data reliability is the utmost requirement. These are the fundamental prerequisites that are required to be executed easily by an effective E-wellbeing framework. The creators depict how there is consistently an opportunity of danger assault from both inside and outside the organization. Thus, they have zeroed in their examination on an assault scientific categorization, which shows various types of assaults looked in changed regions of security. They have isolated existing and potential dangers based on the data and network-explicit trade off. The author had described a shared security model to decrease the security issues across the medical care frameworks. The security model has been planned with dynamic properties to oblige future inconspicuous dangers and assaults. The model plainly portrays what happens when another sort of danger happens. The current model gets wasteful to avoid such assaults. Thus there is a need for dynamic calculations to manage these eccentric circumstances. The model gives an approach to a solid joint effort between administrations with the goal that the impacts because of the present, conceivable, and inconspicuous assaults can be decreased and disposed of. Likewise, it shows the effect of huge information, encompassing insight and wearable across different E-wellbeing settings. It gives strategies and guidelines to improve IoT-based E-wellbeing frameworks and characterizes the arrangement of difficulties and exploration holes across the IoT-based E-wellbeing frameworks.

The utilization of cloud worldview in E-medical services frameworks is defined, which clarifies in a nutshell the benefits of utilizing distributed computing in biomedicine. As we have examined previously, progressively wellbeing observing and the measure of information gathered from different patients are huge to such an extent that it can't be put away by utilizing customary methods. Distributed computing stockpiling administrations assume a significant job in the examination of biomedicine innovations. A protected cloud design for IoT and medical services frameworks is given in [4]. It calls attention to the security issues in both distributed computing and portable telecommunication. It proposes an effective model that permits specialists to distantly screen their patients through versatile application by utilizing the cloud. It consolidates cell phone, bluetooth, and cloud to share quiet information in a safe and secret way.

In [3] the author has depicted that the diabetes impact millions of people around the world. Notwithstanding, diabetes finding is yet a strenuous measure. The advancement of wearable clinical sensors and AI centers aims a way ahead to address this test. With the increasing demand of wearable clinical sensors and AI, these devices empower a constant, client straightforward component for gathering information and then breaking down anatomical signs. The author had proposed a system known as DiabNN, which joins productive neural organizations and wearable smart devices, which help in diabetes determination. It also includes sidesteps that include the extraction stage and acts straightforwardly on wearable devices and consolidates off-the-rack. A DiabNNs by leveraging slope-based development and size-based pruning calculations is also being prepared. Thus, we have indicated that DiabDeep can be used in an unavoidable style, while offering high adequacy and accuracy.

In [5] the author proposes IoT-based system framework for perceiving falls of elderly people in indoor conditions, which takes ideal conditions of low-power far off sensor organizations, savvy appliance, enormous information, and distributed computing. For this reason, a 3D-pivot accelerometer inserted into a 6LowPAN gadget wearable is utilized, which is answerable for gathering information from developments of older individuals progressively. To give high productivity in fall discovery, the sensor readings are prepared and examined utilizing a choice trees-put together Big Data model running with respect to a Smart IoT Gateway. On the off chance that a fall is distinguished, an alarm is initiated and the framework responds consequently by sending warnings to the gatherings answerable for the consideration of the old individuals. At long last, the framework offers types of assistance based on cloud. From clinical viewpoint, there is a capacity administration that empowers medical services proficient to admittance to falls information for perform further examination. Then again, the framework offers a support utilizing this information to make another AI model each time a fall is recognized. The aftereffects of investigations have demonstrated high achievement rates in fall recognition regarding exactness, accuracy, and gain.

In [6] the examination is identified with build up a smart watch-based structure for ongoing and online appraisal and portability checking (ROAMM). The proposed ROAMM system will incorporate a smart watch application and worker. The smart watch application will be utilized to gather and preprocess information. The worker will be utilized to store and recover information, distant screen, and for other authoritative purposes. With the incorporation of sensor-based and client announced information assortment, the ROAMM system takes into consideration information representation and rundown insights in genuine time. The strategy presently leads to biological flashing evaluation, which was initially created for mental purposes to survey what exercises individuals do and how they feel, and their opinion about during their day-by-day lives. The technique requests people to give precise journals from their encounters at intermittent or framework-characterized events. It was achieved by the way that individuals are poor at reproducing their mental experience after it has happened. When oftentimes and haphazardly inspected, biological appraisals are regularly viewed as "reality" since they gauge an impartial normal that tends to one or the other overestimate or disparage the state. The ROAMM structure meets a portion of the significant prerequisites for the up and coming age of the IoT for mHealth. ROAMM offers an intelligent interface (e.g., inciting for detailing indications) and far-off application arrangement (e.g., altering information assortment rates and sorts of factors to be determined), just as worker highlights for making it adaptable for online customization. Furthermore, the smart watch accelerometer equipment furnishes profoundly connected outcomes with an approved, research-grade accelerometer.

10.3   CHALLENGES IN DIGITAL HEALTHCARE ADOPTION

Computerized medical services frameworks use advances, for example, IoT and enormous information that are utilized to associate patients and suppliers across medical services frameworks. These frameworks are likewise being progressively associated by means of the web to different sorts of clinical wearable innovations that are being worn for constant medical services observing shows the populace embracing the clinical wearable technology [2]. Investigating the information about different patients from the sources like medical clinics, homes, facilities, office additionally turns into an incredible concern. The record of unstructured clinical information turns into another issue and dealing with an enormous volume of clinical information and mining the helpful information in a compelling way additionally turns into an extraordinary issue. The principal work is that everybody should be profited in the wellbeing framework, to be specific the supplier, patient, payer, and the board. Another significant factor establishes is that analyzing hereditary information is a computational danger undertaking and joining with standard clinical information adds more layers increment the odds of multifaceted nature. Ultimately protection of information has become the greatest issues, and the conduct of the patient is taken through different sensors with different social associations and interchanges.

10.3.1   WHAT CAN IoT DO FOR HEALTHCARE

IoT and digital gadgets empowered gadgets have made observance in the medical care area so that the records of the patients can be kept secured. With this procedure the far away checking of the patient's prosperity helps in reducing the data loss, and the length of center prevents re-affirmations and improving results. It has led to a decrease in the cost of medical services costs, which collectively results in improving the results. IoT has applications in clinical administrations that benefits patient, families, specialists, crisis facilities, and protection organizations.

IoT for patients—Wearable devices like fitness bands and other devices which are wirelessly connected monitors body measures such as blood pressure, heart rate, and glucose levels. These gadgets can be tuned to remind carbohydrate level, practice check, arrangements, circulatory strain varieties, and much more. IoT has transformed people, particularly old patients, by empowering steady following of ailments.

IoT for physicians—The physicians can also keep track of patients' health more effectively by using wearable and other home monitoring equipment embedded with IoT. With this technology they can track patients' adherence to treatment plans or any need for immediate medical attention. It makes healthcare profession under an eye and can connect with them any time. Through the data collection from IoT devices best treatment process for patients will be provided.

IoT for hospitals—Aside from observing the patient's health, there are numerous different zones where IoT gadgets are helpful in clinics. IoT gadgets labeled with sensors are utilized for following constant area of clinical gear like wheelchairs, defibrillators, nebulizers, oxygen siphons and other observing hardware. Implementation of the medical staff at various areas can likewise be broken down in genuine time. The spread of diseases is a significant worry for patients in hospitals. IoT-empowered cleanliness-observing gadgets help in keeping patients from getting contaminated. IoT gadgets likewise help in resource the executives like drug store stock control, and ecological observing, for example, checking cooler temperature, and moistness and temperature control.

IoT for medical coverage organizations—There are different entryways for prosperity and with IoT-related devices. Protection agencies can utilize data to get secured. This data will enable them to perceive distortion states and recognize opportunities for supporting. IoT devices get straightforwardness among security net suppliers, and customers support, assessing, claims dealing with, and with examination measures. Security net suppliers may offer persuading powers to their customers for using and sharing prosperity data. IoT devices can moreover enable protection offices to support claims through the data got by these devices.

10.4 WEARABLE HEALTH DEVICES

Wearable Health Devices (WHDs) are continuously helping people with better screening and their prosperity status both at an activity/health level with a potential for earlier insightful and course of treatment. The advancement change in the downsizing of electronic devices is enabling to design more reliable and flexible wearable devices, contributing for a general change in the prosperity checking approach [7,8].Wearable innovation alludes to the data innovation (IT) empowered gadgets that can be carried on the client body, for example, wrist, arm, or head WHD and late logical improvements on the territory (electrocardiogram, pulse, circulatory strain, breath rate, blood oxygen immersion, blood glucose, skin sweat, capnography, internal heat level, movement assessment, cardiovascular implantable gadgets, and encompassing boundaries). Wearable gadgets and network between these gadgets and PCs are key ideas behind the innovative changes in healthcare [9,10]. These capacities include: following and checking of patients through wearable gadgets, far off help through telemedicine and far off analysis, which are key in giving crisis location, data the executives identified with drug, treatment, and clinical exhortation, and cross authoritative mix of emergency clinic data frameworks [4].

10.5 SECURITY ISSUES IN WEARABLE DEVICES

The way that all types of wearable gadgets are put away from person body and the information is transmitted into nearby capacity gadget without encryption. Likewise it does not give any stick and secret key insurance. So the unapproved individuals can undoubtedly get to your own information. The wearable gadgets are associated with PC, advanced mobile phone utilizing using features of bluetooth and Wi-Fi [11]. It makes security a serious issue but our goal is to protect the data. The wearable gadgets that resemble watches and smart bands contain the latest data about clients. With the absence of encryption all minute information like ledger subtleties, federal retirement aide number, and individual body data by programmers [12] (Table 10.1).

As indicated by Statist, the wearable gadgets market is at present having an overall income of around $26 billion, and is required to reach nearly $34 billion of every 2020. In order to enhance the security the protection information need to accomplish gadget code and guidelines. Additionally the administration of protection information is facing future difficulties in wearable gadgets since inaccessibility of security code and PIN, secret phrase during the transmission of those information to neighborhood gadgets like PC, advanced cells are found.

TABLE 10.1
Conjecture for wearable gadgets around the world

Devices	2017	2018	2019	2022
Smart watch	34.80	34.97	21.23	128.50
Wristband	41.50	44.10	21.43	150.00
Sports watch	48.20	48.84	21.65	168.00
Bluetooth headset	80.96	63.86	22.31	206.00

10.6 VITAL SIGNS—MOST IMPORTANT TO BE MONITORED

The human body has numerous distinctive physiological signs that can be estimated: from electrical signs to biochemical, human signs are removed and be utilized to more readily comprehend for the wellbeing status. They can be obtained utilizing wearable sensors and gadgets. These days innovation and wearable situations arrange WHDs as per three perspectives: situation of utilization (home/far off or clinical climate); the kind of checking (disconnected or on the web); and the sort of client (solid or patient).

10.6.1 VALUABLE VITAL SIGN

Electrocardiogram (ECG)—ECGs are among the most generally utilized bio signals, as an indicative apparatus in medical services climate, giving data of the heart electrical cycle. The ECG waveform is described by five pinnacles and valleys (named P, Q, R, S, T, U), where everyone speaks to an adjustment in the electrical capability of the heart bringing about muscle action and ensuring in heart development. The most separated pinnacle of the ECG is the R-top remembered for the QRS complex that speaks to the ventricles depolarization where there is a higher differential potential. The ECG waveform is utilized to dissect the cardiovascular system and to anticipate coronary infractions. The examination of the ECG waveform designs assumes a significant job in analyzing of cardiovascular illnesses (CVD).One of the upsides of WHDs for clinical purposes and with accreditations in the ECG checking.

10.6.2 PULSE (HR)

Heartbeat (HR) is a standard fundamental sign and has become an ordinary assessment in both clinical administrations and wellbeing/sport works out. The checking of this sign gives information about the physiologic status by exhibiting changes in the heart cycle. This basic sign can be helpfully isolated from the ECG (R-top) or photo plethysmography (PPG) signals. Regardless of the way that these two physiological signs have particular morphologic information in their waveforms and are from two different physiological origins, they contain tantamount heartbeat information. There are substitute ways to deal with measure heartbeat, for example, using inertial sensors or scales, named ballistocardiogram (BCG), anyway are procedures that don't have attainable assessment when differentiated and the

HR eliminated from the ECG and PPG. It is critical in game and development settings to evaluate or instruct how the heart reacts during action and recovery. Heartbeat vacillation examination is getting thought as a fundamental marker of the prosperity status of the cardiovascular system. It is in like manner a human psychophysiological status pointer, for instance, in pressing factor and exhaustion measurements. Medical specialists propose beat signal as an assessment related to beat that can substitute it. It is portrayed as the generous melodic augmentation of a vein conveyed by the development of volume of blood crashed into the vessel achieved by the pressure and loosening up of the heart. This assessment gives more information than HR, like strength, adequacy, and consistency of heartbeat. An issue implied in the composing is the reducing of blood volume in case of an inconsistent heartbeat. Heartbeat sign should not be seen as comparable to heartbeat and it will in general be evaluated using beat oximetry principles, methodology also used to measure blood oxygen immersion [13].

10.6.3 BLOOD PRESSURE

Blood pressure (BP) is viewed as the main cardiopulmonary boundary, showing the pressing factor applied by blood against the blood vessel divider. BP gives circuitous data about the blood stream when the heart is contracting (systole) and unwinding (diastole) and can likewise demonstrate cell oxygen conveyance. It is affected by a few human physiological attributes: cardiovascular yield; fringe vascular opposition; blood volume and thickness; and vessel divider versatility. Wandering BP observing permits getting BP readings a few times each day, which is ideal to checking (hypertension), probably the best danger to the worldwide weight of infections, improving cardiovascular sicknesses forecast.

BP is generally estimated utilizing inflatable pressing factor sleeves with a stethoscope on the patient's arm. This strategy was adjusted to perform independent BP estimation, including a completely computerized inflatable sleeve that measure BP by relating outside pressing factor with the greatness of blood vessel volume pulsations. Continuous observing with a sleeve can bring about undesirable results, for example, rest disturbance, skin aggravations and an expansion in feelings of anxiety. To tackle this issue, new innovations for walking BP observing have been created. One is to appraise BP dependent on heartbeat wave travel time between the beat wave got by photoplethysmography (PPG) and ECG (R-top), both estimated on the chest or with the PPG signal obtained on the wrist. All the more as of late researcher proposed an exploratory watch-type model which utilizes a pressing factor sensor close to the outspread vein, giving exact pulse estimation on an individual advanced cell, an ongoing persistent checking BP wearable gadget.

10.6.4 RESPIRATION RATE

Respiratory rate wandering observing is significant in the discovery of indications of respiratory infections, for example, respiratory disorder, persistent obstructive pneumonic illness and asthma, improving the organization of medicines is necessary. This consistent observing is especially significant in kids with pneumonic diseases [14].

This imperative boundary is regularly determined from the procured respiratory waveform that mirrors the chest volume variety during the motivation and lapse. The examination of this information is mostly in serious competitors which can help in the accomplishment of a superior respiratory presentation.

10.6.5 BLOOD OXYGEN SATURATION (SpO2)

Blood oxygen immersion (SpO2) is an incredibly significant crucial boundary and simple to quantify utilizing photoplethysmography (PPG) innovation and heartbeat oximetry standards. The PPG technique empowers to gain vein variety waveform, and when estimated utilizing two frequencies (typically 660 nm and 905 nm) it is conceivable to appraise blood oxygen immersion. This is because of the hemoglobin absorbance range change when it limits with oxygen. Utilizing oximetry standards, it is conceivable to gauge the measure of oxygen that is being conveyed by platelets (ordinarily: 95–100%). This measure may prompt distinguish persistent condition change that in any case could be missed, for example, lower level of oxygen (<95%) which demonstrates hypoxia and causes deficient oxygen supply to the human body. Other than clinical use, beat oximeter walking observing has a specific interest in the assessment of vigorous effectiveness of an individual endeavor a standard exercise. There are a few non-intrusive innovations to gauge blood oxygen immersion that can be applied to wearable gadgets; however PPG stands apart being exceptionally well known in clinical climate. Finger is the most utilized spot to get blood oxygen immersion levels and is the most ordinarily utilized in facility conditions. Ring PPG sensors are being worked on because of its all the more wearing-ease and effectively adaptation [15]. Mobile associations lead these sensors to a substantially more autonomous and wearable gadget. Ear projection can likewise be utilized and a new exploration introduced an exceptionally little chip (3 × 6 mm) equipped for measure blood oxygen immersion.

10.6.6 SKIN PERSPIRATION

Skin sweat is a clinical boundary yet a physiological sign used to break down human response to a few circumstances. Life circumstances can cause neurological responses from the autonomic sensory system (ANS) invigorating an expansion of skin perspiring. This dampness changes the electrical conductance of the skin, permitting estimating the amount of sweat delivered by sweat organs, named as galvanic skin reaction (GSR). As ANS is dependable to control other physiological boundaries like pulse, breath and circulatory strain, GSR has been utilized close by the acquisitions of a portion of these signs. For instance, skin sweat and pulse fluctuation can be utilized to group mental states, helping in the qualification, as likewise in the discovery of mental stress [16]. In games, skin sweat ceaseless checking is viewed as a significant physiologic sign with colossal applications around there and human conduct. From skin sweat, it is conceivable to get data about the physiological state of the subject because of the few particles and atoms that comprises it. For instance, actual pressure can be utilized in psychophysiological assessment of militaries going through extreme preparing.

There are two principle kinds of sensors in skin sweat observing: epidermal-based sensors and Fabric/adaptable plastic-based sensors:

- Epidermal-based have a conformal contact between the anodes surface and the biofluid, as elastomeric stamps to print terminals straightforwardly on human epidermis for ceaseless observing.
- Fabric/adaptable plastic-based sensors, the most utilized, having a fundamental favorable position of steady contact with a huge surface zone of the skin. These can be installed into texture or screen-printed into it, acquiring particulars estimations like pH and particles fixation as $NH4+$, $K+$ and $Cl-$.

10.6.7 Capnography

Blood oxygen immersion estimation by beat oximetry is a generally utilized technique to get to blood vessel oxygenation yet it's anything but a decent strategy for human ventilation appraisal. Capnography is a non-obtrusive and savvy technique to assess human ventilation, demonstrating the carbon monoxide levels present in the breath cycle, being extremely valuable to dodge clinical issues and guarantee tolerant safety. Capnography is fundamentally utilized external the clinical climate to screen rest apnea disorder. Ordinarily this issue is analyzed and checked utilizing polysomnography or cardio-respiratory polygraphy (can likewise incorporate capnography observing, however not as a solitary

10.6.8 Internal Heat Level

Internal heat level (BT) is the result of the harmony between heat creation and warmth misfortune in the body, being its estimation indispensable to maintain a strategic distance from numerous components DE functionalization because of high temperatures (e.g., proteins denature and lose work over specific temperatures). BT partitions in two measures: center temperature (CT) and skin temperature. Skin temperature changes inside a more extensive scope of temperatures than center temperature, as the body's thermoregulation components direct center temperature. Skin temperature is influenced by blood flow and is likewise related with HR and metabolic rate. Outside components, for example, air dissemination, surrounding temperature and dampness additionally assume a significant part in this internal heat level guideline mechanism [17]. Diverse wearable frameworks have been created to quantify the two temperatures, for example, skin-like varieties of exactness temperature sensors or wearable glue gadgets to ceaselessly gauge temperature. An exceptionally ongoing model is a re-usable remote epidermal temperature sensor a battery-less RFID thermometer that is demonstrating to be a promising gadget to appraise CT.

10.6.9 Cardiovascular Implantable Devices

With climate sensors it is conceivable to gauge the inhabitance action of subjects, effectively assessing metabolic rate, chiefly in inside conditions because of the non-commitment of outside components. The increment of implantable heart gadgets is prompting an advancement of long haul reconnaissance, to improve persistent security and care. These gadgets are mostly implantable pacemakers, cardioverter defibrillators and heart resynchronization treatment frameworks. A far off observing of these gadgets will limit the need of parental figures in a few circumstances, permitting an early recognition of unfriendly occasions and brief restorative measure, getting to modern data put away in the gadget's memory. The fuse of new correspondence innovations will give a day by day, far off, remote, tolerant autonomous mobile observing of clinical and specialized information. Feeling boundaries are the ecological boundaries in each subject environmental factors and have a high pertinence in a few human body observing territories. The most utilized sensors are temperature, light, stickiness and sound level. The nonstop observing of air toxins is additionally significant because of its relationship with cardiovascular and pneumonic illnesses. Open air every day exercises ought to likewise be consistently observed with atmosphere sensors to examine climate qualities that the human body is oppressed during sport exercises or essentially restoration works out, being temperature and mugginess imperative to assess dehydration [18].

10.7   IOT AND AI AS TOGETHER

Both IoT and man-made intelligence is dependent on one another. The web of things suggests dealing with enormous volumes of information. Since IoT is most recent innovation that associates the large number of keen gadgets, speed and precision are the measures that are yet to be improved [19]. Though AI not just emulates the human method of performing errands however it additionally gain from what the example is all about.AI programming implanted inside IoT gadgets and enlarging mist or edge processing answers for carry insight to IoT. Thus, brilliant gadgets produce quite an immense measure of quickly dissected sensor information [20].

10.8   AI AND IOT IN HEALTHCARE

With regards to joining computer based intelligence and IoT in medical services, will improve operational productivity in this field. Following dissecting, control, advancement, preparing, and mechanization, demonstrating, foreseeing are the key advances that accommodate the keen and productive use of simulated intelligence calculations in IoT gadgets. Consequently, the primary use instances of AI empowered IoT are the accompanying:

• Medical staff, patients, and stock following
• People suffering from Chronic Disease
• Drug the board
• Emergency room stands by time decrease
• Remote wellbeing control

The most ideal approach to disclose why one necessities to utilize simulated intelligence empowered IoT in medical services is to give a more itemized investigation of the IoT operational standards empowering a more nuanced comprehension of possible fields of its application in the medical care framework [21,22].

10.8.1 GADGETS WITH ACTUAL INTERFACES TO/FROM THIS PRESENT REALITY

On a very basic level, in medical care, any help a customer demands are identified with the actual world. Also, the utilization of administrations includes the actual association of parental figures, patients, and the gadgets as these are associated gadget and as advanced mechanics in medication it communicate with the actual climate through different actual interfaces.

10.8.2 ORGANIZED INFORMATION CONTRIBUTION THROUGH SENSORS

IoT innovation produces remote sensor organizations. As recently expressed, these organizations are effectively crossing over the physical and computerized universe. Information is gathered by the sensor gadgets and then shipped off the information to the control place for additional input.

10.8.3 MINUSCULE INFORMATION/YIELD GADGETS

There are sure prerequisites for the appearance and size of the actual IO gadgets. Additionally, the necessities should be changed in accordance with the ecological conditions in which the gadget is working. Thus, rather than human interfaces that need moderately enormous information/yield gadgets, actual interfaces of IoT gadgets get contribution through sensors (which are small because of the utilization of miniature electromechanical frameworks (MEMS) innovation) and send information back to versatile/cloud PCs through wired or remote interfaces. Consider such cases as embedded heart-cadence screens and gadgets constantly estimating and observing biochemical information [23].

10.8.4 HUMAN–MACHINE–CLIMATE FRAMEWORK DRIVERS

Obviously, human-machine cooperation alludes to the cycle of correspondence among individuals and computerized frameworks. In any case, the web of things is based on the establishment of a more perplexing relationship among the human, machine, and climate. In medical care, the climate is a profoundly significant boundary that infers the amount of physical and social factors and the ongoing observing of the ecological factor is significantly more basic for this industry once the IoT innovation is in activity [24].

10.8.5 CONTINUOUS ACTIVITY AND CHOICE CONTROL

One of the principle favorable circumstances the interoperability of AI and IoT is bringing is that there is an opportunity to monitor what is happening and to respond upon it on the spot. It implies the move toward dynamic patient association, altered treatment designs ongoing change and a more shrewd way to deal with information. Ongoing examination is just conceivable when a surge of information is ceaseless. In any case, it is not really conceivable that a framework doing complex handling activities can adapt to the almost ceaseless information stream from various sensors. It is a constant computer based intelligence framework that can decrease the measure of information and empower insightful information in the executives.

10.9 IMPACTFUL UNIQUENESS OF IOT ASSOCIATED WITH MEDICAL FIELD

There are different highlights of the IoT application. Here we can contemplating of those highlights due to which IoT applications is firmly suggested in clinical documented appeared in Figure 10.1. With consistent availability gave by IoT applications/gadgets, clinical staff can screen Covid-19 patient just as self-isolate people remotely [25,26]. As there are number of the clinical staff who are not accessible contrasted with the absolute number of tainted or suspected Covid-19 infection. With information security gave by IoT applications, clinical staff can gather the fundamental boundary these patients at one place and choose further action [6]. IoT applications are definitely not hard to use so the patients can manage these applications all alone. With less usage cost, IoT application gives incredible degree of exactness. IoT application will successfully confine the individual to individual contact which will at last lessen the spread of the Covid-19. Additionally with utilization of such applications we can save an existence of our clinical staff. The wellbeing boundaries which are checked by IoT gadget are transferred on cloud which will be helpful for any specialist to investigation the patient history. Alongside observing wellbeing boundary, IoT gives the crisis administrations which incorporate following the area (GPS) of patient by wellbeing station, setting up compensation among specialist and patient, sending rescue vehicle from closest emergency clinic to tolerant. For observing this boundary, diverse biosensors will be interfaced with various sheets like Node MCU, Android and Raspberry Pi [27] (Figure 10.2).

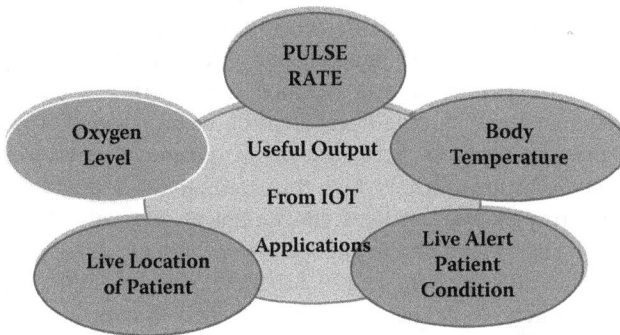

FIGURE 10.1   IoT in COVID-19 pandemic situation.

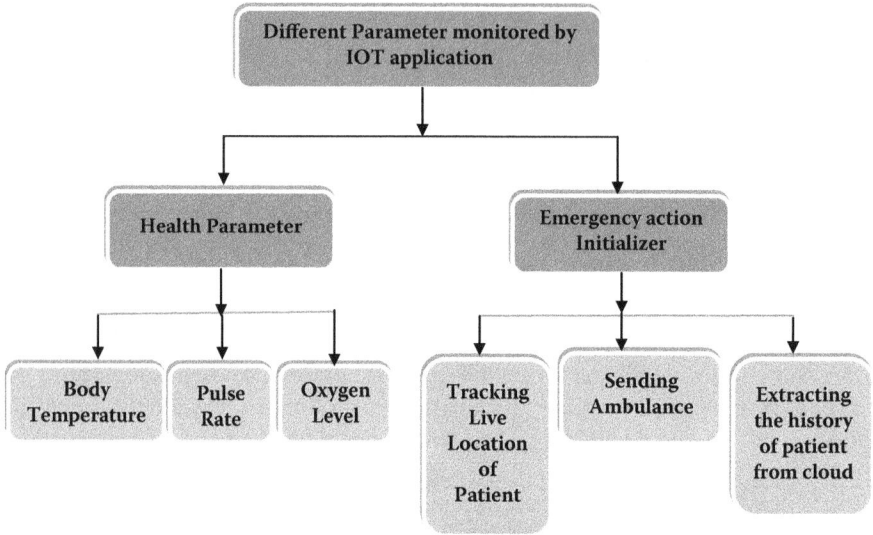

FIGURE 10.2 Different parameters monitored by IoT.

Likewise we can set a caution framework for quiet reminding to screen the wellbeing boundaries which will be ship off the clinical officials and close by wellbeing station. For detecting the pulse in the IoT-based framework applications ROHM's BH1790GLC optical sensor screens, pulse rate sensor, BM-CS5R pulse screen wearable heart observing inductive sensor are used for detecting the internal heat level in the IoT-based medical services application. Also LM35, MAX30205, G-TPCO-033, NTC indoor regulators and RTD sensors are utilized [28].

10.10 FUTURE MODEL OF HEALTHCARE BASED IOT AND MACHINE LEARNING

The information from the sensor network is gathered and handled by the microcontroller. The proposed results are put in the cloud storage. From the cloud the handled information can be recovered and analyzed. The investigated information is again put in the cloud which can be recovered (Figure 10.3).

The whole framework can be sectored into three significant parts. Wellbeing checking framework, Health state expectation framework and emergency ready framework which are the three significant areas of the proposition. The information gathered and measures must be kept secretly. To guarantee privacy and security, encryption components are utilized which adds credit to the drafted framework. The wellbeing monitoring module involves the equipment segments of the framework that makes it IoT empowered and is utilized to record the wellbeing boundaries of the patient utilizing different sensors [29,30]. Here, Raspberry Pi goes about as a focal worker to which all the sensors are associated through the GPIO pins or utilizing MCP3008 simple to-computerized convertor if their yield is in the simple structure as Raspberry Pi works just on advanced signs. Wellbeing state forecast is

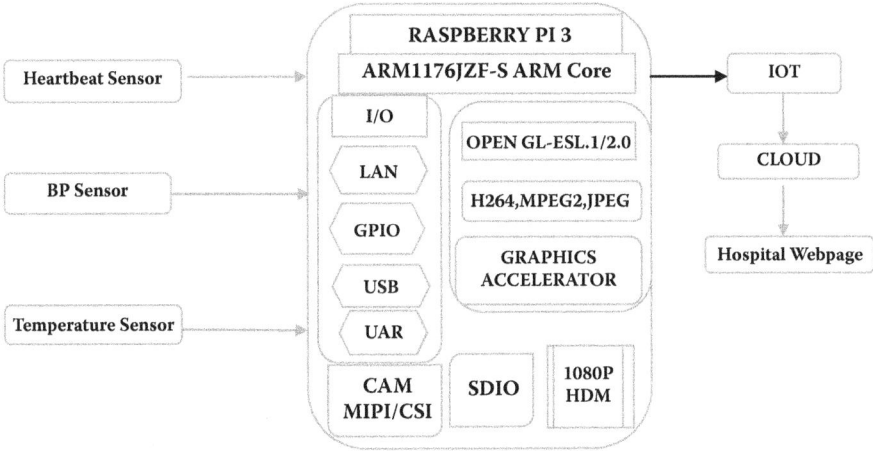

FIGURE 10.3 Architecture of IoT and Machine Learning.

quite possibly the most encouraging modules of the proposed framework. In this module, the patients' wellbeing information are gathered from the tangible hubs and put away in the database [31]. The information put away in the data set is exposed to be tried in the KNN classifier which arranges different conditions of the individual's wellbeing. The precise order is made by the classifier which barely needs manual reviewing

10.10.1 IoT ARCHITECTURE FOR DISEASE DETECTION

This framework gives a stage to observing and regulating patients by the use sensor organizations. The plan comprises of both equipment and programming areas. The equipment area incorporates heart rate sensor, temperature sensor, blood pressure sensor, and Raspberry Pi board. The phases of the cycle incorporates assortment of sensor esteems, stockpiling of information in the cloud and the investigation of the information put away in the cloud to check for anomalies in the medical issue (Figure 10.4).

The assortments from the standard regularly happen when there is an undetected action in the body parts [32]. The beat can be assessed by using beat sensor. The speed of the heart at every second can be assessed. The sensor is interfaced with Raspberry Pi board to picture the resultant characteristics. The characteristics can be envisioned by using either persistent screen or by interfacing a LCD show. Since the volume of data is enormous, all the data accumulated are delivered off the cloud. The data transport off the cloud is penniless down in the close by side. All things considered, the speed of heart beat will as a rule increase persistently for any sporadic conditions. A couple of open source cloud stages maintain Raspberry Pi board [33]. It is an open source and the data assembled are moved in the cloud by selecting the real area. The examination of the characteristics accumulated for the presence of any varieties from the standard is done by using AI figuring's. The characteristics accumulated in the cloud are then imported with the ultimate

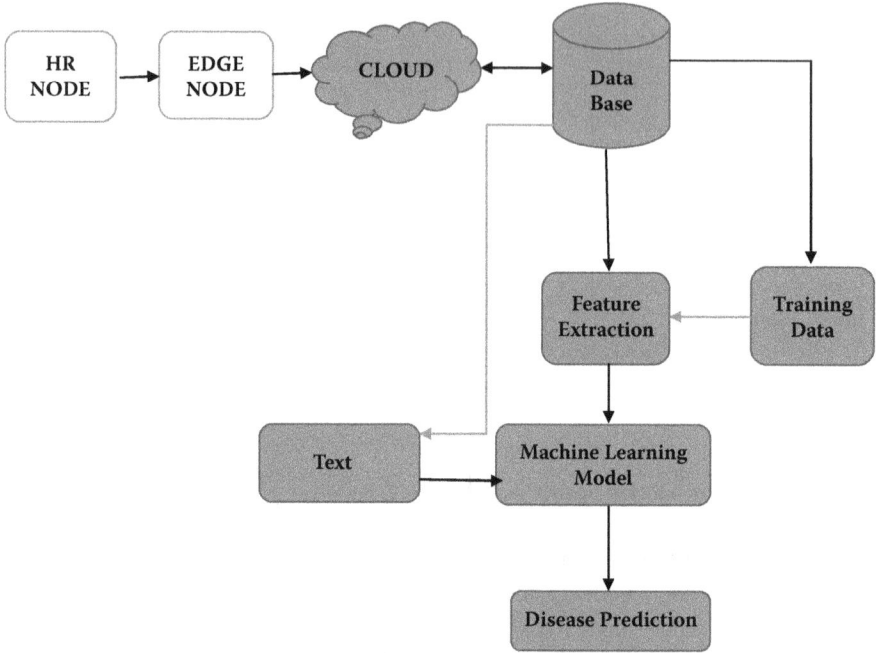

FIGURE 10.4 Block diagram for disease detection.

objective of examination. To get accurate assumptions, tremendous entirety data ought to be prepared [34]. Stage Larger the data readied, higher the precision. The dataset that will be prepared should comprise of the information gathered from different people under numerous conditions. Additionally, the dataset ought to have the information gathered from people of various age and it ought to have the information of both solid and unfortunate people. The information that is tried till the past meeting should be remembered for the preparation dataset and the information that is gathered at the prompt second is the information to be tried. By the utilization of the information prepared at first and the down to earth information that is incorporated, expectation is made [35]. The Health Fog model is an IoT-based haze empowered distributed computing model for medical services, which can deal with the information of heart patients adequately and analyze the wellbeing status to distinguish coronary illness seriousness. Health Fog coordinates assorted equipment instruments through programming segments and permits organized and consistent start to finish incorporation of Edge-Fog Cloud for quick and precise conveyance of results [36].

10.10.2 IMPROVING APPROPRIATION OF MEDICAL CARE SYSTEM WITH IOT AND MACHINE LEARNING

The field of AI is developing consistently, alongside the development of the IoT. Sensors, nano cameras, and other such IoT components are presently pervasive PCs, stopping stations, traffic light focuses and even in home machines. There are a huge number of IoT gadgets on the planet and more are being fabricated each day [37]. They gather tremendous measures of information that is taken care of machines by means of the Internet, empowering machines to 'learn' from the information and make them more productive. Today, the IoT interfaces a few areas, for example, fabricating enterprises, medical care, structures, vehicles, traffic, malls, etc. Information assembled from such assorted areas can unquestionably cause the foundation to adapt seriously to work all the more productively. Let us take an illustration of brilliant leaving it adequately takes care of vehicle leaving issues. IoT observing today can find void parking spots and rapidly direct vehicles to parking spaces. Today, savvy structures can computerize focal warming, cooling, lighting, lifts, fire-wellbeing frameworks, and the kickoff of entryways, kitchen apparatuses, and so forth, utilizing the IoT and AI (ML) strategies. Another significant issue looked by brilliant urban areas is vehicle flocking [38]. This circumstance can be kept away from by the development of mechanized interstates and by building shrewd vehicles. IoT and ML together offer better answers for keep away from vehicle running. This will bring about more prominent efficiency, diminished blockage and less car accidents. Today, drones in military activities are modified with ML calculations. This empowers them to figure out which bits of information gathered by IoT are basic to the mission and which are definitely not. They gather continuous information when in-flight. These robots survey all approaching information and naturally dispose of superfluous information, successfully overseeing information payloads issues at a quicker speed. Patients will likewise have more control of their own data. During the pandemic, it has been imperative for clinical offices to use or put more in new advanced medical services advances. The medical services area benefits massively from going more computerized, particularly for advancing social removing. Clinical experts are additionally improving their associations with patients by offering more reasonable choices through advanced administrations. Rather than patients visiting emergency clinics for minor occurrences, looking for quicker arrangements online is getting more prudent and advantageous. Customers can arrange drugs on the web and get remedies at a neighborhood drug store. Computerized and portable innovations are carrying immense advantages to the medical services area. By grasping these advances, medical services associations can see better achievement rates [39]. Today, keen, helped living conditions for locally established medical services for ongoing patients are exceptionally basic. The climate joins the patient's clinical history and semantic portrayal of ICP (singular consideration measure) with the capacity to screen the day to day environments utilizing IoT advances. In this way the Semantic Web of Things (SWOT) and ML calculations, when consolidated together, bring about LDC (less separated guardian). Telemedicine can be viewed as a `crude' type of an IoT in medical services model. With IoT, a patient can be noticed and now and again treated distantly through camcorders and other electronic actuators [32].The resultant incorporated medical care system can give huge investment funds while improving general wellbeing. In protection frameworks today, self-mending drones are gradually picking up broad acknowledgment. Each robot has its own ML calculation as it flies on a mission. Utilizing this, a gathering of robots on a mission can recognize when one individual from the gathering has fizzled, and afterward speak with different robots to pull together and proceed with the military mission without interference.

In this time of correspondence and network, people have various advancements to help their everyday prerequisites. In this situation, IoT along with Machine Learning is arising as a reasonable answer for issues [40]. Block chain IoT and Machine Learning is an astounding threesome of Emerging advancements. Block chain innovation makes information safer, Machine Learning investigates the information, and IoT makes information safer. In the coming not many years, a block chain-based environment will arise. Block chain would decrease a few issues like applications, development openings, identity management,

10.11 CONCLUSION

Wellbeing variables of human whenever left unnoticed will bring about difficult issues and even reason threat to their life. Computerizing the ceaseless observing of heath boundaries through IoT is talked about as novel arrangement. Innovation assumes the significant job in medical care for tangible gadgets as well as in correspondence, recording and show gadget. It is critical to screen different clinical boundary sand post operational days. Henceforth the most recent pattern in healthcare specialized strategy utilizing IoT and Machine Learning strategies. Web of things fills in as an impetus for the medical services and assumes conspicuous job in wide scope of medical care applications. Starting preparing and approval of AI calculations are performed by utilizing the UCI dataset. Testing stage appraises the expectation of anomalies from the sensor information gathered through the IoT structure. Factual investigation is performed from information collected into the cloud from IoT gadget to appraise the precision in forecast rate and for this sort of IoT, stage based persistent checking of human heath boundaries, AI calculations had assumed a critical job.

REFERENCES

[1]. M. Darrell, Improving health care through mobile medical devices and sensors. *Brookings Institution Policy Report*, 10, 1–13 (2013).

[2]. P. S. Sousa, D. Sabugueiro, V. Felizardo, R. Couto, I. Pires and N. M. Garcia, mHealth sensors and applications for personal aid. in *Mobile Health*, S. Adibi, Ed., Berlin, Germany: Springer (2015), Springer Series in Bio-/Neuroinformatics, vol. 5.

[3]. Kheirkhahan, M., et al., A smartwatch-based framework for realtime and online assessment and mobility monitoring. *Journal of Biomedical Informatics*, 89, 29–40 (2019).

[4]. S. Majumder and M. J. Deen, Smartphone sensors for health monitoring and diagnosis. *Sensors*, 19 (9), 2164, (2019).

[5]. Yacchirema, D., de Puga, J. S., Palau, C. and Esteve, M., Fall detection system for elderly people using IoT and ensemble machine learning algorithm. *Personal and Ubiquitous Computing*, 23, 801–817 (2019).

[6]. Yin and N. K. Jha. A health decision support system for disease diagnosis based on wearable medical sensors and machine learning ensembles. *IEEE Transactions on Multi-Scale Computing Systems*, 3 (4), 228–241 (October 2017).

[7]. L. Xavier, R. Thirunavukarasu and R. Thirunavukarasu, A distributed tree-based ensemble learning approach for efficient structure prediction of protein. *International Journal of Intelligent Engineering and Systems*, 10 (3), 226–234 (2017).

[8]. Vembandasamy, R. Sasipriya and E.Deepa, Heart diseases detection using Naive Bayes algorithm. *International Journal of Innovative Science, Engineering & Technology*, 2(9), 441–444 (2015).

[9]. T. Huang, L. Lan, X. Fang, P. An, J. Min and F. Wang, Promises and challenges of big data computing in health sciences. *Big Data Research*, 2 (1), 2–11 (2015).

[10]. H. Asri, H. Mousannif, H. Al Moatassime and T. Noel, Big data in healthcare: Challenges and opportunities, in *Proceedings of the international Conference on cloud Technologies and applications (CloudTech)*, pp. 1–7, Marrakech, Morocco (June 2015).

[11]. O. Akmandor and N. K. Jha. Smart health care: An edge-side computing perspective. *EEE Consumer Electronics Magazine*, 7 (1), 29–37 (January 2018).

[12]. Dai, H. Yin and N. K. Jha, NeST: A neural network synthesis tool based on a grow-and-prune paradigm. arXiv preprint arXiv:1711.02017 (2017).

[13]. Ahmadi, H., Arji, G., Shahmoradi, L., Safdari, R., Nilashi, M. and Alizadeh, M., The application of internet of things in healthcare: A systematic literature review and classification. *Universal Access in the Information Society*, 18(4), 837–869 (2019).

[14]. Simblett, S., et al., Barriers to and facilitators of engagement with remote measurement technology for managing health: Systematic review and content analysis of findings. *Journal of Medical Internet Research*, 20 (7), e10480 (2018).

[15]. Raja, K., Saravanan, S., Anitha, R., Priya, S. S. and Subhashini, R., Design of a low power ECG signal processor for wearable health system-review and implementation issues. In: 2017 11th International Conference on Intelligent Systems and Control (ISCO). IEEE (2017), 383–387.

[16]. A. M. Rahmani, et al., Exploiting smart e-health gateways at the edge of healthcare internet-of-things: A fog computing approach. *Future Generation Computer Systems* 78 (2018), 641–658 (2018).

[17]. Milenkovic, M. J., Vukmirovic, A. and Milenkovic, D., Big data analytics in the health sector: Challenges and potentials. *Management: Journal of Sustainable Business and Management Solutions in Emerging Economies*, 24(1), 23–33 (2019).

[18]. Ullah, K., Shah, M. A. and Zhang, S., Effective ways to use Internet of Things in the field of medical and smart health care. in 2016 International Conference on Intelligent Systems Engineering (ICISE), 2016, 372–379 (2016).

[19]. Vallabh, P. and Malekian, R., Fall detection monitoring systems: A comprehensive review. *Journal of Ambient Intelligence and Humanized Computing* 9 (6), 1809–1833 (2018).

[20]. Anand, P., Pinjari, H., Hong, W. H., Seo, H. C. and Rho, S., Fog computing-based IoT for health monitoring system. Journal of Sensors, 2018 (2018), Article ID 1386470, 7 pages. 10.1155/2018/1386470.

[21]. Yacchirema, D., de Puga, J. S., Palau, C. and Esteve, M., Fall detection system for elderly people using IoT and ensemble machine learning algorithm. *Personal and Ubiquitous Computing*, 1–17 (2019).

[22]. Shahid, N., Rappon, T. and Berta, W., Applications of artificial neural networks in health care organizational decision-making: A scoping review. *PLoS ONE*, 14 (2), 1–22 (2019).

[23]. Zemouri, R., Zerhouni, N. and Racoceanu, D., Deep learning in the biomedical applications: Recent and future status. *Applied Sciences*, 9 (8), 1526–1546 (2019).

[24]. Soleimani-Roozbahani, F., Ghatari, A. R. and Radfar, R., Knowledge discovery from a more than a decade studies on healthcare Big Data systems: A scientometrics study. *Journal of Big Data*, 6 (1), 1–15 (2019).

[25]. R. Y. Kim, The impact of COVID-19 on consumers: Preparing for digital sales. in *IEEE Engineering Management Review*. doi: 10.1109/EMR.2020.2990115.

[26]. Aleem A., Javaid M., Vaishya R. and Deshmukh S. G., Areas of academic research with the impact of COVID-19. *AJEM (American Journal of Emergency Medicine)*, 38(7), 1524–1526 (2020).

[27]. Hegde, N., Bries, M., Swibas, T., Melanson, E. and Sazonov, E., Automatic recognition of activities of daily living utilizing insolebased and wrist-worn wearable sensors. *IEEE Journal of Biomedical and Health Informatics*, 22 (4), 979–988 (2018).

[28]. Park, E., Park, E., Kim, K. J., Kim, K. J., Kwon, S. J. and Kwon, S. J., Understanding the emergence of wearable devices as nextgeneration tools for health communication. *Information Technology & People*, 29 (4), 717–732 (2016).

[29]. Rajput, D. S. and Gour, R., An IoT framework for healthcare monitoring systems. *International Journal of Computer Science and Information Security (IJCSIS)*, 14 (5), 451 (2016).

[30]. H. Jamaladin, Mobile apps for blood pressure monitoring: Systematic search in app stores and content analysis. *JMIR mHealth and uHealth*, 6, 11 (2018).

[31]. Wu, J., Li, H., Cheng, S. and Lin, Z., The promising future of healthcare services: When big data analytics meets wearable technology. *Information & Management*, 53, 1020–1033 (2016).

[32]. Mutlag, A. A., Khanapi, A. M., Ghani, N. Arunkumar, Mazin Abed Mohammed, Othman M. and Enabling technologies for fog computing in healthcare IoT systems. *Future Generation Computer Systems, Elsevier Science Direct*, 90, Jan. 2019, 62–78 (2019). 10.1016/j.future.2018.07.049.

[33]. Ahmed, S., El Seddawy, A. I. and Nasr, M., A proposed framework for detecting and predicting diseases through business intelligence applications. *International Journal of Advanced Networking and Applications*, 10 (4), 3951–3955 (2019).

[34]. Malik, M. M., Abdallah, S. and Ala'raj, M., Data mining and predictive analytics applications for the delivery of healthcare services: A systematic literature review. *Annals of Operations Research*, 270 (1–2), 287–312 (2018).

[35]. M. Hauskrecht, Visweswaran S., Cooper G. and Clermont G., Outlier detection of patient monitoring and alerting. *Journal of Biomedical Informatics*, 46(1), 47–55 (2015).

[36]. Birnbaum M. L., Ernala S. K., Rizvi A. F., et al. A collaborative approach to identifying social media markers of schizophrenia by employing machine learning and clinical appraisals. *Journal of Medical Internet Research*, 19 (8): e289 (2017).

[37]. Marin~elarena-Dondena L., Ferreti E., Maragoudakis M., et al., Predicting depression: A comparative study of machine learning approaches based on language usage. *Cuad Neuropsicol/Panam J Neuropsychol*, 11 (3), 42–54 (2017).

[38]. Puliafito, C., Mingozzi, E., Longo, F., Puliafito, A. and Rana, O., Fog computing for the internet of things: A survey. *ACM Transactions on Internet Technology*, 19 (2), Article 18 (April 2019), 41 pages (2019).

[39]. George, A., Dhanasekaran, H., Chittiappa, J. P., Challagundla, L. A., S.S. Nikkam and O. A., Internet of Things in health care using fog computing, 2018 IEEE Long Island Systems. Applications and Technology Conference (LISAT) (2018). 10.11 09/LISAT.2018.8378012.

[40]. S. S. Kazi, G. Bajantri and T. Thite, Remote heart rate monitoring system using IoT. *International Research Journal of Engineering and Technology (IRJET)*, Volumemac_mac 05 (04) (April 2018).

Shweta Agarwal and Chander Prabha

CONTENTS

DOI: 10.1201/9781003171829-11

11.1   INTRODUCTION

Artificial intelligence is so impactful in the field of healthcare as its purpose is to make systems more powerful in handling healthcare challenges, and by using different techniques, data can be interpreted, which is collected by diagnosing various chronic diseases like cancer, diabetes, Alzheimer's disease, and cardiovascular diseases. It helps in improving clinical intervention, disease prediction, early detection, and disease progression. Machine learning (ML) techniques play a vital role in the healthcare sector, including the advancement of analytical model. These models can provide immediate benefit to clinical decision support system and healthcare service applications. To classify behavioral characteristics and health symptoms of the patient, these models examine the acquired data from different sources and sensor devices. ML and Internet of Things (IoT) have been widely used in healthcare.

Here, we'll discuss different ML algorithms that are useful in healthcare for the diagnosis and prediction of diseases, along with an importance of IoT in Healthcare.

11.1.1   STUDY OF ML ALGORITHMS FOR DISEASE PREDICTION

Today's computing era is the era of the ML. ML is something in which a machine or system is able to learn from certain algorithms and make predictions on the basis of it. ML algorithms are implemented everywhere. Its implementation is popular in so many applications. In online customer support, recommendation system, self-driving car, etc., ML algorithms are widely used [1,2].

One such implementation of ML is in the field of healthcare, where it is useful in disease prediction and diagnosis that helps doctors for easier and better diagnosis of diseases. Most common three ML algorithms are:

  i. Supervised Learning (Train Me)
 ii. Unsupervised Learning (I'm self-sufficient in Learning)
iii. Reinforcement Learning (My life My rules, Hit and Trial)

Some of the commonly used Supervised ML techniques [3], which are useful for the prediction and diagnosis of diseases are mentioned below:

a. **Decision Tree**—It is a tree-like representation of decisions and all their possible solutions based on certain conditions. It is a type of classification which is helpful for physicians as well as doctors in diagnosing patients with higher risk of particular diseases. Earlier disease prediction is possible with the help of decision trees.

b. **Logistic Regression**—It is a supervised classification method based on linear regression [4]. It is known as regression but not logistic classifier because logistic regression uses linear models. This model can be used for binary classification as well as for multi-class classification problem. This model is useful to find a certain class of an independent variable; it can also find the possibility that a new instance belongs to or does not belongs to a new class by using an outcome that lies in range zero and one. Hence, to use the model for binary classification, and to make predictions, threshold the classifier output to 0.5. If the hypothesis returns a value $>= 0.5$, it is classified as "1," otherwise as "0." In healthcare, LR model helps in finding whether the tumor is malignant or not.

c. **Support Vector Machine**—It is capable of performing outlier detection, regression and classification. Support Vector Machine is a discriminative classifier that is formally designed by a separative hyperplane. It can classify linear as well as non-linear data. It works by first mapping every data item into an n-dimensional feature space where n is the number of features, and then identifies the hyperplane that separates the data items into two classes while maximizing the marginal distance for both classes and minimizing the classification errors [5]. To perform the classification, we then need to find the hyperplane that differentiates the two classes by the maximum margin.

d. **Random Forest**—It is a collection or ensemble of DTs [6], where decision trees are build using the whole dataset by considering all features but RF only a fraction of rows are selected randomly and particular number of features also selected at random for training. In this way, DTs are grown and each DT will result in a final outcome and RF will just compile the result of DTs to bring the final result. In RF, the use of multiple trees reduces the risk of overfitting along with less time required in training. Its main advantage is that when a large portion of data is missing, then also it produces high accurate predictions and efficiently runs in large databases.

  e. **Naïve Bayes**—NB is simple and powerful predictive modeling classification technique on the basis of Bayes theorem [7]. Alternatively known as Bayes law or Bayes rule, this theorem describes the possibility of an occurrence based on previous knowledge of the circumstances that may be related to an event. In simple terms, if feature depends on each other [8], then also it assumes that the presence of particular feature in a class is unrelated to the presence of any other feature. This model is useful and easy to build for large datasets.

  f. **K-nearest neighbor**—On the basis of similarity of features, classification can be performed using KNN classifier [9]. For classification, it is used as one of the simplest supervised ML algorithm. Based on how its neighbors are classified, it classifies data points. All available cases are stored and new cases are classified on the basis of a similarity measure. K in KNN is a parameter referring to the number of nearest neighbors to be included in the majority voting. A process called parameter tuning is to choose the correct value of k, and it is necessary for better accuracy.

11.1.2 IoT in Healthcare

IoT performs a crucial role in healthcare. There exists so many definitions of IoT, but it can be defined as a network of interconnected devices that communicate and exchange data through M2M (machine to machine) communications [10–12]. Healthcare generally faces issues in research, devices and treatment.

Medical research lacks data from the real world that is helpful to solve crucial conditions; hence for medical examination, they have to rely on left-over data. Via real-time testing and research, IoT provides a solution to access useful data and improves the standard of treatment. By designing systems rather than equipment, it bridges the gap between reading devices and providing healthcare. It completely transforms the patient healthcare by making it more technologically advanced.

11.1.2.1 Applications of IoT in Healthcare

There are so many IoT applications in healthcare. Some of the IoT applications are shown in Figure 11.1 and are listed below:

  a. **Blood pressure monitoring**—It is the most significant physiological parameters of the human body. There are many blood pressure devices popular that are safe and simple to use [11]. Healthcare systems when linked with sensors, makes easy communication between doctors and patients. To collect the patient's BP in real time, electronic BP monitor is attached to an IoT sensor.

  b. **Rehabilitation system**—A rehabilitation system will enhance and recover physical abilities and improve the life of individuals in order to mitigate challenges related with elderly populations and wherever there is a shortage of health providers [11]. Some smart care systems are there that is community-based and offers successful therapy. It is possible to use an ontology-based automation modeling methodology approach connected to the

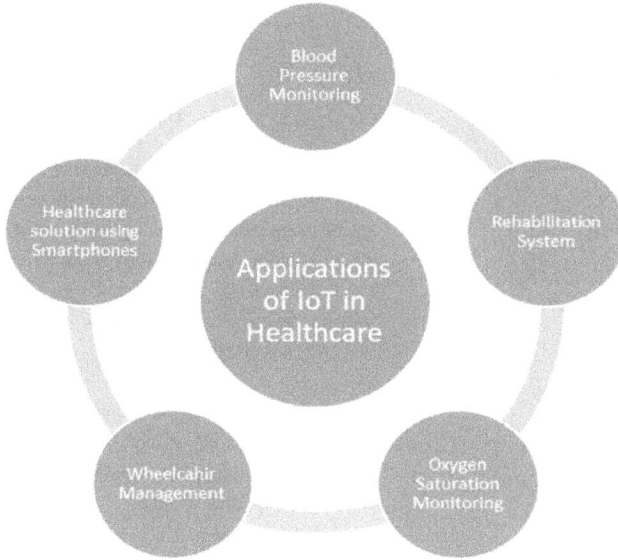

FIGURE 11.1   Applications of IoT in healthcare.

IoT-based smart recovery system to easily interact and distribute medical services according to patient needs [10].

c. **Oxygen saturation monitoring**—To continuously monitor the saturation of patient's blood oxygen in a non-invasive manner, a device named as pulse oximeter is used [11]. Many developments are there in communication technology, such as wireless networks, and because of low power consumption and low loss, medical sensors are already booming. Continuous pulse oximeters are used in many medical procedures to consider the levels of oxygen in the blood and also the heart rate (HR). IoT sensors, which are attached to the body of the patient, regulate and monitor the patient's pulse rate and oxygen levels, which can restrict patient activity [13].

d. **Wheelchair management**—People who suffer from physical disease or disability and unable to walk, use wheelchair. In order to be used as a human-centric sensing (sensor) system for wheelchair users, WBANs (Wireless Body Area Networks) will connect smart objects to the Internet. There will be a resistive pressure sensor that will sense when the human body falls off the wheelchair. There is another accelerator sensor in a smart wheelchair that senses the fall of the wheelchair [14].

e. **Healthcare solutions using smartphones**—Smart healthcare applications and devices offer healthcare professionals (HCPs) with many benefits. There are many medical healthcare apps that are currently accessible and ready for use in many areas, such as proper clinical decision making, patient continuous monitoring as well as consultation with doctors, communication, information and time, health record [15]. The treatment has been speed up with the use of mobile applications and sensors that support in improving patient outcomes.

TABLE 11.1

Healthcare apps for smartphones [11]

Healthcare Apps	Description
Heart rate monitor	It is useful in continuously monitoring the heart rate and also gathers all related information in real-time.
Fall detector	As the name indicates, this app keeps track of person's activity and generates an alert at the time of falling.
Pedometer	This is a commonly used app which records our footsteps at the time of walking, and stores the information about total calories burned per unit time.
Water your body	This is very useful for those persons whose water intake is very low. As it tracks our drinking habits and reminds us to drink water in every hour.
Skin vision	It helps in identifying skin disorder earliest by tracking the skin condition time to time.
Calorie counter	It is helpful in keeping track of the food consumed by us and also calculates fat, cholesterol as well as weight present in our body.
Blood pressure monitor	This app helps in collecting real-time data of the patient's BP level and analyzes it.
Body temperature	It keeps track of the temperature of the body and provides notification when the temperature of the body is increased.
Eye exercises—eye care Plus	It helps in monitoring eye vision and provides training as well.
Asthma trackers and log	This app is for Asthma patients to track their information of real-time.
Cardio mobile	This app helps in monitoring real-time data of cardiac rehabilitation in a person.
Pill reminder	It is very useful to remind a patient about taking the pills on time.

As seen in Table 11.1, few common healthcare applications for smartphones.

11.2 HEALTH MONITORING USING IOT AND MACHINE LEARNING

IoT, AI, ML, and big data help physicians in finding the root cause of diseases in patients and also predict its seriousness using various technological tools and algorithms. IoT is a solution in reducing the burden on healthcare. Health monitoring system is a system useful to track health of a patient with the aid of sensors. It keeps track of the pulse rate of the patient, heart rate, pressure level rate, temperature, and so on. The system mechanically warns a user when the device senses any sudden changes in patient pulse or temperature and even displays description of patient temperature and heartbeat live on an internet [16].

11.2.1 Materials and Methods Used for Health Monitoring

11.2.1.1 Heartbeat Rate Sensor

The pulse sensor is one of the active heartbeat sensors for Arduino fitting and attachment play. It cuts to a fingertip and quickly expands in an Arduino, also provides an open-source tracking program that, diagrams the pulse. The sensor's front part is checked by the heart shape logo that is typically at the side of the skin that produces contact. A little low round hole can be seen on the front that is a spot from which LED originates from back. The LED gleams light into the fingertip or ear ligament or other thin tissue, and the sensor scans the proportion of light bouncing back. It is a way to learn the beat. Opposite side of sensor is location where majority of the components are mounted.

11.2.1.2 Dataset

Dataset is a perception that comes from space. A dataset is a set of examples and we typically require a few datasets for different reasons when dealing with AI techniques. Using AI calculations, the data is then prepared and tried. To prepare our model, a dataset is used to authorize the accuracy of the model and to feed the data into AI calculation.

11.2.1.3 Information Pre-processing

Pre-processing of information is a structure that turns into an impeccable educational record over grungy information. For example, Random Forest estimation does not improve invalid attributes, so from chief unpleasant educational record to perform flighty backwoods check, invalid qualities must be administered. In a predefined position, some specified AI model requires data. Another opinion is that the enlightening spectrum should be structured in order to perform more approximation of ML and DL (Deep Learning) in a record to choose the best one.

11.2.1.4 Machine Learning Classifiers

Some well-known characterizations are utilized in ML algorithms like—Decision Tree, LR, NB, SVM, and K-nearest neighbor. Any such algorithm can be used to diagnose whether the disease is present or not. A smart intelligent system to predict the disease is shown in Figure 11.2.

By incorporating this through the functionality of a wearable sensor system that has sensors installed on it, IoT has been used in making systems that alert the patient's peers in case of abnormality. ML is helpful in medical diagnosis field by using models that are equipped to recognize any abnormality in patient's condition [18].

UCI dataset is used on which initial level training as well as testing of various ML algorithms is performed. Testing phase helps in estimating the prediction of different abnormalities obtained by an IoT system from the collected sensor data. To estimate the accuracy of prediction percentage, statistical analysis is carried out from data accumulated from the IoT system in the cloud. ML algorithms are much helpful in this type of IoT platform that focuses on continuous monitoring of human health parameters [19].

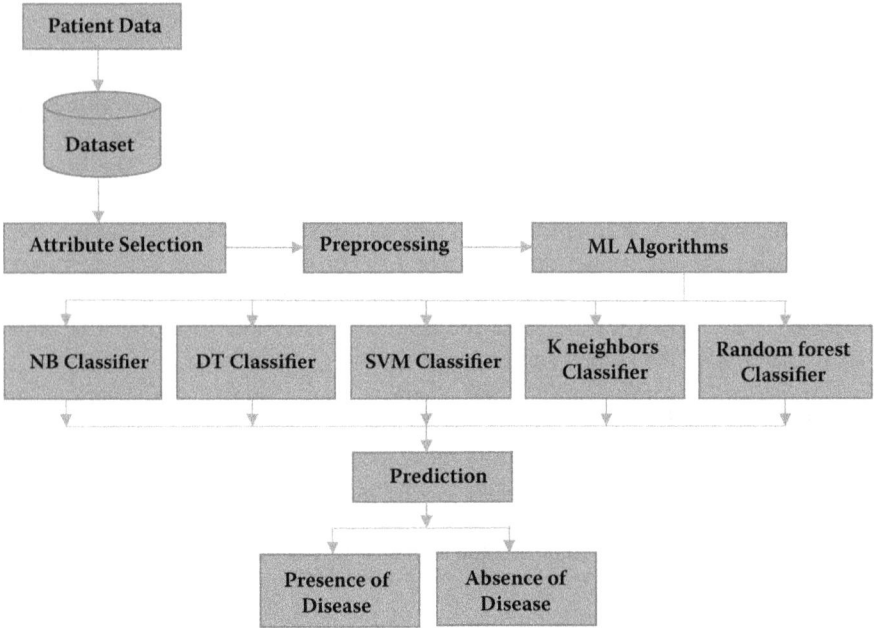

FIGURE 11.2   A smart intelligent system for predicting disease [17].

11.3   APPLYING MACHINE LEARNING IN IOT DATA FOR DISEASE PREDICTION AND DIAGNOSIS MODEL

Health care prediction and diagnosis system based on IoT comprises of "internet on health sensor things." ML techniques help in predicting various medical applications like brain tumor, diabetes, and cancer [20]. It involves big data, which is problematic for physicians to handle, but they need such historical data to predict patient's health, in which ML algorithm will be useful.

Data mining techniques are used such as MLP, RF, DT, SVM, and KNN, and their efficiency is compared to confirm healthcare industry's quality of service. Manual health related facilities are often unable to meet on time due to remote physical locations and thus causes significant life hazards. To support medical emergencies, real-time monitoring, early diagnosis and chronic disease, the main reason for using the IoT-based health care system is to use updated health care networks powered by wireless technology. In addition, IoT offers effective scheduling of scarce resources by ensuring the best utilization and facilities for patients.

Out of global population, 12.3% aged greater than and equal to 60 years, according to the United Nations Population Fund report, and by 2050, that figure will grow to nearly 22%. Thus, in such a situation in which the IoT-based health care system plays a critical role in bridging the gap between patients and doctor, there will be a tremendous need for medical assistance for the elderly.

Hence, in this section, various methodologies using IoT and ML to predict and diagnose various diseases will be discussed.

11.3.1 Brain Tumor Classification Using Machine Learning and Role of IoT in Providing Solution

One of the deadliest diseases caused by uncontrollable and irregular partitioning of cells is the Brain Tumor. Various kinds of brain tumor exist, but the following types can be identified specifically as brain tumors [21,22]:

- Benign tumor
- Pre-malignant tumor
- Malignant tumor

A tumor which does not affect the healthy tissues, does not spread to non-adjacent tissues, and does not grow unexpectedly known as benign tumor. Moles are one of its examples, while a pre-malignant tumor is a pre-carcinogenic stage and, can be identified as a cancer, if not treated.

Malignant neoplasm is also a kind of tumor that worsens with time and the death of the infected individual is eventually the outcome. Within the skull, tumor cells are present and develop within the skull, which is considered as the primary tumor.

Incipient brain tumors are malignant brain tumors. Outside a skull, the tumor emerges and reaches to region of the skull called secondary tumor. One of the examples of secondary tumors are metastatic tumors. In the skull, the tumor takes its place and interferes with the brain's normal functioning. The tumor switches to skull and raises brain pressure. First step towards treatment is the detection of the tumor [21,22].

"Detection of the brain tumor is one of the most challenging tasks in the medical image segmentation, since brain images are complicated and tumors can be analyzed only by expert physicians. In brain tumor diagnosis, the important task is to determine the exact location, orientation, and area of the abnormal tissues" [23]. "The important task of brain tumor diagnosis is the exact location, orientation and area of abnormal tissues" [23]. In computer integrated surgery, presurgical planning and analysis of pathology, brain's MRI may be useful [23,24].

A software system based on IoT Thingspeak platform's support SVM classifier that deals with brain cancer detection has been developed. It helps in detecting the tumor in brain by using MRI images of infected brains. SVM classifier is an enhanced SVM ML algorithm which is used for regression and classification purposes. The primary purpose of SVM classifier is to analyze and classify the collection of inputs accordingly.

11.3.1.1 IoT Thingspeak Platform

IoT cloud platform that is open source is Thingspeak. It was introduced for IoT applications as a supporting service by ioBridge in 2010. Thingspeak provides an immediate simulation of device-aggregated data and is also used to prototype and prove the IoT framework principle that involves analytics.

Following features are included in some of the main capabilities of Thingspeak:

- Easy configuration: Using general IoT protocols, it configures devices to send data.
- Visualization: In real time, it visualizes collected sensor data.
- Aggregation: This feature aggregates data from third party's sources on request.
- Analysis: On events or schedules basis, it runs an automatic IoT analytics.
- Prototyping: It develops IoT systems and prototypes without developing web applications or setting up servers.
- Automation: Using Twilio or Twitter that is third party providers, it automatically manipulates the data and communicates.

Thingspeak allows the user either to submit notification or to trigger the IP-connected thing in the environment to run on the environment.

11.3.1.2   Required Model and its Stages

The model consists of many stages [25]:

- Collecting MRI images of brain
- Sharing MRI images on the website of secure database
- Using Thingspeak platform, reading data from website's database

Implementation of above stages helps doctor to monitor patient's health through cloud. This procedure is much helpful for a doctor to check as per tumor location that which part of the brain to be moved at the time of pre surgery.

The representation of brain tumor detection model is shown in Figure 11.3. Usually, the field of medical monitoring requires greater manual capability to track the health of the patient. These are the most important concerns in the medical industry. It leads to destructive situations in case where medical situation is not examined in sufficient time.

11.3.1.3   Implementation and Result

This brain tumor detection model via Thingspeak platform consists of three major components: the computerized MRI imaging device is the first part, in which images are compiled and stored as a JPG file and (second part) sent to a central broker of the website. A website from TMDHosting with domain name audaymohamad.com is developed for experimental research. The third part of the proposed framework is the platform of Thingspeak; the analytical power of the Matlab program is applied in this part.

The SVM classifier algorithm is used with a set of preprocessing operations. At the cloud level, these algorithms are implemented based on cloud Matlab features installed within the Thingspeak platform. With the Matlab software R2017a and the Thingspeak platform, local implementation of tumor detection using SVM algorithm is done. The results therefore conclude that, in comparison to the same

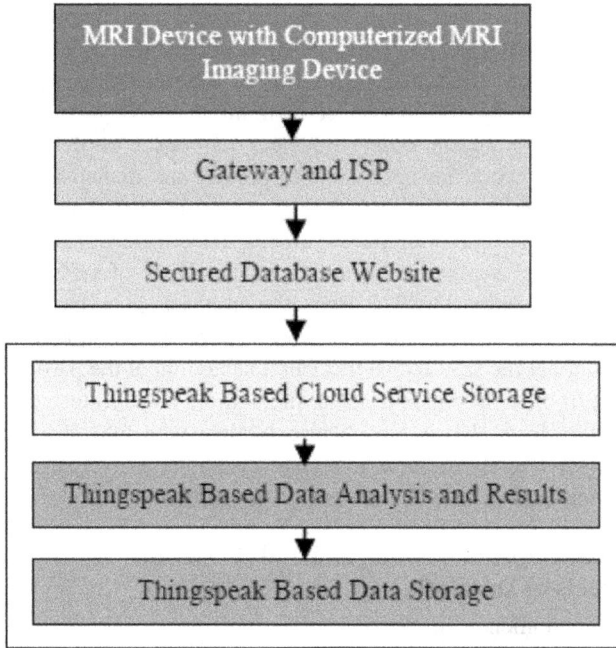

FIGURE 11.3 Model of detecting brain tumor [25].

algorithm which was implemented locally, this classifier has excellent processing results. Testing done on only three infected brains MRI images, and all of them identified as brain tumor and thus we can say that proposed system's accuracy is 100%.

Three MRI photographs of affected brains have been analyzed and all these images have been identified as brain tumors, so the reliability of the proposed method is 100%.

11.3.2 Early Detection of Dementia Disease Using Machine Learning and IoT Based Application

Dementia is a disease that typically causes difficulties with a person's memory, language, perception, problem solving, and thinking, these symptoms are enough to affect their everyday lives. This disease is caused by nerve cell destruction due to which brain starts to shrink and problems arises which can sometimes be seen in a brain scan.

It is a challenging job, especially for elderly people who live in residential care, to identify the signs of the early stages of dementia. The smart environments and IoT will help with early detection via non-intrusive monitoring of the everyday activities of elderly people. The smart IoT sensor-based environment may help control the everyday activities of elderly people and can advise neurological drop in the person. It is also possible to warn older adults or caregivers, and seeing a geriatrician could be suggested. In this way, IoT based remote monitoring can also allow older adults to advice on the potential signs of dementia as a friend and advice them to see a clinician. Additionally, in terms of smarter living, this will increase the caregivers and elderly people's peace of mind.

By passive monitoring, in order to detect the onset of dementia, different methods exist. Some work has been done to predict and diagnose dementia using image-based deep learning techniques from patient's EEG datasets and MRI scans [26–29]. In addition, several attempts have been made to recognize the dementia's onset from behavioral symptoms of adults on the basis of GPS and wandering accelerometer identification [30–32]. Here, the emphasis is on creating a model in order to predict dementia's onset on the basis of publicly available datasets, which includes details about the selected instrumental behaviors of the participants in their everyday lives. In order to create models, the authors have collected and analyzed the characteristics from the dataset. These models take into account the users' gestures and selected task's duration in recognizing cognitive impairments linked to forgetfulness, confusion and other actions of dementia patients.

11.3.2.1 Characteristics of Dementia and Its Adverse Effects of Dementia

A widespread phenomenon in elderly people is dementia which is also a leading cause of death among individuals over an age of 70 [33]. Dementia is normally caused by degeneration of the cerebral cortex, the portion of the brain that is responsible for personality, behavior, perceptions and emotions [34].

In specific region, patients with dementia die as a result of the loss of brain cells in a specific area. The cognitive impairment that characterizes dementia results in these dead cells. In many parts of the world, the well-being of the ageing population is a considerable concern. For their caretakers and families, remote monitoring of elderly people's health and well-being is helpful.

Five major symptomatic areas linked to dementia have been identified by the Alzheimer's Association are shown in Figure 11.4. In addition, these five forms of core dementia symptoms may be sub-categorized further into sub-symptoms [35].

Behavioral and psychological symptoms of dementia (BPSD) may provide multiple signs for predicting the dementia's onset along with above key symptomatic areas. Any of these dementia sub-symptoms can fit very closely into the signs of BPSD. A clinical phenomenon of heterogeneous collection is BPSD. BPSD symptoms are present in around 80–90% of people having dementia [37]. The phenomena of BPSD include changes in personality, deregulated patterns of sleep and wake-up, irregular motor behavior, vision and thinking changes, altered mood, and impaired feelings [37]. In dementia patients, the below list shows some common BPSD symptoms:

a. Apathy
b. Repeated vocalization
c. Change in personality
d. Sleeping disorder
e. Inappropriate behavior
f. Spitting

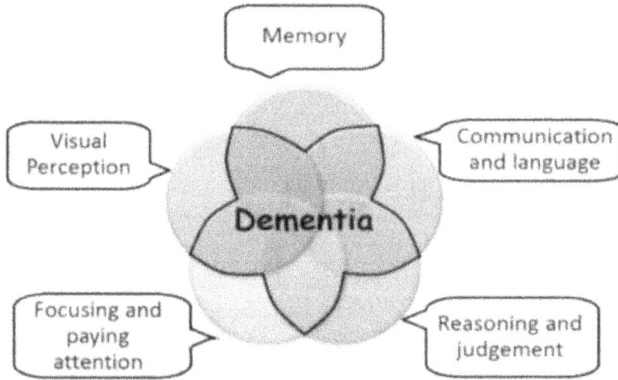

FIGURE 11.4 Dementia-related five main symptomatic areas [36].

g. Biting
h. Wandering
i. Aggression
j. Psychomotor agitation
k. Delusions
l. Hallucinations
m. Depression
n. Anxiety
o. Screaming

The behaviors in the dataset relate to the symptomatic fields, as well as to the domains of BPSD. As such, the presence of symptoms signifies a cognitive impairment in an elderly people may be detected using IoT-based systems, leading to the diagnosis of the development of dementia.

11.3.2.2 Identifying Dementia Onset

It is difficult to recognize the early signs of dementia since the symptoms develop steadily for a patient, and the changes are not recognized by those around them. Therefore, the MRI scan, which is also under progress, is increasingly involved in detecting dementia phases. The Mini-Mental State Test (MMSE) is the most common clinical diagnosis carried out by geriatricians to diagnose cognitive impairment [38]. If this score continues to drop, it can mean that dementia is developing in a person. Typically, many elderly people live without understanding that their cognitive condition is declining, so they do not pursue medical treatment.

Related to five main categories of BPSD symptoms, ambient sensors may be used to track and assemble data on behaviors. Intelligent models can be developed by tracking the everyday activity and routine task as well as behavioral patterns via IoT devices to predict the development of dementia. Techniques such as AI and ML can help classify cognitive-state patterns. Within a residence, restlessness, wandering behavior can produce irregular sensor fire which helps to implement an intelligent model. As a result, movement detection using presence and motion sensors, as well as recognition and completeness of action, are essential components of input data.

In addition, performing a task properly and with less recurrence, compared to wandering, forgetfulness and anxiety, would decrease residential sensor activation. As a model building source, the sensor activation counter is therefore considered. Completing ADL is a positive indicator of an older adult's well-being. The repeated loss of the critical ADL can lead caregivers to feel worried about their cognitive wellbeing. The ML approach is therefore employed in this model to analyze the ADLs from the dataset. In order to recognize the onset of dementia, this method can help to assess the duration and completeness of each ADL.

11.3.2.3   Model Development and Performance Analysis

The overall system's flowchart is represented in Figure 11.5. All user actions will be tracked from the smart environment, as per the flow displayed in diagram. Then, to prepare for extracting the functionality, such data would be filtered and pre-processed. Among all the features, between rooms and corridors entry-exit sensors, task completion time and sensor firing events are important for this function. In addition, an IoT-enabled smart environment can provide important features such as the total completion counter for IADL operations and the period of each IADL. The features will be obtained and chosen using the ranking method, also the validity as well as importance of an application will be assessed. After that, dataset would be prepared for usage in the study of ML to construct a model.

CASAS dataset [39] is used in this model. This is a commonly used dataset that Washington State University has provided. The dataset contains ADL and IADLs of different participants with low-level sensor information.

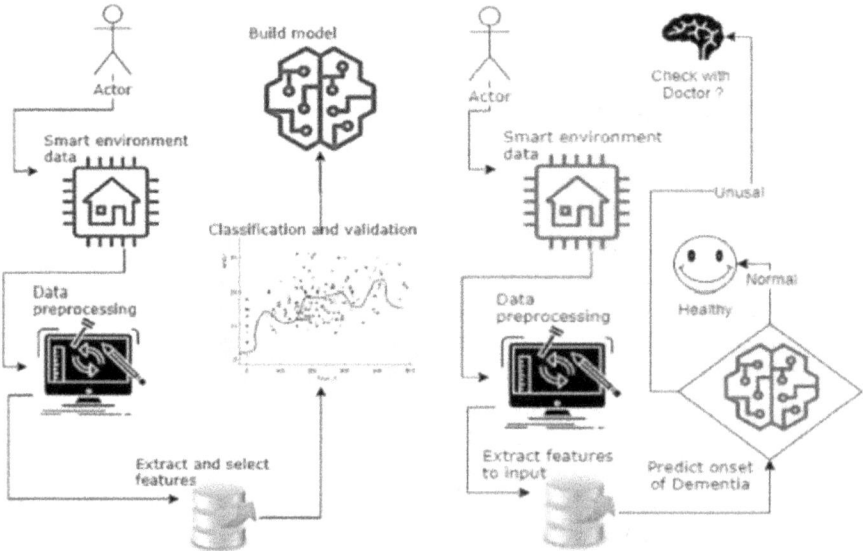

FIGURE 11.5   System flowchart to classify the onset of dementia [36].

On the basis of series of sensor activation, sensor activity logs are auto-generated. All the relevant and extractable features linked to this work are based on the details in log files. A significant aspect that is possible to obtain from the data is the time of completing every ADL and IADL. It is also possible to collect deactivation events and motion sensor activation reflecting a participant's behavior. Moreover, starting information and task completion can also be extracted. For each sensor, the cumulative number of motion sensor firings is taken as a characteristic for each participant. The algorithm used for extracting characteristics from log files is defined in the next section.

11.3.2.4 Features Extracting Algorithm from CASAS Dataset

Feature extracting algorithm from CASAS dataset is mentioned below:

Step 1. Equal to cumulative number of files for data samples, start a loop. For each loop, features will be extracted and stored as a row of records.

Step 2. To maintain the appropriate sensor data for tasks 1–8, trim the loaded file in each loop.

Step 3. Calculate each task's duration (in total, eight tasks) and store the record using inner loop.

Step 4. Count the sensor firing events using an inner loop for each appropriate sensor (51 sensors) and save the record.

Step 5. Repeat all above four steps until complete features of the data file are not extracted. Then, export the output to a feature matrix table for ML.

In order to identify the patterns within the classes, features are extracted from the dataset. It is mandatory to have focus on the data to explore interrelated parameters until building of real model is not completed. The cognitive disabled individual will have difficulty in completing a given task. Hence, on certain tasks, they could lose out. It is predicted that even though they have completed a task, it will take a lengthier time to complete it. It is an original assumption of the dataset before any model is developed. These essential patterns can appear in the results from the point of view of feature analysis. After close review, it is noted that certain participants have not completed certain tasks that fall under either classification: cognitively disabled or cognitively healthy. The algorithm placed straight "0 seconds" for these unfinished tasks to complete a particular task. In the dataset, these zeros indicate missing values. Rather, it would be a large sum that would reflect non completion of task. Hence, this Zero was exchanged by double of maximum value of that feature during data preprocessing.

11.3.2.5 Discussion and Result

The above model has an ability to predict the dementia disease, with an accuracy of 90.74% by using DT model in comparison to previous work with 88% accuracy. By achieving 89% and 87.38% F-Score, respectively, optimal results for the balanced and imbalanced dataset are produced by RUSBoosed Ensemble-based model. Only 50 features, which are very few, are used in this model, but better F-score and precision can be achieved. It would also help to provide predictive treatment for older adults to successfully predict the cognitive impairment of a person with dementia. This therefore adds to their cognitive well-being and better independent living.

11.3.3   A SEGMENTATION AND CLASSIFICATION IoT MODEL FOR PREDICTING LUNG CANCER

An IoT Model for predicting lung cancer will be discussed in this section by using medical images presented as an input to the real-time framework created as a prediction method.

11.3.3.1   System Architecture

A new Predictive Modeling based on IoT that predicts lung cancer via images which are uploaded by public. For efficient image segmentation, new transition region extraction process based on the fuzzy c-means clustering approach is defined here. The Otsu thresholding approach is used in this work to extract the transition region efficiently from images of lung cancer. In addition, on edge lung cancer images, the image area filling method and morphological cleaning method are done. An incremental classification algorithm, that combines existing ARM (Association Rule Mining), current DT (Decision Tree) algorithm with temporal features and the standard CNN [40], is also used to make an algorithm efficient to make decisions over lung cancer images. The representation of Architecture is presented in Figure 11.6.

11.3.3.2   Results and Discussion

As an online application using classification, clustering and transitional extraction to predict lung cancer diseases, a new Predictive Modeling based on IoT has been developed. The efficient transition region extraction method is used by this model to efficiently perform image segmentation. In addition, current Fuzzy C-Means Clustering algorithm has been used for segmentation that integrates thinning, morphological cleaning and extraction process of transitional region-based feature from the lung cancer image feature. To improve precision of the classification, mentioned segmentation method is used. In addition, a new incremental classifier is implemented to make successful decisions about an image of lung cancer to predict the images affected by lung cancer using ARM, current DT, with temporal characteristics and the CNN.

In comparison to the other existing models, the experimental findings revealed that the prediction precision of this model is greater. 85% precision was achieved by this model, which is 2% more than other models. Future work can be done on the introduction of fuzzy rough set principle for decision-making over the images affected by lung cancer.

11.4   HEART DISEASE PREDICTION MODEL USING IOT AND ML ALGORITHMS

In this section, using healthcare sensors and UCI Repository dataset an accurate system is developed to predict the patient suffering from heart disease. In addition, to identify the data of patients for heart disease identification, classification algorithms are used.

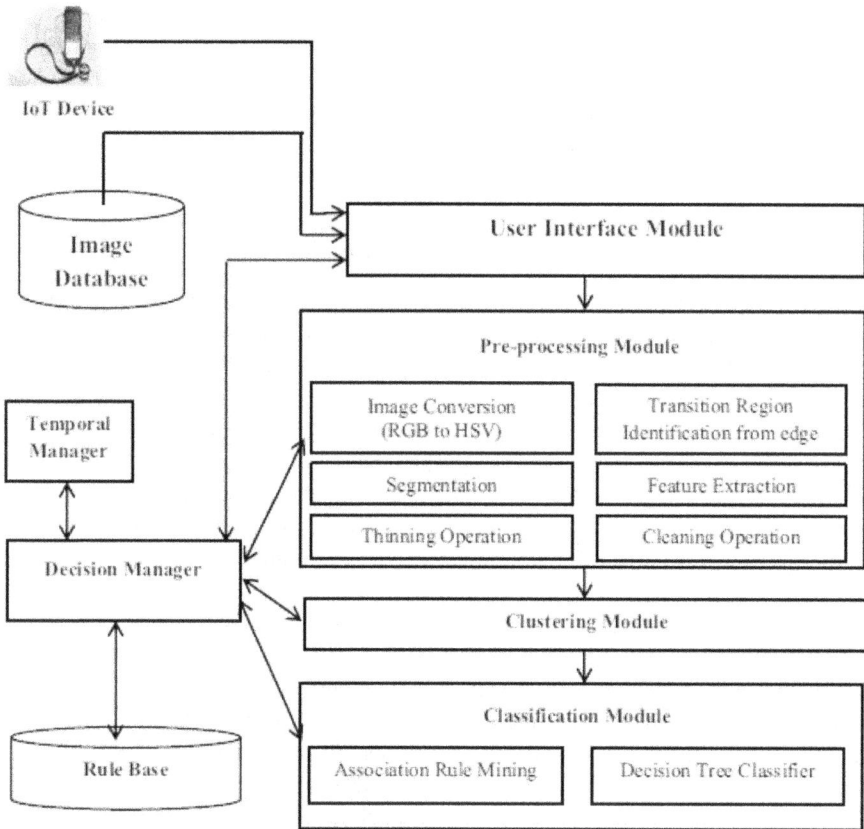

FIGURE 11.6   System architecture [41].

11.4.1 Introduction

From last few years, healthcare monitoring is increased significantly because of technological advancement in the field of sensing devices, IoT and Internet. Many hospitals use mobile apps to schedule an appointment, search medical records and review reports. However, to track ECG, blood sugar, blood pressure as well as other physiological symptoms, healthcare wearable gadgets (such as ECG machine, 3G BP measuring system, etc.) can be used. There are more advantages to the advancement of smart devices in healthcare, such as reduced workload of clinical staff, increased patient medical awareness, and decreased costs[42]. Moreover, it is still a major problem to connect the intelligent devices to each other to attain this intention. The biggest problem lies in the protocol of communication [43]. Since traditional wired communication is not applicable to mobile transmission, a large number of studies have been carried out to link intelligent items via short and long-range wireless transmissions.

IoT and cloud-based disease diagnosis model will be discussed in this section for diagnosing, predicting and monitoring heart disease. In such case, in addition to healthcare sensors, the use of the UCI Repository dataset to predict patient suffering from heart disease. In addition, classification algorithms are used to classify patient's data for heart disease detection. Using data from the benchmark dataset, the classifier will be trained in the training process. During testing method, the actual patient data to classify the disease were used to determine the existence of disease. Using a collection of classifiers including SVM, MLP (multilayer perceptron), LR, J48, a benchmark dataset is evaluated for experimentation.

11.4.2   IoT-Based Disease Diagnosis Model

The diagnosis model is represented in Figure 11.7. It consists of five major components via ML based heart disease prediction system, Cloud Database, patient data, heart disease dataset and Medical IoT sensors. Wearable and embedded IoT gadgets are known to be IoT gadgets, which are used to collect data from remote areas. Such measurements collect data using human body-linked IoT devices.

The UCI repository's dataset is used, which contains previous patient's data logs obtained from healthcare centers. In the cloud, all these datasets are saved. For accessing it anytime, the necessary data will be stored in the cloud. Heart disease prediction model is liable for predicting heart diseases with the help of classification algorithms of ML. This model presented functions in three steps. Data is collected in first step using human body IoT devices, benchmark dataset, and patient records. All collected data will be stored in the cloud storage in next step. The prediction of heart disease takes place in the last step, by classifying the results. Using dataset for training classifier to determine the existence of heart disease, classification algorithm initially conducts the training process. Then, to accurately predict whether the patient suffers from heart disease, the trained classifier is able to test the medical records. The report would be produced and made available to the user.

11.4.3   Results and Conclusion

Results of several classifiers against heart disease dataset are shown in Figure 11.8. It is obvious from the figure that MLP presented worse results with minimum precision. Competitive efficiency was shown by the SVM and LR, greater than the accuracy obtained by MLP. Although MLP is superior to LR and SVM, but fails to deliver good results in comparison to J48 classifier. Then, MLP attained minimum precision in terms of F-score, which indicates poor performance in classification. At the same time, better classification efficiency than MLP is obtained by the SVM and LR. In addition, the J48 received better F-score results in classification. Higher

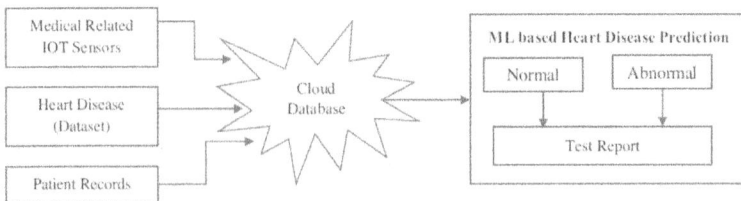

FIGURE 11.7   IoT based disease diagnosis model [44].

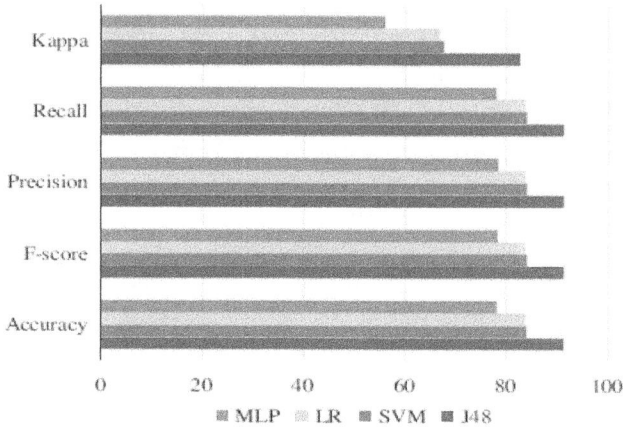

FIGURE 11.8   Various classifier's comparison on the dataset of heart disease [44].

accuracy value shows better efficiency of classification. With a minimum accuracy value, the MLP classifier showed bad performance, while the SVM and LR classifier obtained a better accuracy value, respectively. Interestingly, the J48 classifier, with a maximum accuracy value, achieved better classification efficiency. MLP obtains minimum recall value and J48 classifier achieves the highest recall value. At the same time, with a recall value, the LR and SVM classifiers shows approximately same output. It is stated that with a kappa value, the LR and SVM classifiers indicated good results than MLP. It is noteworthy that the maximum kappa value was obtained by the J48 classifier. Perhaps surprisingly, in terms of overall performance, J48 classifier has been found to be effective heart disease diagnosis model.

11.5   AUTOMATED NUTRITION MONITORING SYSTEM USING IOT AND DEEP LEARNING

A correct balance of nutrient intake is very important, particularly in infants. When the body is deprived of essential nutrients, it can lead to serious disease and organ deterioration which can cause serious health issues in adulthood. Automated monitoring of the nutritional content of food provided to infants, not only at home but also in daycare facilities, is essential for their healthy development. To address this challenge, this section presents a new IoT based fully automated nutrition monitoring system, called Smart-Log, to advance the state-of-art in smart healthcare.

11.5.1   INTRODUCTION

One of the critical concerns in healthcare is tracking daily food intake. Tracking devices or wearables are introduced to retain a healthier lifestyle in smart healthcare, by focusing on monitoring calorie output or calorie input [45]. Monitoring calorie output and intake both are essential [46]. An objective of such system could vary from weight loss monitoring to healthy balanced diet, resolving nutrition imbalances is an underlying inspiration. This can be caused by both overeating and

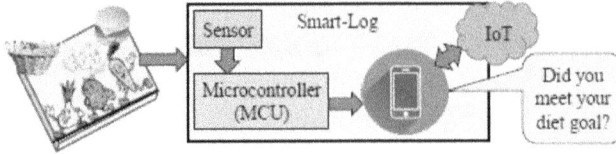

FIGURE 11.9   View of smart log system [52].

malnutrition, in which not enough nutrients are consumed, resulting in a high consumption of non-nutrient fats, salt, and foods. In today's major cities, overeating can lead to obesity, which is a significant health issue. Nutrition imbalances in babies and children that can occur in various adult modalities, like bleeding gums, thinning hairlines, weak physical structure, cognitive disorders, and weak immune system, are few names.

The conceptual view of a Smart-Log system is provided in Figure 11.9, which can be part of any household. The IoT is the key facilitator in this research. The IoT is used as the link between cloud-based analytics and sensor-derived data [47]. It is a physical network in which each device can be recognized within the network [47]. In the IoT, each recognizable part is a 'thing' that can link to the Internet. It helped developers and researchers in building smart systems, with a broad range of business spectrum protected by IoT [48]. It is one of an enabling technology for smart cities where different components (such as cars, utilities, homes, traffic, hospitals, and houses) of infrastructure are interconnected [49]. IoT has facilitated remote assistance in context of healthcare and has improved the life of people [50,51].

11.5.2   SMART LOG SYSTEM

It is possible to consider the device architecture as a product that includes a smart sensor board along with a smart phone application. A module for measuring food is included on the sensor board. The weight of a food ingredient or product, co-ordinated by a wireless module-integrated microcontroller, is transmitted through wireless to the cloud over an Internet. In an IoT network, the device is thus converted to a 'thing'. The corresponding nutritional data of the food item is acquired through the smart phone application with the help of the smart phone camera. A value of an overall consumed nutrient is then given by system. Using smart phone application, the forecast and measured nutrient values are accessed by customer. The DFD of Smart-Log system is depicted in Figure 11.10.

11.5.3   RESULT AND CONCLUSION

With high precision in diet control, the implemented design of a self-sufficient food's data logging system is cost effective. The nutrient feature extraction algorithm based on Bayesian network and five-layer perceptron neural network can work to evaluate the nutritional balance. Some products logged several times were included in the input dataset. To solve this, in the case of duplication, alternative options are provided to the customer to correct a data entry with a corresponding

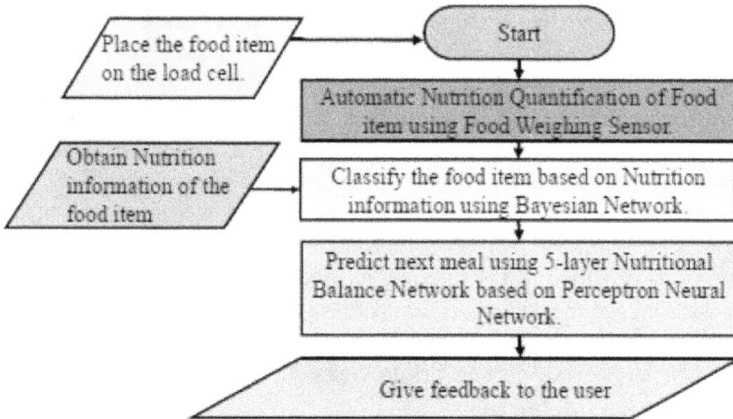

FIGURE 11.10   DFD of smart log system [52].

improvement in final accuracy. Along with an overview of nutritional quality of the meal, the device makes recommendations to minimize the risk of imbalanced diet. For household or child care use, this device may become an important product. The Smart-Log reach is seen in this section in the sense of infant food preferences, can be used by adults by extending the database in cloud storage.

11.6   MONITORING OF ARRHYTHMIA PATIENTS IN REAL TIME VIA IOT AND ML

Cardiac arrhythmia (also known as dysrhythmia) is an abnormal heartbeat disorder that causes the patient to suffer sudden loss of life [53]. In order to overcome this unexpected loss of life, the cardiac activity of patients with arrhythmia needs to be constantly controlled to include an effective medical procedure. Today, the IoT is used in tracking new healthcare domain in real time. The main support of m-health (medical health) is supervision and access to medical services, with a major decrease in the cost of early detection and preventive monitoring [54]. In order to monitor patients' well-being, IoT devices such as pulse oximeter, electrocardiogram (ECG) monitor, blood pressure monitors, blood glucose monitor, etc. facilitate remote health care management. ML algorithms are currently applied to facilitate predicting the conditions of m-health. Many classification techniques in healthcare make detection and diagnosis of disease, psychoanalysis, survival analysis and even hospital management much simpler. In several leading countries, an automated diagnostic device for earlier disease detection is being implemented. ML techniques are used to evaluate data obtained from different medical tests to provide automated disease diagnosis [55]. ML thus becomes a supporting method with a trained algorithm in the medical field that involves different characteristics and classes of disease.

Several causes of arrhythmia are there, such as irregular heartbeat, blood potassium or sodium deficiency, heart muscle changes, various coronary disorder, post-operative healing processes, etc. Irregular ECG is crucial in arrhythmia prediction. If not diagnosed, then the sudden condition can cause cardiac arrest [56]. Supraventricular tachycardia, atrial fibrillation, atrial flutter, and ventricular tachycardia are the ECG-based classifications for retrospective data analysis of resuscitation cardiac rhythms [57]. An automatic arrhythmia categorization will save many patients lives [58]. A random forest classifier is intended for the diagnosis of arrhythmias in 16 types [59]. The efficiency of the classifier may be affected by excessive datasets and several feature choices. To overcome this problem, SRS (simple random sampling) and CFS (correlation-based feature selection) classification methods are used. CFS filtering method [60] conducts the most suitable feature selection, and the data collection is re-sampled by SRS to obtain a uniformly distributed class data set. This work employs ML method for classifying the arrhythmia data set is used in this work to create a real-time arrhythmia monitoring system using sensors and IoT devices.

11.6.1 ARRHYTHMIA PATIENT MONITORING AND CLASSIFICATION

The main purpose of this method is to offer a mechanism for monitoring patients with arrhythmia and classifying arrhythmia to enhance diagnosis. In hospitals, this device will be used to expand health services to patients. A specific number is given to patients with abnormal heartbeats to access the application in this concept. For physicians and patients with limited access, the application has various views. This concept continuously tracks the patients using wearable sensors, then transfers their details to iOS/android applications that are used by both patients as well as doctors. The patient suspected of having arrhythmia is checked continuously for physiological parameters such as heart rate and temperature via wearable sensors. The iOS/android program alerts the patient to wear the wearable ECG sensor in case of irregular heartbeat detection. The software automatically classifies patient status into 16 classes of arrhythmias [61] by using ML. It helps patients and physicians to have two separate opinions.

With enhanced security and privacy, the mobile app is made using which doctors could see the records of all patients whereas patient can see their own medical record only. There are five key components of this architecture: visualization, classification, cloud storage, data transfer and data sensing which are shown in Figure 11.11.

- The method of data sensing includes tracking patients for temperature monitoring, ECG and pulse rate using wearable sensors. To provide emergency medical care, the location of patients is often tracked using the GPS (Global Positioning System). Generally, sensors are combined into a microcontroller that reads sensor data. The sensing of information consists of GPS and wearable sensors.
- The component for transmission of data contains Wi-Fi module that collects data from microcontroller and transfers it through cloud to mobile app. In order to achieve data protection, this transition must be performed in a safe way.
- The main part of device storage is cloud storage. The method is structured such that patients' biomedical data is preserved longer. Such long-term storage helps health professionals to detect arrhythmias disease.

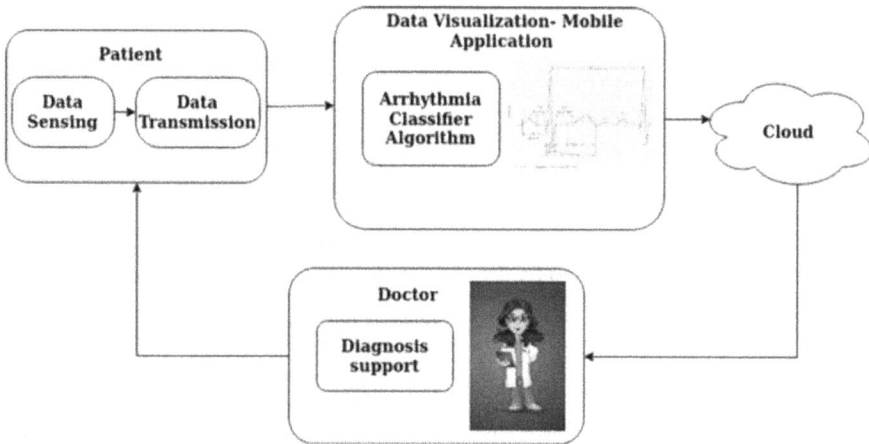

FIGURE 11.11   Arrhythmia patient monitoring and classification architecture [62].

11.6.1.1   Data Sensing

It is done with design qualities using wearable sensors that doesn't affect the lightweight, mobility and easy to operate for patient. To form WPAN, wearable sensors are aggregated. The biological data obtained by the wearable devices are temperature and heart rate. ECG data is collected when irregular heartbeat detection is observed by the application. With the aim of providing care during medical emergencies, location of patients is also monitored. The patient's ECG, temperature and heart rate are continuously acquired from the BAN, and GPS is used to monitor the location. The values are collected by the microcontroller from the sensors. This phenomenon is identified as an energy-efficient sensing mechanism [63]. In [64], with 93.75% accuracy, continuous status monitoring of wounds. This is done in the segmented regions by classifying wound tissues. Whereas the telewound technology network (TWTL) proposes to remotely track wounds using smartphones in such a way that rural and urban people benefit from a remote monitoring system.

Using the mobile application, decision making process is developed and informed. In real time, patient is presumed to be in normal condition. The microcontroller controls the temperature and heart rate in this state, which can be programmed to periodically compare heart rate values on a regular basis. When the value falls below the threshold range, a signal is transmitted to the application that instructs the patient to wear ECG monitor, and data from the microcontroller is obtained by ECG sensor. In addition, as stated in wearable sensors [65], this technique overcomes major problems such as reliability, privacy problems and user interface.

11.6.1.2   Classification and Visualization

The cloud data is accessed by a mobile application that makes sensor decisions and classifies arrhythmias. The mobile application analyses sensor data and makes a decision about the use of sensors and informs the patients. Using random forest classifier and resampling process along with the chosen characteristics, arrhythmia classification is done. This method of arrhythmia classification requires classifier's training with dataset from clinical reports and previous data from the ECG sensor. After training phase, classifier is equipped with the latest sensor data that classifies arrhythmia into 16 groups and has 96% precision. Visualization is important access to the voluminous data and data will be convenient for both patients and doctors. Data visualization is recognized as a distinct and significant field of research. Using an interactive smartphone application, the visualization of data is accomplished. Different colors are used to display the categorized data. This approach is fitted with color categories and distance to facilitate the recognition and comprehension of data differences.

11.6.2 Results and Discussion

The framework is implemented using TensorFlow program. Import a suitable library and create an application that will be able to identify arrhythmia. From UCI repository, the sample dataset is collected. This database has 452 samples and 274 characteristics. Using the methods indicated in, the sample data set is resampled. To achieve precision over a limited collection of samples, data resampling is required. The number of patients varies, but it is important to ensure the accuracy of the application such that the choice of features is taken out. There are many arrhythmia classification algorithms, but this one is chosen to preserve the consistency and durability of various data volumes for the method. Patient's heart rate is constantly tracked, and with respect to various heart rates, type of arrhythmia can be analyzed.

The testing and training dataset are the two subsets of UCI repository's original dataset and are selected independently. In comparison, training dataset train the classification algorithm, and by measuring the classifier rate, the dataset is tested for the output. The confusion matrix tests classifier's efficiency. To increase the classifier's precision, this technique of data resampling is used. The result shows that the scheme's accuracy is 97.2%. Thus, the approach more reliably classifies patients with arrhythmia efficiently from a distance away.

11.6.3 Conclusion

The monitoring system of arrhythmia patients in real-time helps in reducing risk of human life with the help of ML techniques and wearable sensors.

11.7 IOT IN HEALTHCARE: AN OVERVIEW OF BENEFITS AND CHALLENGES

11.7.1 Benefits of Applying IoT

Several benefits of applying IoT are:

    i. **Simultaneous monitoring and reporting**—Real-time monitoring of smart devices will save a million lives in the case of a medical emergency such as asthma attacks, diabetes, cardiac disease, etc. With real-time monitoring of the situation in place, enabled devices will collect useful medical and health-related data via a smart medical system linked to a mobile app. Data like ECGs, weight, oxygen, blood sugar, and blood pressure are retrieved and transmitted by the connected IoT device. The data is stored in the cloud and may, as per the sharing access authority, be shared with an authorized user.

ii. **End-to-end affordability and connectivity**—IoT will aid to simplify the workflow of patient and healthcare through mobility solutions. This solution enables machine to machine connectivity, interoperability, data movement and knowledge exchange, making it incredibly cost effective to provide healthcare services. This technology-driven set-up will reduce costs by minimizing unwanted visits and using higher performing services. This would strengthen the method of allocation and resource preparation.

iii. **Data assortment and analysis**—Handling large amount of data for healthcare professionals is not easy. Real-time collected data through mobile devices enabled by IoT can be separated and analyzed by mobility solutions powered by IoT. To reduce errors and speeding up decision-making, this can minimize raw data processing and will accelerate health care analytics and data-driven insights.

iv. **Tracking and alerts**—In life-threatening conditions, real-time tracking and alerts will turn into a blessing to safeguard the health of a serious patient with continuous updates and alerts for careful diagnosis, analysis, and monitoring. IoT-powered mobility solutions allow tracking, alerting, and monitoring in real time. This helps doctors to hands-on interventions, improve accuracy and suitable intervention, while enhancing the results of patient's care delivery.

v. **Remote Medical Support:** A situation could come in patient's life in which he/she is seeking medical help, but because of barriers such as location and lack of expertise, unable to communicate with a doctor. The issue has solution in IoT-enabled mobility systems which can assist patients with appropriate medical support. Via healthcare delivery chains which are interconnected to patients through IoT devices, patients can take medical medications right at home. This coin has two sides. Healthcare IoT applications have also faced some challenges along the way.

11.7.2 CHALLENGES OF IoT IN HEALTHCARE

As there are major benefits to IoT in healthcare, still some challenges are there that need to be addressed. Without understanding these challenges, healthcare technologies of IoT could not be considered for deployment.

i. **Security and privacy**—IoT-enabled healthcare provides various advantages, but also produces numerous vulnerable security spots. There may be several possible consequences, connected devices such that sensors, smartphones, etc., could be hacked. Hackers might log into Internet-connected medical devices and can access or steal personal health information or even change it. They must be encrypted if there is data transfer from one system to another. Hackers can also go a step further and hack a whole hospital network, infecting the notorious Ransomware virus on the IoT computers. This ensures that patients and their heart rate monitors, blood pressure readers, and brain scanners are kept hostage by hackers. False health statements, fake IDs creation for selling and buying drugs are few examples of misuse of IoT device data.

ii. **Integration**—Another significant task for implementing effective IoT in healthcare is integrating various devices and protocols within the network. There are many network-connected smartphones that collects the data actively. Several communication protocols are there which complicate an information aggregation method. The implementation of IoT in healthcare industry is impeded by the incorporation of various types of devices.

iii. **Technology adoption**—In the healthcare system, the product that is developed should also be monetized because it is not sufficient to invest for new technology to develop new app with creative ideas that benefit doctors and patients.

iv. **Data overload and accuracy**—Because of communication protocols and non-uniformity of data, aggregation of data for analysis and critical insights is difficult. For improved results and accurate precision, IoT gathers data in bulk. In the longer run, data overloading can impact the decision-making process in the hospitality sector in the longer run.

v. **Cost**—Cost is one of the challenges in planning of IoT applications for healthcare mobility solutions. However, if the implementation of IoT could solve major problem, then costs are absolutely worthy. When the organization saves time and manpower by spending a massive amount of resources and capital on developing an IoT app, the returns will be similarly enormous, all while optimizing sales operations, attracting more revenue sources and providing more IoT business prospects.

vi. **Massive inputs of generated data**—It would produce massive quantities of data by getting numerous sensors in a healthcare facility and having more transmitting information from distant areas, all in real-time. From Terabytes to Petabytes, the data is generated by IoT in healthcare would make higher storage requirements. Cloud and AI-driven algorithms help in organizing and making sense of data if used properly, but it requires more time. Hence, it will take lot of time and effort to create a large-scale IoT healthcare solution.

11.8 ML APPLICATIONS TO IOT

ML is the main method among computational applications to IoT. There are lots of ML-enabled IoT applications, some of them are listed in Table 11.2.

11.9 CONCLUSION AND FUTURE SCOPE

ML, and the development of the IoT, is growing gradually. In the planet, there are millions of IoT devices and more are being manufactured every day. They gather enormous amounts of data over the Internet that is fed to machines, allowing

TABLE 11.2
Healthcare applications of ML and IoT

Applications	Description	Use Case	Advantages
Wearable Devices	This application helps users gather health status and vital signs. In addition, it also maintains users connected to the cloud so that they transmit data. After analyzing and collecting huge amounts of cloud data, the necessary decision can be taken by the provider.	Occupancy Control Mass Screening Admitted Patient's Data	• Quick decision making with edge computing • Faster response time with data analysis on cloud • Large amount of data collection on cloud • Real-time monitoring
Remote Diagnostic and Telemedicine	It may be difficult sometime to reach clinic for medical care and routine check-ups. Hence, remote diagnostic and telemedicine assistance can provide virtual visit via text, voice, video like different medium of communication using which doctors can easily diagnose patient and can prescribed medicines by capturing patient's data like body temperature, heart rate, etc., via IoT devices and without exposing workers to direct patient interactions.	3D handled scanner design remote drug dispensing	• Data collection via IoT devices • Medical assistance without direct contact of patient and doctor.
Automation and Robotics	From providing medicines to conducting advanced surgery, this application helps in multiple healthcare facilities. The robotic cart provides patients with food, medicines and other essential helps to reduce close contact.	Da Vinci Surgical System Smart air purifiers	• Improves medical staff's efficiency • Identifies whether patient has consumed medicine or not.
Drones	This application is useful in various tasks like sanitizing hospital areas, remote monitoring, spraying disinfectants, and many others. Any discrepancies in such region can be reported by its ML enabled camera. For further decision-making and analysis, these drones with IoT sensors report and collect different data to the cloud platform.	Post COVID-19	• Reduces medical staff's burden. • Useful in traffic route clearing

machines to 'learn' from the data and making them more effective. Healthcare IoT systems include nano sensors attached to the patient's body's skin to monitor blood pressure, sugar levels, heartbeat, etc. This raw material is sent to the servers of the patient residing on the highly encrypted cloud network. Using advanced ML algorithms, the doctor may access raw data, prior prescriptions, etc., to prescribe new medications to patients in distant areas if appropriate. It is also possible to rescue people from life-threatening health problems such as sudden heart attacks, tumors, etc.

The aging population needs immense medical assistance, in which the IoT-based health care system, along with ML, plays a crucial part in bridging the distance between patients and doctor. Hence, various ML techniques are discussed in this chapter with customized IoT data techniques for disease prediction that can be applied with greater precision to ML models of healthcare. Various models were described on the accurate prediction system for life threatening diseases such as heart diseases, Lung Cancer, Dementia, Arrhythmia and Brain Tumor using different datasets, and their experimental results are also discussed using various algorithms. IoT applications in healthcare have faced both advantages and obstacles along the way.

For images affected by lung cancer, fuzzy rough set theory may be a potential work in this direction. It is also possible to add a Smart-Log with tracking tools to monitor user activities used for precise automatic diet prediction of adults. In case of arrhythmia disease, to enhance earlier detection and correct diagnosis of arrhythmic patients, certain other factors such as blood pressure should be controlled.

REFERENCES

[1]. K. Rishav, Epidemic outbreak prediction using artificial intelligence. *International Journal of Information Technology and Computer Science*, 10, 49–64 (2018).

[2]. M. Nilashi, O. b. Ibrahim, H. Ahmadi and L. Shahmoradi, An analytical method for diseases prediction using machine learning techniques. *Computers & Chemical Engineering*, 106, 212–223 (2017). ISSN 0098-1354, 10.1016/j.compchemeng.201 7.06.011.

[3]. S. Uddin, A. Khan, and M.Hossain et al., Comparing different supervised machine learning algorithms for disease prediction. *BMC Medical Informatics and Decision Making*, 19, 281 (2019). 10.1186/s12911-019-1004-8.

[4]. D. W. Hosmer Jr, S. Lemeshow, and R. X. Sturdivant, Applied logistic regression. Wiley, (2013).

[5]. T. Joachims, Making large-scale SVM learning practical. SFB 475: Komplexitätsreduktion Multivariaten Datenstrukturen, Univ. Dortmund, Dortmund, Tech. Rep. 28 (1998).

[6]. L. Breiman, Random forests. *Machine Learning*, 45 (1), 5–32 (2001).

[7]. D. V. Lindley, Fiducial distributions and Bayes' theorem. *Journal of the Royal Statistical Society: Series B (Statistical Methodology)*, 1, 102–107 (1958).

[8]. Rish, An empirical study of the naive Bayes classifier, in *IJCAI 2001 Workshop on Empirical Methods in Artificial Intelligence*, 3 (22), 41–46: IBM New York (2001).

[9]. T. Cover, and P. Hart, Nearest neighbor pattern classification. *IEEE Transactions on Information Theory*, 13 (1), 21–27 (1967).

[10]. Y. J. Fan, Y. H. Yin, L. D. Xu, Y. Zeng and F. Wu, IoT-based smart rehabilitation system, *IEEE Transactions on Industrial Informatics*, 10 (2), 1568–1577 (May 2014).

[11]. S. M. R. Islam, D. Kwak, H. Kabir, M. Hossain and K.-S. Kwak, The Internet of Things for health care: A comprehensive survey, *IEEE Access*, 3, 678–708 (2015).

[12]. D. V. Dimitrov, Medical Internet of Things and big data in healthcare, *Healthcare Informatics Research*, 22 (3), 156–163 (Jul. 2016). [Online]. Available: http://www.ncbi.nlm.nih.gov/pmc/articles/PMC4981575/.

[13]. C. Rotariu and V. Manta, Wireless system for remote monitoring of oxygen saturation and heart rate, Federated Conference on Computer Science and Information Systems (FedCSIS), Wroclaw, Poland, 193–196 (2012).

[14]. L. Yang, Y. Ge, W. Li, W. Rao and W. Shen, A home mobile healthcare system for wheelchair users, IEEE International Conference on Computer Supported Cooperative Work in Design (CSCWD), Hsinchu, China, 609–614 (2014).

[15]. C. Lee Ventola, MS mobile devices and apps for health care professionals: Uses and benefits. PT.2014; 39 (5): 356: 364. [Online] https://www.ncbi.nlm.nih.gov/pmc/articles/PMC4029126/. [Accessed: 04-05-2017].

[16]. H. N. Saha et al., Health monitoring using Internet of Things (IoT), 2017 8th Annual Industrial Automation and Electromechanical Engineering Conference (IEMECON), Bangkok, 69–73 (2017) doi: 10.1109/IEMECON.2017.8079564.

[17]. H. Pandey and S. Prabha, Smart health monitoring system using IOT and machine learning techniques, 2020 Sixth International Conference on Bio Signals, Images, and Instrumentation (ICBSII), Chennai, India, 1–4 (2020). doi: 10.1109/ICBSII4 9132.2020.9167660.

[18]. K. Srivardhan Reddy et al., IoT based health monitoring system using machine learning. *International Journal of Advance Research and Innovative Ideas in Education*, 5, 381–386 (2019).

[19]. D. M. J. Priyadharsan, K. K. Sanjay, S. Kathiresan, K. K. Karthik, and K. S. Prasath, Patient health monitoring using IoT with machine learning. *Irjet*, 6(3), 7514–7520 www.irjet.net.

[20]. P. Kaur, R. Kumar, and M. Kumar, A healthcare monitoring system using random forest and internet of things (IoT). *Multimedia Tools and Applications* 78, 14 (July 2019), 19905–19916 (2019). doi: https://doi.org/10.1007/s11042-019-7327-8

[21]. P. Katti and V. R. Marathe, Implementation of classification system for brain tumor using probabilistic neural network. *International Journal of Advanced Research in Computer and Communication Engineering*, 4(10), 188–192 (2015). doi:10.17148/IJARCCE.2015.41038.

[22]. D. B. Birnale and S. N. Patil, Brain tumor MRI image segmentation using FCM and SVM techniques. *International Journal of Engineering Science and Computing*, 6(12), 3939–3942 (2016).

[23]. J. Li, D. Joshi and J. Z. Wang, Stochastic modeling of volume images with a 3-D hidden markov model, US National Science Foundation, USA.

[24]. S. H. Talpur, The appliance pervasive of internet of things in healthcare systems. *International Journal of Computer Science Issues*, 10(1), 419–424 (2013) http://arxiv.org/abs/1306.3953.

[25]. N. Jumaa, A. Mohamad and S. Majeed, Internet of things mathematical approach for detecting brain tumor. *International Journal of Engineering & Technology*, 7, 2779–2783 (2018). 10.14419/ijet.v7i4.16283.

[26]. E. Moradi, A. Pepe, C. Gaser, H. Huttunen, and J. Tohka, Alzheimer's disease neuroimaging initiative. Machine learning framework for early MRI-based Alzheimer's conversion prediction in MCI subjects. *Neuroimage*, 104, 398–412 (2015).

[27]. H. Adeli, S. Ghosh-Dastidar, and N. Dadmehr, A spatio-temporal wavelet-chaos methodology for EEG-based diagnosis of Alzheimer's disease. *Neuroscience Letters*, 444, 190–194 (2008).

[28]. A. Cichocki, S. L. Shishkin, T. Musha, Z. Leonowicz, T. Asada, and T. Kurachi, EEG filtering based on blind source separation (BSS) for early detection of Alzheimer's disease. *Clinical Neurophysiology*, 116, 729–737 (2005).

[29]. C. R. Jack, R. C. Petersen, Y. C. Xu, P. C. O'Brien, G. E. Smith, R. J. Ivnik, B. F. Boeve, S. C. Waring, E. G. Tangalos, and E. Kokmen, Prediction of AD with MRI-based hippocampal volume in mild cognitive impairment. *Neurology*, 52, 1397 (1999).

[30]. K.-J. Kim, M. M. Hassan, S.-H. Na, and E.-N. Huh, Dementia wandering detection and activity recognition algorithm using tri-axial accelerometer sensors. In Proceedings of the 4th International Conference on Information Technologies & Applications, Fukuoka, Japan, 1–5 (20–22 December 2009).

[31]. Q. Lin, D. Zhang, X. Huang, H. Ni, and X. Zhou, Detecting wandering behavior based on GPS traces for elders with dementia. In Proceedings of the 2012 12th International Conference on Control Automation Robotics & Vision (ICARCV), Guangzhou, China, 672–677 (5–7 December 2012).

[32]. T. Qassem, G. Tadros, P. Moore, and F. Xhafa, Emerging technologies for monitoring behavioural and psychological symptoms of dementia. In Proceedings of the 2014 Ninth International Conference on P2P, Parallel, Grid, Cloud and Internet Computing, Guangdong, China, 308–315 (8–10 November 2014)

[33]. ABO Data Statistics. Causes of death, Australia. Statistics; Canberra, ACT, Australia: Australian Bureau of Statistics (2018).

[34]. G. Blessed, B.E. Tomlinson, and M. Roth, The association between quantitative measures of dementia and of senile change in the cerebral grey matter of elderly subjects. *British Journal of Psychiatry*, 114, 797–811 (1968).

[35]. F. Ahamed, S. Shahrestani, and H. Cheung, Identification of the onset of dementia of older adults in the age of internet of things. In Proceedings of the 2018 International Conference on Machine Learning and Data Engineering (iCMLDE), Sydney, Australia, 1–7 (3–7 December 2018).

[36]. F. Ahamed, S. Shahrestani, and H. Cheung. Internet of things and machine learning for healthy ageing: Identifying the early signs of dementia. *Sensors (Basel)*, 20(21), (2020).

[37]. J. Cerejeira, L. Lagarto, and E. Mukaetova-Ladinska, Behavioral and psychological symptoms of dementia. *Frontiers in Neurology*, 3, 73 (2012).

[38]. T. N. Tombaugh and N. J. McIntyre, The mini-mental state examination: A comprehensive review. *Journal of the American Geriatrics Society*, 40, 922–935 (1992).

[39]. D. J. Cook, A. S. Crandall, B. L. Thomas and N. C. Krishnan, CASAS: A smart home in a box. *Computer*, 46, 62–69 (2012).

[40]. C. Rangaswamy, G. T. Raju, and G. Seshikala, Novel approach for lung image segmentation through enhanced fuzzy C-means algorithm. *International Journal of Pure and Applied Mathematics*. 117 (21), 455–465 (2017).

[41]. D. Palani, K. Venkatalakshmi, An IoT based predictive modelling for predicting lung cancer using fuzzy cluster based segmentation and classification. *Journal of Medical System*, 43(2), 21 (2018). doi: 10.1007/s10916-018-1139-7.PMID:30564924.

[42]. G. Yang, S. He, Z. Shi and J. Chen, Promoting cooperation by social incentive mechanism in mobile crowdsensing, *IEEE Communications Magazine*, 55 (3), 86–92 (2017).

[43]. J. Liu, N. Kato, J. Ma and N. Kadowaki, Device-to-device communication in LTE-advanced networks: A survey. *IEEE Communications Surveys and Tutorials*, 17 (4), 1923–1940 (2015).

[44]. M. Ganesan and N. Sivakumar, IoT based heart disease prediction and diagnosis model for healthcare using machine learning models, 2019 IEEE International

Conference on System, Computation, Automation and Networking (ICSCAN), Pondicherry, India, 1–5 (2019). doi: 10.1109/ICSCAN.2019.8878850.

[45]. J. Wang, Z. Zhang, B. Li, S. Lee and R. Sherratt, An enhanced fall detection system for elderly person monitoring using consumer home networks, *IEEE Transactions on Consumer Electronics*, 60 (1), 23–29 (February 2014).

[46]. J. Wei and A. D. Cheok, Foodie: Play with your food promote interaction and fun with edible interface, *IEEE Transactions on Consumer Electronics*, 58 (2), 178–183 (May 2012).

[47]. S. M. R. Islam, M. N. Uddin, and K. S. Kwak, The IoT: Exciting possibilities for bettering lives, *IEEE Consumer Electronics Magazine,*5(2), 49–57 (April 2016).

[48]. B. K. Kang, S. H. Park, T. L. Lee and S. H. Park, IoT-based monitoring system using tri-level context making model for smart home services, in: Proc. IEEE Int. Conf. Consum. Electron., no. 198–199, (2015).

[49]. S. P. Mohanty, U. Choppali and E. Kougianos, Everything you wanted to know about smart cities, *IEEE Consumer Electronics Magazine*, 5 (3), 60–70 (July 2016).

[50]. P. Sundaravadivel, E. Kougianos, S. P. Mohanty and M. Ganapathiraju, Everything you wanted to know about smart healthcare, *IEEE Consumer Electronics Magazine*, 8 (1), 18–28 (January 2018).

[51]. S. Bounyong, S. Adachi, J. Ozawa, Y. Yamada, M. Kimura, Y. Watanabe and K. Yokoyama, Fall risk estimation based on cocontraction of lower limb during walk. In: Proceedings of the 2016 IEEE International Conference on Consumer Electronics (ICCE), 331–332, 2016. doi: 10.1109/ICCE.2016.7430634

[52]. P. Sundaravadivel, K. Kesavan, L. Kesavan, S. P. Mohanty, E. Kougianos, Smart-Log: A deep-learning based automated nutrition monitoring system in the IoT. *IEEE Transactions on Consumer Electronics*, 64(3), 390–398 (2018). doi:1 0.1109/TCE.2018.2867802.

[53]. V. Krasteva and I. Jekova, QRS template matching for recognition of ventricular ectopic beats. *Annals of Biomedical Engineering*, 35 (12), 2065–2076 (2007).

[54]. D. Niewolny, How the internet of things is revolutionizing healthcare, freescale semiconductors. In Proceedings of International Conference on Healthcare (pp. 211–219) (2013).

[55]. J. Hayashi, T. Kunieda, J. Cole, R. Soga, Y. Hatanaka, and M. Lu, et al., A development of computer-aided diagnosis system using fundus images. In Proceedings Seventh International Conference on Virtual Systems and Multimedia (pp. 429–438) (2004). IEEE.

[56]. S. Raj and K. C. Ray, ECG signal analysis using DCT-based DOST and PSO optimized SVM. *IEEE Transactions on Instrumentation and Measurement*, 66 (3), 470–478 (2017).

[57]. A. B. Rad, T. Eftestøl, K. Engan, U. Irusta, J. T. Kvaløy, and J. Kramer-Johansen, et al., ECG-based classification of resuscitation cardiac rhythms for retrospective data analysis. *IEEE Transactions on Biomedical Engineering*, 64 (10), 2411–2418 (2017).

[58]. Luz, E. J. Da S., Schwartz, W. R., Cámara-Chávez, G. and Menotti, D. ECG-based heartbeat classification for arrhythmia detection: A survey. *Computer Methods and Programs in Biomedicine*, 127, 144–164 (2016).

[59]. S. K. Mohapatra and M. N. Mohanty Analysis of resampling method for arrhythmia classification using random forest classifier with selected features. In 2018 2nd International Conference on Data Science and Business Analytics (ICDSBA) (pp. 495–499) (2018, September). IEEE.

[60]. A. Ozcift and A. Gulten, Classifier ensemble construction with rotation forest to improve medical diagnosis performance of machine learning algorithms. *Computer Methods and Programs in Biomedicine*, 104 (3), 443–451 (2011).

[61]. H. A. Guvenir, B. Acar, G. Demiroz and A. Cekin, A supervised machine learning algorithm for arrhythmia analysis. Computers in Cardiology, 1997 (pp. 433–436). IEEE (1997, September).

[62]. C. Chakraborty, A. Banerjee, M. kumar, H. Kolekar and L. Garg, Internet of things for healthcare technologies, Book Chapter. Springer: Singapore. 10.1007/978-981-15-4112-4.

[63]. T. Torfs, V. Leonov, C. Van Hoof and B. Gyselinckx, Body-heat powered autonomous pulse oximeter. In SENSORS, 2006 IEEE (pp. 427–430). IEEE (2006, October).

[64]. C. Chakraborty, Computational approach for chronic wound tissue characterization. *Informatics in Medicine Unlocked*, 17, 1–10 (2019).

[65]. T. Martin, E. Jovanov, and D. Raskovic, Issues in wearable computing for medical monitoring applications: A case study of a wearable ECG monitoring device. In Digest of Papers. Fourth International Symposium on Wearable Computers (pp. 43–49) (2000, October). IEEE.

12 Challenges and Solution of COVID-19 Pandemic Based on AI and Big Data

Meenu Gupta, Rachna Jain,
Kashish Garg, and Kunal Jain

CONTENTS

12.1 INTRODUCTION

The year 2020 should have marked the commencement of an exhilarating decade in the fields of medicine and science with digital technological growth. These

DOI: 10.1201/9781003171829-12

229

technologies could be used to approach and examine the scientific difficulties and diseases such as the recent coronavirus (COVID-19) disease, which is caused by the severe acute respiratory syndrome coronavirus 2 (SARS-CoV-2 virus) [1,2]. The disease was first observed in the province of Wuhan, China, and is rapidly outspreading across the globe. The virus causes symptoms like cough, cold, fever, and, in more severe cases, difficulty breathing [3]. As the novel coronavirus has been expanding its impact from China to other regions and countries across the globe, many measures are being taken at both national and international levels to control the sudden outburst of the deadly virus. Lockdown measures have been taken all over the world, but they are affecting the modern economies in every way, including social and economic impacts. The pandemic has created a worldwide health emergency, and a collaboration at the global level is essential to fight against it [4]. Table 12.1 discussed the ten most-affected countries from this deadly disease around the world. This table displays the details of the total number of infected cases and deaths. The number of causalities from this virus is continuously increasing, as shown in Figure 12.1, and there is an urgent need to stop these deaths to protect the world [5].

So far, 376,005 have died so far from the novel coronavirus worldwide as of June 01, 2020. The fatality rate is still continuously increasing despite several measures being taken by the government and the public. The pandemic has affected around 213 nations and different territories worldwide [6].

So here are the best opportunities for emerging digital technologies including artificial intelligence (AI) and Big Data Analytics to benefit human society that could be used while fighting against the novel coronavirus and in controlling the number of deaths and finally put an end to the fatal virus. Such technologies may be used for tracking, identifying, detecting, and preventing the disease and further examining the effect of the sickness on humanity and therefore can help in educating the public on health education and its importance. Both of these technologies are highly related to one another [7]. AI can be used for the detection of the disease,

TABLE 12.1

Top ten countries with the highest death cases from COVID-19 along with the total number of positive cases reported as of June 1, 2020 [6]

S. No.	Country	Total cases	Total deaths
1	USA	36,892,215	634,662
2	India	32,040,618	429,313
3	Brazil	20,213,388	564,890
4	Russia	6,512,859	167,241
5	France	6,339,509	112,356
6	UK	6,117,540	130,503
7	Turkey	5,968,868	52,437
8	Argentina	5,041,487	108,165
9	Colombia	4,846,955	122,768
10	Spain	4,643,450	82,227

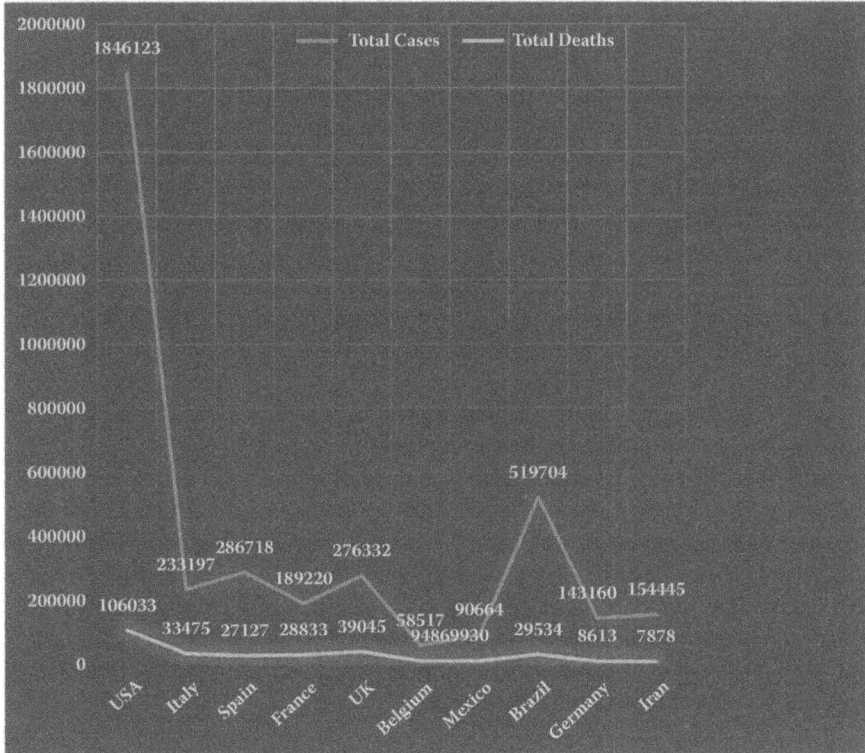

FIGURE 12.1 The total number of deaths is continuously increasing as the number of positive cases is increasing.

predict the outcomes, and addressing the public, while Big Data can be used to model and analyze the disease activity and its growth. AI will boost the identification and diagnosis of COVID-19, since there is an immediate need to have reliable and low diagnostic tests because many countries at present do not have the necessary tests or tools to differentiate COVID-19 from the "common flu." Certain AI algorithms could be used as a primary screening method for suspected infections, to send the high-risk patients to a laboratory for further examination and tests and finally to isolate and quarantine them if required. Big Data Analytics offers a great number of opportunities to check and analyze the performance of the viral activity and in return to direct the health workers to better plan for the pandemic [8].

This chapter is classified into the following subsections. Section 12.2 discusses the role of AI in COVID-19 disease. This section mainly focuses on medical chatbot, chest imaging X-ray, and monitoring of social distancing through robots and drones. The role of Big Data technique in COVID-19 is further discussed in Section 12.3. In Section 12.4, challenges faced with AI and Big Data in COVID-19 have been discussed. The analysis of COVID-19's impact on different countries, along with the proposed solutions, is presented in section 12.5. Finally, at the end of Section 12.6, conclusion and future scope are discussed.

12.2   ARTIFICIAL INTELLIGENCE IN COVID-19

Artificial intelligence simply means to simulate human intelligence in machines such that these are programmed to think like human beings or mimic their actions. In recent days, digital technology has been very helpful in tackling various situations during the COVID-19 spread across the world. Taking into account the problems relating to the COVID-19 pandemic, AI can offer sophisticated solutions that are capable, together with modern technology, of managing the strength of human knowledge, intelligence, and creativity. The existing form of AI can be tried to identify a different pattern for COVID-19 databases, establishing some different machine learning and deep learning algorithms and techniques. It can deliver enough results in case one has enough data to test different systems with many approaches in a less amount of time [7].

AI technique uses a CT scan methodology to detect viruses and is also helpful in assisting the medical professionals in identifying the components of the vaccine for the virus. It is also being used for creating medical chatbots so that people can take an assessment of their body, and one's condition can be analyzed [9]. One of the most important things to protect oneself from the virus is social distancing and sanitization. AI, through robots and drones, plays a very important role in this domain [4]. Authors [10] discussed the case of the manufacturing of masks by the charity and their problem faced in production. The authors further focused on the benefit of the blockchain and AI in the creation of the mask by charity and tracking, verifying the receiving of masks in hospitals by blockchain technique.

12.2.1   Detecting COVID-19 from Chest Imaging Technique (X-Ray)

In more critical cases of COVID-19, disease symptoms such as cough, cold, and faintness can also lead to pneumonia, organ failure, and even death. In people with COVID-19 pneumonia, respiratory problems spread faster in comparison with healthy people. The Chinese government released various new guidelines and recommendations for diagnosing and detecting COVID-19 through blood samples and reverse transcriptase or polymerase chain reaction (RT–PCR), a special indicator. The procedure of gene sequencing with RT–PCR takes a lot of time, and the individual should be admitted to the hospital immediately.

Through the use of an automatic chest CT scanning system, people who have been tested positive with coronavirus and have developed pneumonia can be detected. Therefore immediate isolation and treatment should be considered in the department concerned. A critical person may suffer permanent lung damage even if he or she is not dead. According to the World Health Organization (WHO), COVID-19 creates similar lung holes to SARS, which cannot be recovered. The technique of computed chest radioscopy is also helpful for the detection of pneumonia. An AI automated detection system can help monitor, quantify, and distinguish contact-free subjective communication [11].

A deep learning technique is utilized to extract the graphical characteristics of coronavirus from CT images. This technique ensures a quick and accurate diagnosis in comparison with pathogenic testing and saves time. The key component in the

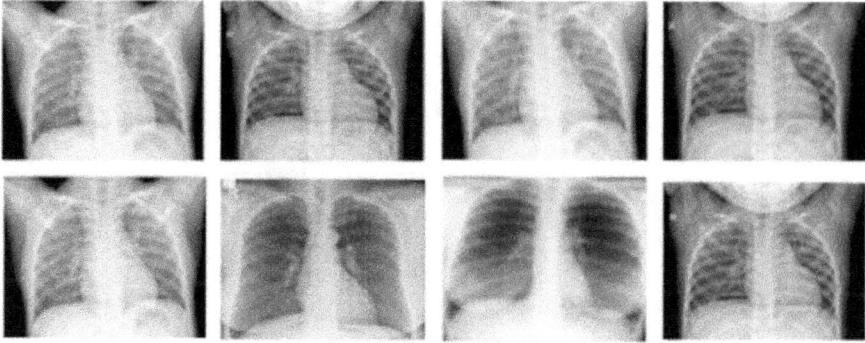

FIGURE 12.2   A normal person's representative chest X-ray images [11].

diagnosis and treatment of the viral disease is chest CT [9]. Some scientists and researchers have said that COVID-19 or coronavirus belongs to the family of SARS-CoV and MERS-CoV viruses. These viruses are formerly existing viruses, and some scientists have also stated that there is an option in chest X-ray and CT imagery to detect SARS-CoV and MERS-CoV. This technique, which includes removal and mining of data, was previously used by doctors to identify pneumonia from MERS-CoV and SARS-CoV.

X-ray machines are used to detect fractured bones, tumors, pneumonia, and lung infections in everyday life. However, the CT scan is a more advanced, complex system to examine different parts of the body, organ, and tissue more clearly and precisely. Figure 12.2 represents the image of an ordinary person's X-ray. The image of an individual with COVID-19 disease is shown in Figure 12.3. Figures 12.2 and 12.3 conclude that the person's lungs are directly impacted by pneumonia caused in COVID-19 or by the novel coronavirus. Using X-ray images is a little less expensive and easier method than the CT imaging, but, in normal X-rays, it is not possible to easily identify the virus, which may lead to an unexpected end [11]. As the number of cases of SARS-CoV 2 virus is continuously rising, a high index of suspicion, exposure to infected persons, and details of travel history are critical for the diagnosis. The radiologists should suggest a proper chest CT designed for COVID-19 as the normal CT scan cannot detect this particular virus [12].

CT scanning using AI is an existing technology for detecting COVID-19 pneumonia using the CT X-ray database. Still, the challenge is how this system can automatically detect COVID-19 pneumonia and not any other viruses or the bacteria and fungi. Various AI algorithms can be used to identify and recognize the condition and spread of the virus into a person in real time. The accurate detection by a well-trained AI model can save many lives and can further help to control and monitor the spread and generation of the deadly virus [9].

Figure 12.4 is a pre-trained prediction model of the COVID-19 affected person. In this model the author [11] applied deep learning techniques for extracting the graphical characteristics of a COVID-19- infected person from the CT image. This technique helps identify the causes of pneumonia and their impact on COVID-19-infected persons.

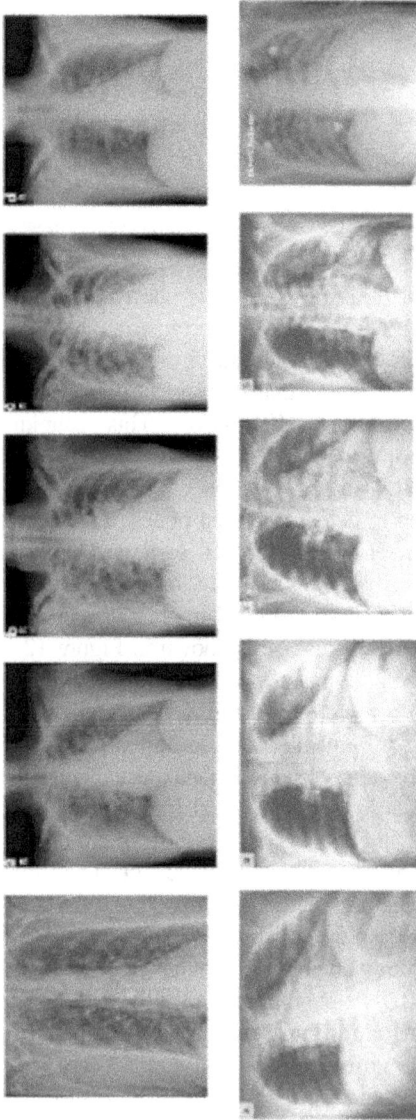

FIGURE 12.3 A COVID-19 patient's representative chest X-ray images [11].

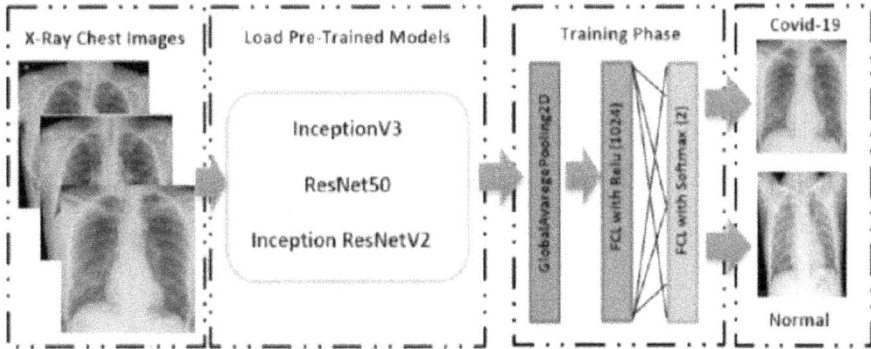

FIGURE 12.4 Prediction of COVID-19 patient using deep learning technique [11].

12.2.2 MEDICAL CHATBOTS TO ADDRESS PUBLIC ENQUIRIES

As the novel coronavirus crisis is continuously accelerating, society needs to keep them updated with the latest facts and figures related to the issue. The professionals need to provide every piece of information to the people so that they can remain healthy in this time of crisis [13]. The traditional media (radio and print channels) have a very limited audience; the younger audience prefers social media, but those are flooded with fake news and are not fully reliable. So, in this case, to address the demand comes to the conversational AI, also known as chatbots, a new technology that provides information access through text or voice. This technology is becoming very important in this time of crisis [14]. Chatbots can be described as the impression of communicating with humans online, while, actually, the person is interacting with computer software, which is put to life by natural language input with the help of AI [15].

The chatbots being used for coronavirus are based completely on the information received from the WHO so that everyone gets the accurate and relevant information. The chatbots are available 24/7, like websites. The data to be searched can be customized based on one's needs and symptoms of the disease. Many companies and organizations are deploying such bots on their websites. Many government bodies provide a facility to their public for seeing bots by either a smartphone or a computer. Microsoft helps fighting against the pandemic by its healthcare bot service, which is powered by its Microsoft Azure to many other organizations to assess the symptoms and risk factors. This service of Microsoft uses AI to help the US Center for Disease Control and Prevention (CDC) to respond to the inquiries of the public and healthcare professionals. The COVID-19 pandemic has been a great platform for the chatbot technology, and its use will continue in the future to provide various benefits in the medicine and healthcare sector and to serve the public [16].

12.2.3 SOCIAL CONTROL THROUGH ROBOTS AND DRONES

The most important factor for keeping oneself safe in the COVID-19 pandemic is practicing social distancing and being quarantined. In this time of crisis, when

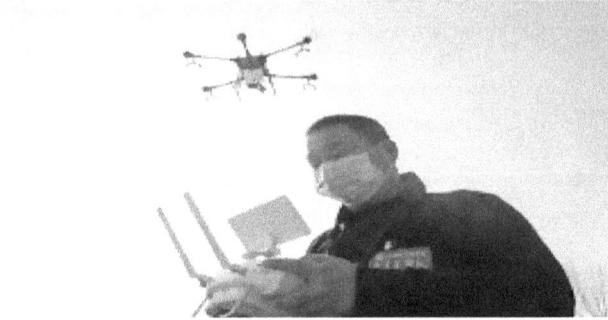

FIGURE 12.5   Human being behavior monitored by a drone during COVID-19 [18].

everyone is isolated, the robots and drones are helping the public, security staff, and medical professionals as the safest and expedient way to grapple with the outbreak.

It is an ideal time to see what drones and robots could do to support humanity in fighting against this viral disease. AI, through the use of thermal imaging, is being used to manage and handle the pandemic for scanning public space, enforcing social distancing and lockdown measures through robots and drones [17]. Drones have been made with installed cameras and GPS tracking systems within them and are being used to track individuals not wearing masks in public spaces, to broadcast information in larger areas, and disinfect the public areas and provide medicines to the needy [7]. Monitoring human activity using a drone is shown in Figure 12.5.

Patient care without the risk to healthcare workers is a matter of concern that is being done through robots using the applications of AI. These robots bring food and medicine to patients when needed. The coronavirus infection not only spreads when an infected person comes in physical contact with the normal person, but it can also spread through respiratory droplet transfer via some contaminated surface. Specifically, for this purpose, robot-controlled no-contact ultraviolet (UV) disinfection is being used [19,20]. Robots are also being utilized for room sanitization and sterilization in isolation wards in the hospitals, as shown in Figure 12.6. The pandemic has prompted more usage of robots and drones worldwide, and this shall increase in the coming future.

In [7], the author concluded that AI is not playing a vital role in the battle against COVID-19, especially in diagnostics, epidemiological, and pharmaceutical point of view. The reason behind this issue is the availability of unbalanced or noisy data. Robots can be treated as a nurse in monitoring the COVID-19- infected patients in the hospital room, as shown in Figure 6. This methodology can save human life because the nurses and doctors handling the COVID-19 patient can also get infected from this disease, and their life can be in danger zone.

12.3   BIG DATA IN COVID-19

Big Data is a field of technology in which there are different ways to analyze, systematically extract information, or deal with a large number of datasets that are

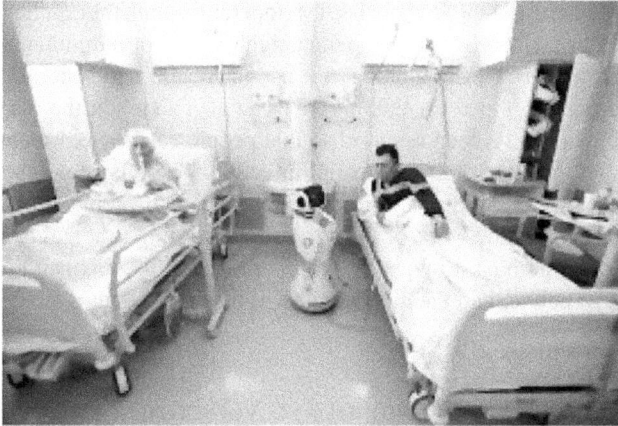

FIGURE 12.6 Robot nurse monitoring a patient during COVID-19 [21].

too complex to handle with the traditional data processing methods. The sudden outbreak of novel coronavirus has brought the advanced Big Data Analytics tool to limelight, seeking to monitor the spread of the disease and its growth and modelling the preparedness and vulnerability of different countries [22]. Data collection and its analysis is a crucial step in assessing the impact of various mitigation strategies during these times. Therefore, there is an urgent need to track the spread of the virus and treat it as soon as possible. In public health, still, the manual systems are used for storing the records and information, but the rise in Big Data has provided an opportunity for the researchers and other professionals to use these modern systems available to them so that time could be saved and lives of people could be saved [1]. The near real-time COVID-19 trackers collect data from various sources worldwide and allow healthcare professionals, scientists, and others to compile and synthesize the data globally.

12.3.1 MODELLING OF DISEASE ACTIVITY, ITS GROWTH, AND AREAS OF SPREAD

Big Data Analytics can play a very important role in the domain of public health in times of crisis. Large volume of electronic health records of patients, monitoring networks, and information from the Internet, from the social media, and through calls are gathered and then analyzed. In the case of infectious and viral diseases, the traditional surveillance systems are of no use because of their time lags, so there is a critical need for such systems that are stable, local, and timely. Monitoring and forecasting of the emergence of the disease, its growth, and the areas to which it is spreading are of particular interest. Viral disease surveillance is one of the most promising tools and an exciting opportunity created by Big Data. The information used for monitoring could be used long after the COVID-19 [23]. Around the world, there are many places where the body temperature is analyzed before entry to some public space. Various governments around the world told their public to enter their information via smartphone on an app and receive a digital pass.

The collected dataset of human body temperature and the applied algorithms helps estimate the probability of any given neighborhood or individual that has been exposed to coronavirus by matching the user's location to that of the infected person. The apps developed for this purpose can also show on the map, where the latest positive cases have been reported so that people could avoid themselves from going there, and thus preventing potential infection. There is some app that allows employers to see where all of his or her employees have been in the past 14 days so that he or she can plan the work of the company according to it and can ensure that they can safely come back to work. A simple program like this can prove of great advantage to the public, and the data stored will be very useful in the coming future for society [8].

12.3.2 MODELLING OF PREPAREDNESS AND VULNERABILITY OF COUNTRIES

Big Data has made the prediction about the novel coronavirus outbreak and the various regions around the world where it would spread. In recent years, various situations and disease outbreaks have shown that a large amount of data of the public can be gathered from diverse places. Presently, in the case of coronavirus, different kinds of information were gathered from airports by methods of screening and tracking and with the utilization of smart sensors mounted at the airport. Besides airports, the data was being taken from bus terminals, market places, and health facilities. This data could be analyzed properly and could be used to find the infected persons and send them in isolation.

This technique will help the government and officials to be prepared accordingly, to handle the situation of a country, if the number of cases increases suddenly. The urban areas generally have Urban Health sensors; these sensors are very light in weight. Hence, they can be carried easily by wearing them as an accessory. These devices are not expressly intended to track the virus outbreak but can help monitoring various other health related parameters, for example, blood pressure, pulse, oxygen level, and body temperature. The data followed by such devices could be used to analyze valuable insights. In another way, sampled data for COVID-19-infected people can be collected using terminal tracking systems and monitored at the time of entry or departure of any person through a particular point.

With the current situation of COVID-19, where everybody is economic and socially affected, it is important to emphasize the adoption of universal standards for data sharing. This will help the country to be prepared for any situation and deal with it [4]. Such techniques have been proved very beneficial in COVID-19; a startup company named "BlueDot" used various methods of data analyzing and predicted the COVID-19 outbreak. Twenty-one days before the government placed travel restrictions in the province of Wuhan, and medical needs had already been reporting signals of the epidemic.

BlueDot startup workers in Canada discovered that their computers had got early warning signals from an online electronic and radio communication device set up across China. BlueDot was the company that notified the WHO, to issue a first virus alert. In this way, all the data that was in their computers—animal disease information, web articles, and travel schedules found patterns of the outbreak and where it might get spread. Countries with less-developed health systems and a low level of preparedness are at a higher risk [24].

12.4 CHALLENGES IN COVID-19 PREDICTIONS USING AI AND BIG DATA

Prediction of COVID-19 is just like fighting with an invisible enemy. This is the biggest viral disease in the history of the world where a substantial number of people have dead so far. Several researchers applied different techniques (i.e., AI, Big Data, etc.) for the detection and prediction of the impact of COVID-19 on a human being and the economy of the country. Researchers also used different datasets such as a total number of casualties vs. infected cases across the globe, or some has considered the impact on the human body like chest X-ray dataset for their analysis on the effect of COVID-19. These techniques and parameters played their different role in the prediction of COVID-19 diseases. Table 12.2 discusses the methods applied to COVID-19-infected cases and their limitations.

AI has been contributing in the health and medicine sector long before the COVID-19 disease, for finding vaccines for different kinds of viral diseases like pneumonia, cold, and plague [26,27]. AI can be used in monitoring the people in crowded areas such as railway stations and bus stands, and infrared camera used in the device can detect the temperature of the human body in the prediction of fever.

In the conclusion of the table, several researchers have given their point of view for Big Data and AI in quest of the vaccine for the deadly COVID-19 treatment.

TABLE 12.2
Techniques and limitations in detection of COVID-19 and health industry

Authors	Technique	Database	Limitations
[11]	AI (a form of Machine learning and deep learning)	Fifty chest X-ray images of COVID-affected patients	Results could be better if provided more dataset for training as well as testing purposes.
[13]	AI	Semi-structured (N-29) interviews and advertised via social media (N-216)	Health chatbot can be used as supplementary rather than replacement of face-to-face interaction with doctors.
[7]	AI	Covid-19	Not effective results received using AI because of a lack of data or a large amount of data. Imbalance of data between privacy and public health AI not able to produce useful results fighting against COVID-19.
[25]	Big Data	Covi-19	Able to predict with descent accuracy but lacking in search related to curing for Coronavirus.

Still, as a result, they concluded that social distancing, wearing masks, isolation, and lockdown played a primary role in fighting against this invisible enemy.

12.5 COVID-19 IMPACTS AND PROPOSED SOLUTIONS

Many countries are affected because of this coronavirus. It has a global impact. Many solutions are proposed by the government to stop future cases of COVID-19, and medical organizations have been intimated to implement these solutions. Let's take a look at the worldwide impact of COVID-19 and measures taken to reduce further transmission.

12.5.1 WORLDWIDE IMPACTS OF COVID-19

The COVID-19 has a global effect, which influences the different sectors like economy and environment. Almost everything got affected due to this pandemic. Some of its implications are discussed in detail here.

12.5.1.1 Impact on the Economy

The most impact of this virus has been on the economy. Many countries have enforced a full lockdown to obstruct more spread of this disease. All domestics, as well as international flights, are cancelled or suspended. Train services have also been stopped. Apart from this, many sectors like tourism and cinema have also come to a standstill. Lockdown leads to the economic recession in many countries. Many private companies have fired half of their employees, and few of them are not getting a full salary due to this lockdown. Some of the powerful countries are facing high inflation and unemployment rate, and due to this, they are unable to provide the best quality service to their people in this crucial time [28]. According to a recent OECD research, 44% of families had at least one person whose employment has been affected by the crisis, such as job loss, layoff, retention scheme, decreased working hours, unpaid leave, or resignation [29].

12.5.1.2 Impact on the Environment

It is rightly said that "God's stick does not make noise." We, humans, have damaged the environment a lot. We only harm nature for our benefits. Environmental concerns include pollution, global warming, climate change, soil erosion, and change in the ecosystem who became the victim of increasing demands of humans [30,31]. Perhaps COVID-19 is the reason where all the human activities are stopped, and nature is healing on its own. Figure 12.7 depicts the commendable improvement in the air pollution level in China. Today, when everyone is in their home, the pollution level decreases drastically. The quality of seawater and the other water bodies has also improved. People have started respecting nature, and they understood the importance of plants and animals to maintain the balance of this nature.

12.5.1.3 Impact on the Society

This virus has had a positive impact on society. Family bonding is getting stronger. Now, families are spending quality time with each other. People are focused on

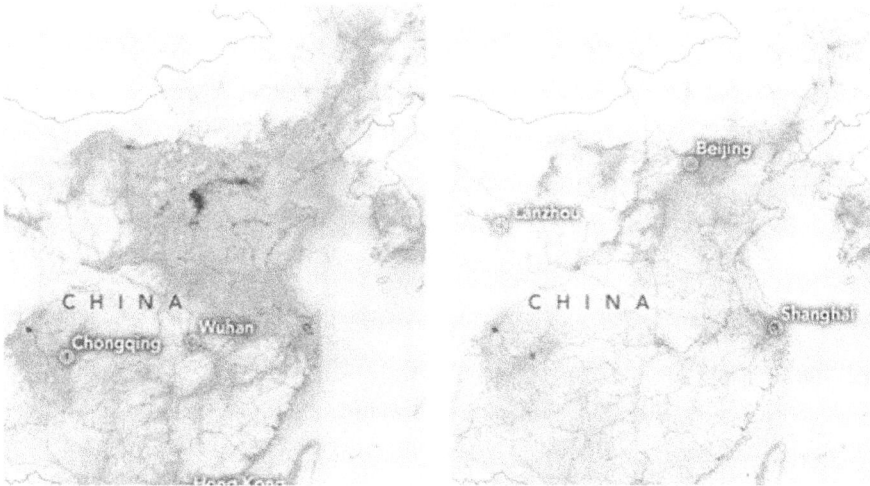

FIGURE 12.7   Pollution level in China before and after the COVID-19.

their health. They realized that money is not everything. Society, in general, is becoming more vegetarian. People understand the importance of nature.

12.5.1.4   Impact on the Functioning of Organizations

Since lockdown is followed in most of the countries, the working of many organizations also gets changed. Many employees are working from home. Educational institutions are also closed, so the teachers are shifted to the online mode of learning. Classes are held through an online platform for college and high school students. In some of the countries, there is a rise in the home delivery business. Now companies are making a huge profit; as people are not allowed to step outside, they are forced to pay high prices for home delivery. Medicines and food industries are using robots for home delivery so that proper distancing is maintained.

12.5.2   PROPOSED SOLUTIONS

The government of different countries proposed many solutions or have taken various steps for containing the virus outbreak. Some of them are given below and discussed in detail.

12.5.2.1   Lockdown and Restriction of Mass Gathering

A person gets infected with the coronavirus only by coming in direct contact with another person or an object carrying this virus. Hence, social distancing is necessary to stop this global pandemic. For controlling COVID-19 situation, the lockdown was imposed by the government of almost every country. There is a restriction on mass gathering in many countries. People are working from home. Despite the government order, it is now the primary duty of every person to maintain the social distancing to stop the spreading of this virus.

12.5.2.2 Afforestation

Million dollars are spent on the vaccination and tests for this COVID-19 virus. But some simple steps like afforestation and protection of wildlife are getting neglected. Forest covers 30% of the entire earth's surface. Forest helps in maintaining the temperature of the earth and also helps in the water cycle. With the growing population, our demands are also increased. Now, we (called humans) cut the trees only for our benefits. This leads to deforestation. Deforestation also gives rise to many diseases related to the birds [32,33], which perhaps would result in a virus pandemic in the future. So there is an urgent need for afforestation. We should plant more and more trees. And we should use only the dead trees as much as possible.

12.5.2.3 Population Control

The growing population has a major impact on the environment [34], which may have an effect on pollution, global warming, deforestation, and many more such negative effects on the environment. China is one of the world's most populated nation. In China, due to the increasing population, people eat frogs, dogs, cats, bats, and almost every animal inhabited there [35]. And the COVID-19 virus has also emerged from China because of eating bat. So the control in population is very much necessary in this matter.

12.5.2.4 Ban on Wildlife Trade

This pandemic has made us realized that animals are also an essential part of nature. We have no right to harm this nature's gift. There should be a permanent ban on wildlife hunting and trade by all the countries. One study has proven that 60% of the transmittable diseases are originated from the animals. So protecting wildlife reduces the risk of a new virus outbreak in the future. China has imposed a temporary ban on animal trade. Some other countries had also banned wildlife hunting.

12.5.2.5 Strictness to Personal Hygiene

People should take their hygiene very seriously. It should not be compromised at any cost. Some simple steps that can be made by us are shown here:

- We should wash our hands properly with soap at regular intervals for at least 20 seconds, especially before and after taking a meal or after coming back from outside.
- We should wear a mask when going outside.
- We should maintain a proper distance with the family members too at home.

The above said are the measures (or solutions) proposed by the government to reduce the spread of the novel coronavirus.

12.6 CONCLUSION AND FUTURE SCOPE

Coronavirus is the first big test for all the futuristic technologies that are fighting against this pandemic. Indeed, these technologies will not necessarily save us, but these can help to a great extent. It is an unknown war, in which humanity is facing the same enemy, the novel coronavirus. In this war, the first battlefield is the hospital where the staff is continuously giving service to the patients and to win the war. It should be the primary measure to ensure that the medical staff is healthy and granted the required resources. The world faced an unknown virus. Sharing and collaborating are the keys and the best remedies. Recent advancements in AI have opened the topic for debate, whether AI doctors (robots) will replace human doctors in the future. The idea of replacing a human doctor is slightly absurd, but it can happen soon and is a matter of concern. Big Data has been of tremendous advantage in the field of healthcare and medicine by making successful AI applications. The healthcare workers have to trust the AI algorithms to use them. Using the data, a lot of hidden information in a vast amount of data could be important to the health and medicine industry. Big Data Analytics has the potential to improve the healthcare system. In the future, consumers can expect a better quality of caring and an increase in customer loyalty. Big Data Analytics provides the best opportunity to take files and store all of the data. The world does not have enough healthcare workers to manage everyone's health, so there is a need for such artificial systems to take care of the people and to support them in the time of need.

ACKNOWLEDGMENT

The authors sincerely acknowledge the contribution and cooperation of everyone throughout the research.

REFERENCES

[1]. Callaghan, COVID-19 Is a Data Science Issue, Patterns (2020), Accessed at: 10.101 6/j.patter.2020.100022.
[2]. B. Tang, F. He, D. Liu, M. Fang, Z. Wu and D, Xu, AI-aided design of novel targeted covalent inhibitors against SARS-CoV-2.Preprint. bioRxiv, 2020.03.03.972133. Published 2020 Mar 8. (2020) doi: 10.1101/2020.03.03.972133.
[3]. M. A. Ruiz Estrada, The Uses of Drones in Case of Massive Epidemics Contagious Diseases Relief Humanitarian Aid: Wuhan-COVID-19 Crisis. *Available at SSRN 3546547* (2020).
[4]. Z. Allam and D. S. Jones, On the coronavirus (COVID-19) outbreak and the smart city network: Universal data sharing standards coupled with artificial intelligence (AI) to benefit urban health monitoring and management. *Healthcare*, 8 (1), p. 46 (2020, March). Multidisciplinary Digital Publishing Institute.
[5]. V. K. Deshwal, COVID 19: A comparative study of Asian, European, American continent.
[6]. COVID-19 CORONAVIRUS PANDEMIC (2020), Accessed at: https://www.worldometers.info/coronavirus/?utm_campaign=homeAdUOA?, April, 2020
[7]. W. Naudé, Artificial Intelligence against COVID-19: An early review. IZA Discussion Papers No. 13110 (2020).
[8]. S. Bansal, G. Chowell, L. Simonsen, A. Vespignani and C. Viboud, Big data for infectious disease surveillance and modeling. *Journal of Infectious Diseases*, 214 (suppl. 4), S375–S379 (2016).

[9]. M. Chung, A. Bernheim, X. Mei, N. Zhang, M. Huang, X. Zeng… and A. Jacobi, CT imaging features of 2019 novel coronavirus (2019-nCoV). *Radiology*, 295 (1), 202–207 (2020).

[10]. S, Johnstone, A viral warning for change. The Wuhan coronavirus versus the red cross: Better solutions via Blockchain and Artificial Intelligence. *The Wuhan Coronavirus Versus the Red Cross: Better Solutions Via Blockchain and Artificial Intelligence* (2020) *(February 3, 2020)*.

[11]. M. Ilyas, H. Rehman and A. Nait-ali, Detection of Covid-19 from chest X-ray images using artificial intelligence: An early review (2020). *arXiv preprint arXiv:2004.05436*.

[12]. Jeffrey P. Kanne, Chest CT findings in 2019 novel coronavirus (2019-nCoV) infections from Wuhan, China: Key points for the radiologist. *Radiology*, 295 (1), 16–17 (2020) doi: 10.1148/radiol.2020200241.

[13]. T. Nadarzynski, O. Miles, A. Cowie, and D. Ridge, Acceptability of artificial intelligence (AI)-led chatbot services in healthcare: A mixed-methods study. *Digital Health*, 5, 2055207619871808 (2019).

[14]. D. S. W. Ting, L. Carin, V. Dzau and T. Y. Wong, Digital technology and COVID-19. *Nature Medicine*, 26, 1–3 (2020).

[15]. A. A. A. Weißensteiner, Chatbots as an approach for a faster enquiry handling process in the service industry. *Signature*, 12, 04 (2018).

[16]. B. Hadas, Delivering information and eliminating bottlenecks with CDC's COVID-19 assessment bot. Accessed at: https://blogs.microsoft.com/blog/2020/03/20/delivering-information-and-eliminating-bottlenecks-with-cdcs-covid-19-assessment-bot/, (2020).

[17]. E. Malliaraki, Social interaction with drones using human emotion recognition. In Companion of the 2018 ACM/IEEE International Conference on Human-Robot Interaction (pp. 187–188) (2018, March).

[18]. A. Mark, All the Invasive Ways China Is using Drones to Address the coronavirus. Available at: https://slate.com/technology/2020/02/how-china-is-using-drones-to-contain-the-coronavirus.html (2020).

[19]. G. Z. Yang, B. J. Nelson, R. R. Murphy, H. Choset, H. Christensen, S. H. Collins… and M. McNutt, Combating COVID-19—The role of robotics in managing public health and infectious diseases. Science Robotics, 5(40) (eabb5589) (2020). doi:1 0.1126/scirobotics.abb5589.

[20]. D. Young, Can you use an infrared camera to detect a fever? Accessed at: https://www.wired.com/story/can-an-infrared-camera-detect-a-fever/, April, 2020.

[21]. E. Maria, Tommy the robot nurse helps Italian doctors care for COVID-19 patients. Accessed at: https://www.pri.org/stories/2020-04-08/tommy-robot-nurse-helps-italian-doctors-care-covid-19-patients (2020).

[22]. C. J. Wang, C. Y. Ng, and R. H. Brook, Response to COVID-19 in Taiwan: Big data analytics, new technology, and proactive testing. *JAMA*, 323(14) 1341–1342 (2020) doi:10.1001/jama.2020.3151.

[23]. R. Verity, L. C. Okell, I. Dorigatti, et al. Estimates of the severity of coronavirus disease 2019: a model-based analysis [published correction appears in Lancet Infect Dis. 2020 Apr 15;] [published correction appears in Lancet Infect Dis. 2020 May 4;] *Lancet Infectious Diseases*, 20 (6) 669–677 (2020) doi.10.1016/S1473-3099(20) 30243-7.

[24]. T. Scott, Big data predicted the coronavirus outbreak and where it would spread. Accessed at: https://www.marketplace.org/2020/02/04/big-data-predicted-coronavirus-outbreak-where-it-may-go-next/, (2020).

[25]. R. Bean, Big Data In the time of coronavirus (COVID-19), Forbes. Accessed at: https://www.forbes.com/sites/ciocentral/2020/03/30/big-data-in-the-time-of-corona-virus-covid19/#2d3df60658fc, (2020).

[26]. T. T. Nguyen, Artificial intelligence in the battle against coronavirus (COVID-19): A survey and future research directions. ArXiv, abs/2008.07343, (2020).

[27]. A. S. S, Rao and J. A. Vazquez, Identification of COVID-19 can be quicker through artificial intelligence framework using a mobile phone-based survey in the populations when cities/towns are under quarantine. *Infection Control & Hospital Epidemiology*, 42, 1–18 (2020).

[28]. OECD Interim Economic Assessment, 2 March 2020. Coronavirus: The world economy at risk. oecd.org/economic-outlook.

[29]. OECD annual national accounts; OECD trade in value added database, and OECD calculations; OECD 2020, http://www.oecd.org/coronavirus/en/, Accessed date:08 April 2020.

[30]. S. Bremer, P. Schneider, and B. Glavovic, Climate change and amplified representations of natural hazards in institutional cultures. *Oxford Research Encyclopedia of Natural Hazard Science* (2019) 10.1093/acrefore/9780199389407.013.354.

[31]. A. Coutts, J. Beringer and N. Tapper, Changing urban climate and CO_2 emissions: Implications for the development of policies for sustainable cities. *Urban Policy and Research*, 28, 27–47 (2010).

[32]. A. Afelt, R. Frutos and C. Devaux, Bats, coronaviruses, and deforestation: Toward the emergence of novel infectious diseases?. *Frontiers in Microbiology*, 9, 702 (2018).

[33]. J. Olivero, J. E. Fa, R. Real, et al., Recent loss of closed forests is associated with Ebola virus disease outbreaks. *Scientific Reports*, 7, 14291 (2017).

[34]. D. Shindell, N. Borgford-Parnell, M. Brauer, A. Haines, J. C. I. Kuylenstierna, S. A. Leonard, V. Ramanathan, A. Ravishankara, M. Amann and L. Srivastava, A climate policy pathway for near- and long-term benefits. *Science*, 356 (6337), 493–494 (2017).

[35]. Y. Fan, K. Zhao, Z. L. Shi, et al., Bat coronaviruses in China. *Viruses*, 11, 210 (2019).

13 A Review of Artificial Intelligence Applications for COVID-19 Contact Tracing

Thein Oak Kyaw Zaw, Mani Sehgar, Saravanan Muthaiyah, and Low Jing Hong

CONTENTS

13.1 INTRODUCTION

COVID-19 pandemic that has spread around the globe has ushered countries to make contact tracing to be one of the key components in combating the virus as lockdown measures were lifted gradually [1]. As the name suggests, "contact tracing" is the process of identifying, assessing, and managing people who have been exposed to a disease to prevent onward transmission [2]. This means that contact tracing in the scope of COVID-19 can be broken down into three separate segments: (1) identification of the close contact (case detection), (2) severity assessment, and (3) managing (people and assets). Contact tracing is crucial because COVID-19 is a highly infectious virus that has proliferated to more than 7,145,800 people, with 407,067 deaths by June 9, 2020, since its first emergence in the end of 2019 [3]. Currently, only few countries have achieved to keep the pandemic under control with contact tracing solutions [4]. This reality indicates that there is much needed work to be exerted to make the solutions efficient and comprehensive, as many countries, if not most, are not able to do so. In the early stage of the pandemic, contact tracing was mainly conducted manually through interviews, and it highly demands human resources [5]. With the number of cases rising every day, resources that interview method requires increase tremendously up to a point that contact tracing are being delayed and becoming inefficient. Thus, countries started to adopt smart digital solutions wherein they utilize

DOI: 10.1201/9781003171829-13

technology such as Internet of Things (IoT) and artificial intelligence (AI) in making the solutions to be fast and effective [6].

Apart from that, recent studies have pointed out that machine learning and AI are the promising technologies that have been adopted by various healthcare providers since they offer bigger upscaling, higher processing power, and reliability, which resulted in better performance than the professionals for specific areas [7].

The same scenario has also been happening for COVID-19, where AI has been used in tackling the pandemic in many aspects. However, the majority of AI applications in contact tracing for COVID-19 have been used in the identification of close contacts (case detection) as well as severity assessment and lack in managing people and assets. This gap can be due to the understanding of the institutions that contact tracing is limited to only case identification. This is a crucial problem because many of the countries have seen a sharp rise in the number of daily cases, and the healthcare workforce is getting overwhelmed as the ratio of patient to front liners is getting substantial [8]. Thus, the healthcare providers need a solution to manage them (the patients, front liners, and medical assets) effectively so that the whole healthcare system will not collapse. In this point of view, the AI is found to be lacking heavily, and this study attempts to expose the gap while explicitly stating in-depth the specific areas that are lacking for the management (people and asset) segment. Not just that, this study will also review on the current application of contact tracing with AI in combating human-to-human COVID-19 infection in three separate segments accordingly that none in the literature world has done before.

13.2   CLASSIFYING CONTACT TRACING SEGMENTS

As stated by the World Health Organization [2], contact tracing (with regard to COVID-19) means the process of identifying, assessing, and managing people who have been exposed to a disease to prevent further transmission. From the statement, contact tracing can be separated into three segments: (1) identification of close contacts (case detection), (2) severity assessment, and (3) managing (people and assets). General understanding on contact tracing mainly revolves only around the first two segments, while overlooking the third one, making the solutions for it to be small in number. This, in return, creates many delays and constraints to provide healthcare services when the number of daily cases is at large. The moment the number of front liners is being overwhelmed by the number of cases, the healthcare efficiency in conducting the three segment activities drops significantly. Thus, solutions that can provide closure for managing (people and assets) are critical as they can help in lowering down the workload and strain of the front liners and the overall healthcare system. The first one, which is identification of close contacts (case detection) basically means diagnosing individuals who have been infected from a patient irrespective of whether the patient is symptomatic or asymptomatic.

With many solutions available in this segment, many of the countries, if not most, have been utilizing mobile phones with bluetooth technology for it [9]. Severity assessment means the ability to determine the severity of the infected patients. Not limited to that scope, it also encompasses projecting the severity at the locations of the outbreak and of the groups of the infected. Last but not least is the

TABLE 13.1

Contact tracing for COVID-19 and its segments by World Health Organization (2020)

Item	Segments
Contact tracing	Identification of close contacts (case detection)
	Severity assessment
	Manage (people and assets)

managing (people and assets) segment in which it is aimed toward resource management. It is a common knowledge that many countries that are in the low-to-middle-income (LMIC) group are already facing strains in the capacity and accessibility of their healthcare systems before COVID-19 pandemic [10]. When the pandemic started, the system became much more overloaded as it tried to cater to everyone, and it affected not just LMIC countries but others as well. Thus, it is important to have solutions that can cater to this issue so that matters like the movement of the patients, utilization of hospitals and their tools, patient monitoring, and transport can be handled without burdening the healthcare professionals and the system. Table 13.1 shows the three segments of contact tracing discussed for COVID-19.

13.3 AIMS OF EACH SEGMENT

Identifying the segments of contact tracing alone will not be adequate in determining whether there are enough AI solutions to cater it. This is because the scope in each segment may be big that it requires more elements in it, or the scope can be a rarely occurring area that very less research ventures into it. Thus, it requires aims, in other words, the objectives of each segment to determine whether there are enough solutions in it that are catering the segments. These aims can be grasped from literatures that are discussing on the types of AI with contact tracing for COVID-19 pandemic. A study by Bansal et al. [11] provided seven utility for AI toward battling COVID-19.

They are outbreak detection, prediction of spread, host–vector identification, preventive strategies and vaccine development, early case detection and tracking, prognosis prediction, and, last but not least, management and drug development. These utilities or aims are quite comprehensive as they cover many techniques of AI, which are deep learning, natural language processing, sentiment analysis, and machine vision. Even so, items such as outbreak detection and host–vector identification can be combined as one as they are referring to almost the same scenario [3]. On the other hand, the application of AI is categorized into four categories: screening and treatment, contact tracing, prediction and forecasting, drugs, and vaccination. Even though the categories or the aims are not much in variety, they still provide examples from several of the AI methods such as deep convolutional neural network, vector machine, and random forest algorithm.

Vaishya et al. [12] provided seven aims of AI in COVID-19 pandemic. They are early detection and diagnosis of the infection, monitoring and treatment, contact tracing of the individuals, projection of cases and mortality, development of drugs and vaccines, reducing workload of healthcare workers, and prevention of diseases. It should be noted that reducing the workload is a general category as the objective of AI is to reduce the workload of the people. All these studies show that there are similarities between the aims of all of the studies. In a study by Agbehadji et al. [13] also provided two aims that are similar, and they are: case detection and contact tracing. Thus, after analyzing the available literatures, the elements are coded into nine aims that relate back to the three segments of contact tracing. They are: (1) screening; (2) early warning and alert; (3) tracking; (4) prediction; (5) diagnosis; (6) prognosis; (7) monitoring, treatment, and cure; (8) societal control; and last but not least (9) asset optimization and tracking. Screening is to basically classify people who are COVID-19 positive from the vast amount of people who have come for medical checkups. It is crucial because more than half of the people who are infected by the virus do not display any symptoms. Yang et al.[14] stated that 48% from the infected patients in Wuhan, China, do not exhibit symptoms. Similarly, a study by Nir Menachemi reported 45% of people who are COVID-19 positive are asymptomatic [15]. Not limited to identification, screening also classifies the severity of the infection in a rapid manner from a huge pool of people. As for the early warning and alert, it is where the AI will try to predict early potential outbreaks and its severity. This is important so that if an outbreak occurs, it can be contained in a faster manner.

Apart from that, screening also detects anything virus related to provide warnings, such as the trend and rate of mortality. Tracking is basically the contact tracing solutions in identifying the patients as well as the people to whom they have spread, to stop the outbreak. In addition to that, a solution that is able to cater for symptomatic and asymptomatic cases will be an added value. After this, forecast model helps in the prediction that is based on the consequences arise when patients were infected due to mortality and transmission rate. In a major outbreak situation where everything is in chaos, prediction helps a long way in reducing the resources for random mass testing, which may not be available [16]. Next is the diagnostic, which means to identify the source of infection. Although this item can be combined with tracking, most of the current world contact tracing solutions have separated it since it is hard to do backward tracing or the identification of the source of infection. This is the reason that diagnostic is separated from tracking.

Prognosis in this case can be considered as the higher level of *tracking,* where it analyzes the path of outbreaks by analyzing their trend. The main difference between them is that *tracking* is focused on identifying close contacts of the patients up to a point that the chain of infection is closed theoretically. *Prognosis* predicts the future state of the outbreak by analyzing the patterns, growth rates, and so on. *Monitoring, treatment, and cure* is basically for the AI to be able to provide required medication based on the symptoms and health conditions in easing up the quarantine centers. Not limited to that, it also monitors as well as predicts recoveries, identifies infected regions, and forecasts potential reoccurrences using AI. Next is the *societal control,* where the objective is to help the movements of the people going to specific quarantine centers. When the number of daily cases is high, it becomes complicated to manage and make decisions on where to send the patients for quarantine. Not just that, it is also meant to provide answers for where to send the patients based on the capacities of the centers, its equipment utilization, the number of front liners, medication resources, and many more items. It should be noted that during emergencies, these matters are a critical issue. Last but not least is the *asset optimization and tracking,* which is quite similar to the previous aim where it focuses on humans. This aim optimizes assets utilization with AI during the pandemic period.

As stated previously, pandemic period is where resources are being utilized at the maximum capacity for a prolonged period, and hence it is important to optimize the usage so that there will be less delays and less problems that popped out. The assets can be infrastructure-related such as the number of beds and available ventilators and can be wearable-related such as the availability of PPE suits and washable gowns. With all these aims identified, they are then directed back to the contact tracing segments that they relate to. Table 13.2 shows the aims of contact tracing segments, and Table 13.3 illustrates the relationship between the segments and the aims.

TABLE 13.2
Aims of contact tracing with AI for COVID-19 pandemic

No.	Aims	Objectives	References
1.	Screening	To **classify** individuals who are positive COVID-19 (and its severity) from the vast amount of people according to many indicators such as symptoms and X-ray images	[3], [13]
2.	Early warning and alert	To **predict** potential outbreaks, case severity, trend, and rate of mortality before they happens (or at their early stage).	[12]
3.	Tracking	To **conduct** contact tracing for the patients and identification of the infected individuals as well as groups from the close contacts.	[3], [11], [12], [13]
4.	Prediction	To **forecast** the future of individuals on mortality rate, severity, and others after a person is infected (not an early-case scenario).	[3], [11], [12]
5.	Diagnosis	To **conduct** backward tracing in order to identify the source of infection.	[11], [12]
6.	Prognosis	To **analyze** the path of an outbreak by analysis of transmission, growth rates, and others.	[11]
7.	Monitoring, treatment, and cure	To **provide** required medication (includes vaccine) and care, based on symptoms and health conditions with monitoring as well as **prediction** on recoveries, infected region localization, and potential recurrences.	[3], [11], [12]
8.	Societal control	To **assist** in the overall human resource management.	[11], [12]
9.	Asset optimization and tracking	To **assist** in the overall asset management.	[11], [12]

TABLE 13.3
Relationship between AI aims and contact tracing segments

Contact tracing segments	No.	AI aims
Identification of close contacts (case detection)	1.	Screening
	2.	Tracking
	3.	Prediction
	4.	Diagnosis
	5.	Prognosis
Severity assessment	1.	Screening
	2.	Early warning and alert
	3.	Monitoring, treatment, and cure
Manage (people and assets)	1.	Societal control
	2.	Asset optimization and tracking

13.4 APPLICATIONS OF AI IN THE CONTACT TRACING SEGMENTS

With three contact tracing segments and aims identified, the applications of AI can now be grouped accordingly and comprehensively. These applications should cover all the aims as much as possible, and the lack in any of the aims will be considered as a gap. Not just that, each aim is also set to consist of at least three solutions (does not matter theoretical or have been commercialized) to indicate that a solution does exists for it. Each aim that has less than three solutions will not be considered as a fulfillment of it. The main objective is to see if there are any AI solutions in each of the aims as it is not an easy task to develop one in a short period of time. It should be noted that the applications that are gathered in the list were gained from literatures in major journal databases from Google Scholar, Emerald Insight, Science Direct, and IEEE Explorer. Table 13.4 illustrates the applications of AI with respect to contact tracing segments and aims.

From Table 13.4, it shows that the identification of close contacts (case detection) segment has the most aims, with AI applications covering most of the aims. Only tracking and diagnosis have a wider gap for not completely utilizing AI solutions. Contact tracing can be a solution where whole world is affected due to COVID-19 situation. The solution includes IoT but there will be an absence of AI. Not just that, it also shows that backward tracing has been ineffective and lacking behind that almost no solutions of AI exist for it. Nevertheless, severity assessment segment has its aims fulfilled quite comprehensively. It is manage (people and assets) segment that has only one solution in one of the aims. Finally, one of the ultimate reasons for AI not being fully utilized for contact tracing

TABLE 13.4

Applications of AI with respect to contact tracing segments and aims

Segment	Aims				
Identification of close contacts (case detection)	**Screening**				
	Source	**Method/ technology Used**	**Types of data**	**Validation method**	**Accuracy**
	[17]	Deep convolutional neural network ResNet-101	Clinical, CT images	Holdout	Accuracy: 99.51% Specificity: 99.02%
	[18]	Support vector machine	Clinical, laboratory features, demographics	Holdout	Accuracy: 77.5% Specificity: 78.4%
	[19]	Deep learning models (MobileNetV2, SqueezeNet) with Social Mimic Optimization method and SVM classifier	X-ray images	k-fold cross-validation	Accuracy: 98.89% Specificity: 98.58%
	Tracking				
	Source	**Method/ Technology Used**	**Types of Data**	**Validation Method**	**Accuracy**
	[20]	Machine learning	Bluetooth RSSI	Holdout	–
	Prediction				
	Source	**Method/ Technology Used**	**Types of Data**	**Validation Method**	**Task**
	[21]	Several ML-based approaches (Adaboost Pregressor, Decision Tree, Elastic Net, Huber Regression, Random Forest, SVM, and others)	Textual and time series	Cross-validation	Mortality rate prediction by analyzing impact from atmospheric temperature and humidity toward COVID-19 transmission
	[22]	AdaBoost with fine-tuned Random Forest model	Text	–	Possible outcome (death, recovery) and severity prediction
	[23]	Multiple linear regression (generalized linear model, conditional	CT images and clinical data	Cross-validation	Screening and severity prediction

(*Continued*)

TABLE 13.4 (Continued)
Applications of AI with respect to contact tracing segments and aims

Segment			Aims		
		inference trees, penalized binomial regression, and SVM with linear kernel)			
			Diagnosis		
	Source	Method/ Technology Used	Types of Data	Validation Method	Accuracy
	NIL				
	Prognosis				
	Source	Method/ Technology Used	Types of Data	Validation Method	Task
	[24]	Artificial neural network–based adaptive increment deep learning model	Time series	Holdout	Reduce the number of deaths while monitoring, forecast growth simulation
	[25]	SVM, linear regression, and polynomial regression	Text	–	Transmission rate analysis, growth rates, and migration rate analysis
	[26]	Modified auto-encoders	Time series	–	Estimate pandemic transmission and evaluate interventions
Severity assessment			**Screening**		
	Source	Method/ Technology Used	Types of Data	Validation Method	Task
	[27]	DenseNet201 based transfer learning and CNN	CT images	Cross-validation	Detection and severity assessment
	[28]	3D CNN-based network	CT-images	Holdout	Severity assessment
	[29]	Multi-objective differential evolution-based CNN	CT images	Cross-validation	COVID-19 detection and severity assessment
			Early warning and alert		
	Source	Method/ Technology Used	Types of Data	Validation Method	Task
	[30]	NN3D DL model	CT images	Holdout	Early stage classification

TABLE 13.4 (Continued)
Applications of AI with respect to contact tracing segments and aims

Segment			Aims		
	[31]	COVID-19Net and DenseNet121-FPN	CT images	Test split	Severity forecast and assessment
	Monitoring, treatment, and cure				
	Source	**Method/ Technology Used**	**Types of Data**	**Validation Method**	**Task**
	[32]	Multi-task DL methods: NABLA-N (for region segmentation) and Inception Residual Recurrent Convolutional Neural Network	X-ray images	Holdout	COVID-19 identification and infected region localization
	[33]	Composite hybrid feature extraction (CHFS)–based Stack Hybrid Classification (SHC) composed of CNN and MK models (SVM, RF)	CT images	Cross-validation	Predicting recurrences in no recurrences COVID-19 cases
	[34]	SVM	Text	Cross-validation	Recovery prediction
Manage (people and assets)	**Societal Control**				
	Source	**Method/ Technology Used**	**Types of Data**	**Validation Method**	**Task**
	NIL				
	Asset Optimization and Tracking				
	Source	**Method/ Technology Used**	**Types of Data**	**Validation Method**	**Task**
	[35]	Random forest and linear Regression	CT images	Intervalidation	Hospital stay prediction

under the three segments is all the data captured are not being stored under a centralized hub. Table 13.5 shows the gap analysis for the AI application from the study conducted. Once again, the gap is identified or recognized only if the solutions are less than three for this study. The reason is that COVID-19 pandemic has been around for only one year, which makes the AI solutions for it in less numbers.

TABLE 13.5

Gap analysis for AI application in contact tracing for COVID-19

Segments/aims	Current State	Desired state	Gap identification (normal, severe, and critical)	Remedial actions
Identification of close contacts (case detection)				
Screening	Adequate solutions	Achieved	None	–
Tracking	Solutions inadequate	Solutions with high accuracy, fast and robust	Severe	More research are needed especially in the identification of asymptomatic close contacts with AI.
Prediction	Adequate solutions	Achieved	None	–
Diagnosis	None available	Solutions to conduct backward tracing	Critical	Bigger developments for contact tracing solutions with the ability to do back tracing in which AI will come in later.
Prognosis	Adequate solutions	Achieved	None	–
Severity assessment				
Screening	Adequate solutions	Achieved	None	–
Early warning and alert	Solutions inadequate	More variety on human assessment solutions as current ones are limited in its scope	Normal	More collaborations with hospitals to gain clinical data in order to conduct more forecasting
Monitoring, treatment, and cure	Adequate solutions	Achieved	None	–
Manage (people and assets)				
Societal control	None available	Comprehensive human-resource management solutions for pandemics	Critical	Awareness and efforts in this scope need to be doubled to make researchers and implementors realize its importance
Asset optimization and tracking	Solutions inadequate	Comprehensive asset management solutions for pandemics	Severe	Awareness and efforts in this scope need to be doubled to make researchers and implementors realize its importance

13.5 CONCLUSION

Contact tracing has been around for quite some time in the research and development arena. It is only during COVID-19 pandemic that it has become such a great importance to the society as it helps tremendously in curtailing the pandemic. Thus, it is also with great urgency that AI solutions in it to be developed in a fast manner in order for it to be better. Therefore, it is important to identify AI solution in each of the segments as well as aims to identify which parts are lacking. These identifications enable researchers to direct their efforts toward the gaps as those are the real problems to be solved. Insights gleaned from this study shows that there is much needed work to be exerted in the managing (people and assets) segment for contact tracing with AI solutions. This is to ensure that COVID-19 pandemic can be handled with better efficiency as humans and assets are a great resource. Not just that, it is also to ensure that the whole healthcare system will not collapse due to overload of cases. Apart from that, the study also illustrates that solutions for backward tracing and contact tracing are both lacking heavily in AI-based solutions. Therefore, again, more studies will need to be conducted in these two areas as they are the keys in controlling the pandemic. Finally, the study opens contact tracing view comprehensively in three segments in which none in the literature world has done before.

REFERENCES

[1]. J. Hellewell, S. Abbott, A. Gimma, N. I. Bosse, C. I. Jarvis, T. W. Russell, J. D. Munday, A. J. Kucharski, W. J. Edmunds, S. Funk, R. M. Eggo F. Sun, S. Flasche, B. Quilty, N. Davies, Y. Liu, S. Clifford, P. Klepac, M. Jit, K. Zandvoort, Feasibility of controlling 2019-nCoV outbreaks by isolation of cases and contacts. *The Lancet Global Health*, 8 (2020). doi: 10.1016/S2214-109X(20)30074-7.

[2]. World Health Organization, Contact tracing in the context of COVID-19—Interim guidance (2020).

[3]. S. Lalmuanawma, J. Hussain, and L. Chhakchhuak, Applications of machine learning and artificial intelligence for COVID-19 (SARS-Cov-2) pandemic: A review. *Chaos, Solitons & Fractals*, 139, 110059 (2020).

[4]. A. Kamradt-Scott, *In many countries the coronavirus pandemic is accelerating, not slowing*. The Conversation. https://theconversation.com/in-many-countries-the-coronavirus-pandemic-is-accelerating-not-slowing-141238 (2020).

[5]. H. Cho, D. Ippolito, and Y. W. Yu, Contact tracing mobile apps for COVID-19: Privacy considerations and related trade-offs. *arXiv preprint arXiv*, 2003, 11511 (2020).

[6]. C. Lin, W. E. Braund, J. Auerbach, J. Chou, J. Teng, P. Tu and J. Mullen, Policy decisions and use of information technology to fight COVID-19, Taiwan*Emerging Infectious Diseases Journal*. https://wwwnc.cdc.gov/eid/article/26/7/20-0574_article (2020).

[7]. T. Davenport, and R. Kalakota, The potential for artificial intelligence in healthcare. *Future Healthcare Journal*, 6 (2), 94–98 (2019).

[8]. M. Buheji, and D. Ahmed, 'Lessons from the front-line' facing the COVID-19 pandemic. *Business Management and Strategy*, 11 (1), 192 (2020).

[9]. A. Hekmati, G. Ramachandran, and B. Krishnamachari, Contain: Privacy-oriented contact tracing protocols for epidemics. *arXiv preprint arXiv*, 2004, 05251 (2020).

[10]. W. T. Siow, M. F. Liew, B. R. Shrestha, F. Muchtar, and K. C. See, Managing COVID-19 in resource-limited settings: Critical care considerations. *Critical Care*, 24 (1). 10.1186/s13054-020-02890-x (2020).

[11]. A. Bansal, R. P. Padappayil, C. Garg, A. Singal, M. Gupta, and A. Klein, Utility of artificial intelligence amidst the COVID 19 pandemic: A review. *Journal of Medical Systems*, 44 (9), 1–6 (2020).

[12]. R. Vaishya, M. Javaid, I. H. Khan, and A. Haleem, Artificial intelligence (AI) applications for COVID-19 pandemic. *Diabetes & Metabolic Syndrome: Clinical Research & Reviews*, 14 (4), 337–339 (2020).

[13]. I. E. Agbehadji, B. O. Awuzie, A. B. Ngowi, and R. C. Millham, Review of big data analytics, artificial intelligence and nature-inspired computing models towards accurate detection of COVID-19 pandemic cases and contact tracing. *International Journal of Environmental Research and Public Health*, 17 (15), 5330 (2020).

[14]. R. Yang, X. Gui, and Y. Xiong, Comparison of clinical characteristics of patients with asymptomatic vs symptomatic coronavirus disease 2019 in Wuhan, China. *JAMA Network Open*, 3 (5), e2010182 (2020).

[15]. A. Zeek, and A. Briggs, *COVID-19 study's preliminary findings show spread of virus in Indiana*. News at IU. https://news.iu.edu/stories/2020/05/iupui/releases/13-preliminary-findings-impact-covid-19-indiana-coronavirus.html (2020)

[16]. C. Menni, A. M. Valdes, M. B. Freidin, C. H. Sudre, L. H. Nguyen, D. A. Drew, S. Ganesh, T. Varsavsky, M. J. Cardoso, J. S. El-Sayed Moustafa, A. Visconti, P. Hysi, E. Bowyer, R. C. Mangino, M. Falchi, M. Wolf, J. Ourselin, S. Chan, A. T. Steves C. J. and T. D. Spector, Real-time tracking of self-reported symptoms to predict potential COVID-19. *Nature Medicine*, 26, 1037–1040 (2020).

[17]. A. A. Ardakani, A. R. Kanafi, U. R. Acharya, N. Khadem, and A. Mohammadi, Application of deep learning technique to manage COVID-19 in routine clinical practice using CT images: Results of 10 convolutional neural networks. *Computers in Biology and Medicine*, 121, 103795 (2020).

[18]. L. Sun, F. Song, N. Shi, F. Liu, S. Li, P. Li, W. Zhang, X. Jiang, Y. Zhang, L. Sun, X. Chen, and Y. Shi, Combination of four clinical indicators predicts the severe/critical symptom of patients infected COVID-19. *Journal of Clinical Virology*, 128, 104431 (2020).

[19]. M. Toğaçar, B. Ergen, and Z. Cömert, COVID-19 detection using deep learning models to exploit social mimic optimization and structured chest X-ray images using fuzzy color and stacking approaches. *Computers in Biology and Medicine*, 121, 103805 (2020).

[20]. F. Sattler, J. Ma, P. Wagner, D. Neumann, M. Wenzel, R. Schäfer, W. Samek, K. Müller, and T. Wiegand, Risk estimation of SARS-Cov-2 transmission from Bluetooth low energy measurements. *NPJ Digital Medicine*, 3(1), 1–4 (2020).

[21]. Z. Malki, E. S. Atlam, A. E. Hassanien, G. Dagnew, M. A. Elhosseini, and I. Gad, Association between weather data and COVID-19 pandemic predicting mortality rate: Machine learning approaches. *Chaos, Solitons, and Fractals*, 138, 110137 (2020).

[22]. C. Iwendi, A. K. Bashir, A. Peshkar, R. Sujatha, J. M. Chatterjee, S. Pasupuleti, R. Mishra, S. Pillai, and O. Jo, COVID-19 patient health prediction using boosted random forest algorithm. *Frontiers in Public Health*, 8, 357 (2020).

[23]. J. Matos, F. Paparo, I. Mussetto, L. Bacigalupo, A. Veneziano, S. Perugin Bernardi, E. Biscaldi, E. Melani, G. Antonucci, P. Cremonesi, M. Lattuada, A. Pilotto, E. Pontali, and G. A. Rollandi, Evaluation of novel coronavirus disease (COVID-19) using quantitative lung CT and clinical data: Prediction of short-term outcome. *European Radiology Experimental* 4(1), 1–10 (2020).

[24]. J. Farooq, and M. A. Bazaz, A novel adaptive deep learning model of COVID-19 with focus on mortality reduction strategies. *Chaos, Solitons & Fractals*, 138, 110148 (2020).

[25]. M. Yadav, M. Perumal, and M. Srinivas, Analysis on novel coronavirus (COVID-19) using machine learning methods. *Chaos, Solitons & Fractals*, 139, 110050 (2020).

[26]. Z. Hu, Q. Ge, S. Li, E. Boerwinkle, L. Jin, and M. Xiong, Forecasting and evaluating multiple interventions for COVID-19 worldwide. *Frontiers in Artificial Intelligence*, 3 (2020).

[27]. R. Jaiswal, A. Agarwal, and R. Negi, Smart solution for reducing the COVID-19 risk using smart city technology. *IET Smart Cities*, 2 (2), 82–88 (2020).

[28]. J. Pu, J. Leader, A. Bandos, J. Shi, P. Du, J. Yu, B. Yang, S. Ke, Y. Guo, J. B. Field, C. Fuhrman, D. Wilson, F. Sciurba, and C. Jin, Any unique image biomarkers associated with COVID-19?. *European Radiology*, 30 (11), 6221–6227 (2020).

[29]. D. Singh, V. Kumar, Vaishali, and M. Kaur, Classification of COVID-19 patients from chest CT images using multi-objective differential evolution-based convolutional neural networks. *European Journal of Clinical Microbiology & Infectious Diseases*, 39 (7), 1379–1389 (2020).

[30]. X. Xu, X. Jiang, C. Ma, P. Du, X. Li, S. Lv, L. Yu, Q. Ni, Y. Chen, J. Su, G. Lang, Y. Li, H. Zhao, J. Liu, K. Xu, L. Ruan, J. Sheng, Y. Qiu, W. Wu … L. Li, A deep learning system to screen novel coronavirus disease 2019 pneumonia. *Engineering*, 6(10), 1122–1129 (2020).

[31]. S. Wang, Y. Zha, W. Li, Q. Wu, X. Li, M. Niu, M. Wang, X. Qiu, H. Li, H. Yu, W. Gong, Y. Bai, L. Li, Y. Zhu, L. Wang, and J. Tian. A fully automatic deep learning system for COVID-19 diagnostic and prognostic analysis, *European Respiratory Journal*, 56(2) (2020).

[32]. M. Z. Alom, M. M. Shaifur Rahman, M. S. Nasrin, T. M. Taha, and V. K. Asari, COVID_MTNet: COVID-19 Detection with multi-task deep learning approaches. arXiv:2004.03747 [eess.IV]. https://arxiv.org/pdf/2004.03747.pdf (2020).

[33]. A. A. Farid, G. I. Selim, and H. A. Khater, A novel approach of CT images feature analysis and prediction to screen for corona virus disease (COVID-19). *International Journal of Scientific & Engineering Research*, 11(3), (2020). doi:1 0.14299/ijser.2020.03.02.

[34]. A. E. Hassanien, A. Salama, and Darwsih, Artificial intelligence approach to predict the COVID-19 patient' s recovery. *EasyChair Preprint,* 3223 (2020).

[35]. H. Yue, Q. Yu, C. Liu, Y. Huang, Z. Jiang, C. Shao, H. Zhang, B. Ma, Y. Wang, G. Xie, H. Zhnag, X. Li, N. Kang, X. Meng, S. Huang, D. Xu, J. Lei, H. Huang, J. Yang, J. Ji, H. Pan, S. Zou, S. Ju, X. Qi. Machine learning-based CT radiomics model for predicting hospital stay in patients with pneumonia associated with SARS-Cov-2 infection: A multicenter study. *Annals of Translational Medicine*, 8(14), 859 (2020). doi:10.21037/atm-20-3026 PMID: 32793703; PMCID: PMC7396749.

Index

For Product Safety Concerns and Information please contact our EU
representative GPSR@taylorandfrancis.com
Taylor & Francis Verlag GmbH, Kaufingerstraße 24, 80331 München, Germany